Synopsis of
Otorhinolaryngology
Including Instruments and X-rays

Synopsis of
Otorhinolaryngology
Including Instruments and X-rays

Barin Kumar Roychaudhuri

MBBS (Cal), DLO (Cal), MS (AIIMS), FSMF (WB)

Ex-Professor and Head, Department of ENT
Calcutta Medical College and Hospital

Ex- Professor, Head and Hony. Consultant
Department of ENT and Head-Neck Surgery
Vivekananda Institute of Medical Sciences
Ramakrishna Mission Seva Pratishthan, Kolkata

Undergraduate and Postgraduate Teacher in ENT, Calcutta University

Ex-Member, Undergraduate Medical Council; Undergraduate and Postgraduate Boards of Studies
Calcutta University and WB University of Health Sciences

Ex-Chairman, Editorial Board, and
Editor, *Indian Journal of Otolaryngology and Head-Neck Surgery*
Official Publication of the Association of Otolaryngologists of India (AOI)

Ex-President, AOI, and Association of Otolaryngologists of SAARC Countries

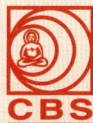

CBS

CBS Publishers & Distributors Pvt Ltd

New Delhi • Bengaluru • Chennai • Kochi • Pune
Hyderabad • Kolkata • Mumbai • Nagpur • Patna

Synopsis of
Otorhinolaryngology
Including Instruments and X-rays

ISBN: 978-81-239-2282-9

First Edition 2013

Published by Satish Kumar Jain for
CBS Publishers & Distributors Pvt Ltd
4819/XI Prahlad Street, 24 Ansari Road, Daryaganj, New Delhi 110 002, India.
Ph: 23289259, 23266861, 23266867   Fax: 011-23243014   Website: www.cbspd.com
e-mail: delhi@cbspd.com; cbspubs@airtelmail.in.
Corporate Office: 204 FIE, Industrial Area, Patparganj, Delhi 110 092
Ph: 4934 4934   Fax: 4934 4935   e-mail: publishing@cbspd.com;
publicity@cbspd.com

Branches

- **Bengaluru:** Seema House 2975, 17th Cross, K.R. Road,
  Banasankari 2nd Stage, Bengaluru 560 070, Karnataka
  Ph: +91-80-26771678/79   Fax: +91-80-26771680   e-mail: bangalore@cbspd.com
- **Chennai:** 20, West Park Road, Shenoy Nagar, Chennai 600 030, Tamil Nadu
  Ph: +91-44-26260666, 26208620   Fax: +91-44-42032115   e-mail: chennai@cbspd.com
- **Kochi:** 36/14 Kalluvilakam, Lissie Hospital Road, Kochi 682 018, Kerala
  Ph: +91-484-4059061-65   Fax: +91-484-4059065   e-mail: kochi@cbspd.com
- **Pune:** Bhuruk Prestige, Sr. No. 52/12/2+1+3/2 Narhe, Haveli
  (Near Katraj-Dehu Road Bypass), Pune 411 041, Maharashtra
  Ph: +91-20-64704058, 64704059, 32342277   Fax: +91-20-24300160   e-mail: pune@cbspd.com

Representatives

- **Hyderabad** 0-9885175004 • **Kolkata** 0-9831437309, 0-9051152362 • **Mumbai** 0-9833017933
- **Nagpur** 0-9021734563 • **Patna** 0-9334159340

Printed at Manipal Technologies Limited, Manipal

to

—————————————————————

my parents

and

my students of
MBBS, DLO, MS and DNB courses
in the golden jubilee year of
my teaching career, 2012

Foreword

Barin is like my younger brother and an excellent teacher in ENT and head-neck surgery. He is a respected ENT surgeon too. He wrote his first book in ENT in 1969 when he was as young as 33 years old. That book was probably the first of its kind written for undergraduate students in medical sciences in our country after independence and became very popular amongst the teachers as well as the MBBS students in our country.

I am glad to know that he has written this book *Synopsis of Otorhinolaryngology* considering the inclusions of development in otorhinolaryngology in the recent past. The colour illustrations and newer chapters on endoscopic sinonasal surgery, endoscopic tympanomastoid surgery, cochlear implantation surgery with posterior tympanotomy, facial nerve exploration and decompression surgery, use of Laser in ENT, etc. will be of immense help for the undergraduate students.

His concept of including the chapters on the instruments and X-rays in a book for the MBBS students in 1969 was of tremendous help for preparation during the final MBBS examinations in ENT.

I hope the MBBS students, the trainees and the practitioners will be benefitted with this concise book in ENT.

Prof. SP Ghosh

BSc, MBBS (Cal), MS (Cal), DLORCS (Eng), FICS (USA)

Ex-Professor
IPGMER and SSKM Hospital
RG Kar Medical College
North Bengal Medical College
National Medical College
Ex-Presidency Surgeon, Govt. of West Bengal
Examiner, Undergraduate and Postgraduate courses
University of Kolkata and Other Universities

Preface

My first book *Diseases of the Ear, Nose and Throat* was published in December 1969 when I was Assistant Professor in the ENT Department, Calcutta National Medical College. It was probably the only ENT book written in independent India for MBBS students. The 5th edition of the book was published in 2001.

I have decided to write another book for the same purpose. The subject of ENT has become more modern and more interesting during the last three decades or more. It provides information about the advanced developments in ENT. The contents of this book, I hope, will be attractive and helpful to the MBBS students. It may also be useful for the trainees in ENT, the ENT practitioners and specialists.

I am grateful to the CBS Publishers & Distributors for the opportunity provided to me and the encouragement given in preparing this book.

The basic information is written as per the requirements of the undergraduate medical students. The advanced information is included in a precise way so that it does not become a burden to the MBBS students. Some figures have been taken from the book *ENT Diseases*, 3rd edition, written by Hans Behrbohm *et al* published by Thieme in 2009. I gratefully acknowledge the authors and publisher of the book for the same.

I profusely thank Dr. Soumitra Ghosh, one of my brilliant students and Assistant Professor, Department of ENT, Vivekananda Institute of Medical Sciences, Kolkata, for his invaluable assistance. I gratefully acknowledge his contribution in this book.

I sincerely acknowledge the teachers in ENT and my postgraduate students of MS, DNB and DLO courses, who have given me impetus and encouragement day in and day out to edit my old book, which was published in 2001. To keep their request and to fulfill their wishes I thought I should write a new book including all the recent developments in ENT and head-neck surgery and newer approaches for the management of deafness, phonation, voice rehabilitation, functional endoscopic sinus surgery, etc.

I request all concerned and my well-wishers and students, many of whom are now the teachers in ENT and head-neck surgery, and some of them are the heads of the Department of ENT and Head-Neck Surgery, to go through this book and send their comments and criticism so that I may enrich the book further to fulfill the relevant requirements for the growth and development of this subject.

Barin Kumar Roychaudhuri

Contents

Section 2: Rhinology (Nose and Paranasal Sinuses)

Otology

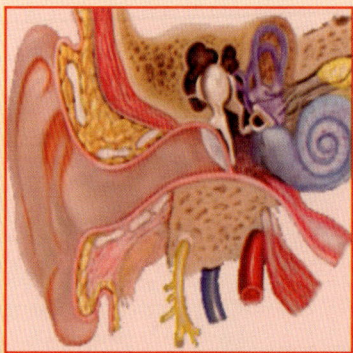

Anatomy of the Ear

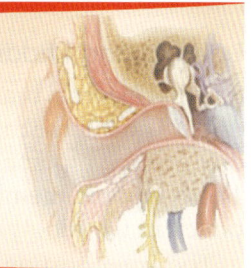

The ear consists of three parts—external, middle and inner. The latter is also named labyrinth, which contains the receptors of hearing and equilibrium (Fig. 1.1).

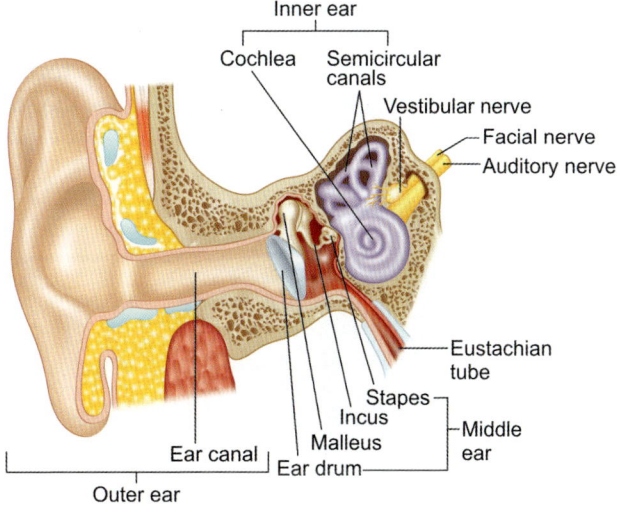

Fig. 1.1: Anatomy of the ear

DEVELOPMENT

Pinna

At six weeks of foetal life six tubercles appear round the dorsal margin of the first external branchial cleft, three on the mandibular arch, and three on the hyoid arch. At the 12th week all the tubercles, except the ventral mandibular tubercle, fuse and become incorporated in a general proliferation of the mesodermal element of the 2nd arch which extends crescentically around the meatal core. In the adult ear the tragus represents the persisting ventral mandibular tubercle. The rest of the auricle is developed from the above-mentioned mesodermal element of the hyoid arch carrying an investment of ectoderm with it, which develops into the covering skin.

External and Middle Ear

The first external branchial cleft or groove is the primordium of the external auditory canal. The internal aspect of the second branchial arch or bar forms part of the wall of the tubotympanic recess, which also contains first and third pharyngeal pouches. The tympanic membrane is formed as a separating membrane between the first pouch in the tubotympanic recess and the first external groove.

The outer portion of the tubotympanic recess develops into the tympanic cavity, while the inner part forms the eustachian tube.

Air spaces and lining membrane of the middle ear below the level of the chorda tympani nerve are developed from the entoderm of the tubotympanic recess. The ossicles are developed from the mesoderm as follows: at first the differentiating ossicles are embedded in the mesoderm above the level of tubotympanic recess. Gradually the investing mesoderm loosens and decreases in cellularity. The lining epithelial membrane of the tubotympanic recess invades the above-mentioned vacuolated mesoderm and wraps itself round the ossicles.

The ossicles start differentiating at 12 weeks and are fully formed in cartilage at 16 weeks when they begin to ossify. Out of all the 3 ossicles, the stapes is the last to ossify (Fig. 1.2).

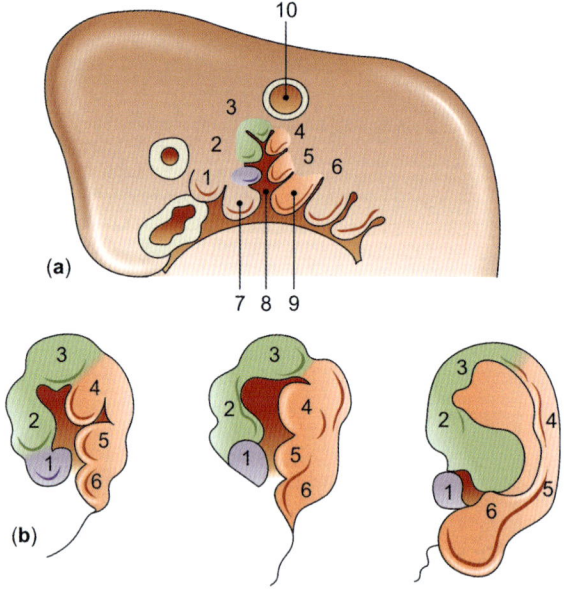

Fig. 1.2: Development of the external ear. (a) An 11 mm embryo, lateral view; (b) Development of the outer ear from 6 hillocks arising from the first and the second branchial arches. 1. Tragus; 2. Crus helicis; 3. Helix; 4. Crus antihelicis; 5. Antihelix; 6. Antitragus; 7. First branchial arch; 8. Branchial cleft; 9. Second branchial arch; 10. Auricular plate

Internal Ear

Immediately above the first external pharyngeal groove, the ectoderm thickens which is called the auditory (otic) placode. The placode gradually invaginates forming a pit, which closes to form a cyst (otocyst) and sinks into the mesoderm underneath the surface ectoderm. Tubotympanic recess grows in between the otocyst and the surface ectoderm. Thus the relationship between the middle and the inner ear is established. The membranous labyrinth or inner ear develops from the otocyst. The mesoderm covering the differentiating auditory vesicle (cochlear duct, utricle, saccule, and semicircular canals) is converted into a cartilaginous capsule to be ossified later on. The ossification begins at the 16th week and is completed by 23rd week of foetal life. The cochlear duct is fully developed by 12th week of foetal life (Table 1.1).

Table 1.1: Different parts of the ear development from different primitive layers

Ear	Primitive layers		
	Ectoderm	Mesoderm	Entoderm
External ear	Auricle External auditory canal Skin and glands	–	–
Tympanic membrane, Middle ear air spaces, Lining membrane and ossicles	Outer layer	Middle layer Malleus and incus from the dorsal end of the 1st arch and the major part of the stapes from the dorsal end of the second arch. The inner aspect of the footplate may be derived from the otic capsule. Upper half of the middle ear, ossicles and mastoid.	Inner layer Entoderm of T.T. recess (1st and 2nd pharyngeal pouch). Lower half of the middle ear below the level of chorda tympani nerve.
Inner ear or labyrinth	Membranous labyrinth, e.g. organ of Corti utricle saccule semicircular canals	Bony labyrinth and petrous temporal bone	–
Pharyngotympanic tube		–	–

CONGENITAL MALFORMATION OF THE EAR

Congenital atresia of the ear occurs in 1 in 10000 births. Unilateral atresia is six times more common than bilateral atresia. Congenital atresia may involve the pinna and/or the external and middle ear (atresia/ microtia). Unilateral cases should be operated on when the child had reached adolescence or young adulthood but there is no hard and fast rule. They may also be operated after a careful selection. In bilateral atresia at least one ear should be operated on much earlier (3 years or older) to render serviceable hearing (15 to 20 dB speech reception threshold), which may be attained in 75 to 80% of patients.

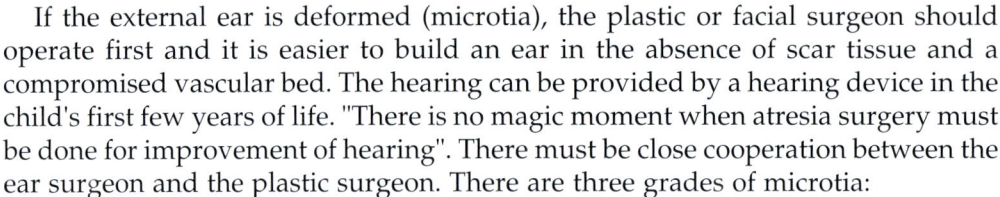

If the external ear is deformed (microtia), the plastic or facial surgeon should operate first and it is easier to build an ear in the absence of scar tissue and a compromised vascular bed. The hearing can be provided by a hearing device in the child's first few years of life. "There is no magic moment when atresia surgery must be done for improvement of hearing". There must be close cooperation between the ear surgeon and the plastic surgeon. There are three grades of microtia:

Grade I: The appearance of external ear is fairly well formed but smaller.

Grade II: The appearance of external ear has some form but is about one-half of a normal size.

Grade III: Poorly formed ear remnant on lateral face.

The plastic surgeon should routinely operate on first in Grade III microtia.

The external ear reconstruction should be delayed until the child is about 7 years of age. This delay is for growth of the rib cage so that sufficient costal cartilage can be harvested for implant. Earliest to operate by the plastic surgeon in Grade III microtia is at the age of 6 or 7 years. The otologist may then plan to open the ear for the hearing purpose, when the patient is 7 to 8 years of age. In unilateral atresia, there is no urgency for repair and the repair can be delayed to suit the convenience of the patient, the parents and the ear surgeon. In Grade I or II microtia, the atresia surgery should be performed as early as 4 years of age.

THE EXTERNAL EAR

The external ear comprises the pinna or auricle and the external auditory canal.

The pinna is composed of a skin-covered yellow elastic, cartilage, the posterior surface of which is convex and smooth. The anterior surface is concave with folds and hollows between them. The skin on the anterior surface is directly adherent to the perichondrium; on the posterior surface the skin is loose. The free anteroexternal margin of the pinna is known as the helix. Towards the bottom the pinna gradually turns into the lobule, which is devoid of cartilage. The lobule consists of well-developed fat and cellular tissue with a small number of vessels and nerves. The protruding cartilage over the external auditory meatus is named the tragus. In front of the helix and parallel to it is a ridge known as the antihelixes, with antitragus at its lower end. The hiatus between the lumina of the tragus and the crus of the helix is named incisura terminalis. An incision here will divide only skin, connective tissue and periosteum (endaural incision) (Fig. 1.3).

The external auditory canal extends from the bottom of concha up to the tympanic membrane. The average length in adult is 24 mm. Its general direction is inwards and slightly upwards and backwards in the outer

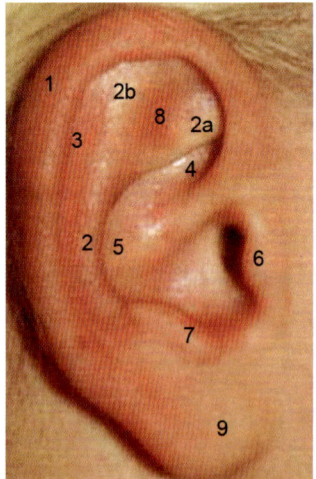

Fig. 1.3: A view of the right auricle with the various anatomical parts named. 1. Helix; 2. Antihelix (a: inferior crus, b: superior crus); 3. Scaphoid fossa; 4. Cymba conchae; 5. Cavum conchae; 6. Tragus; 7. Antitragus; 8. Triangular fossa; 9. Earlobe

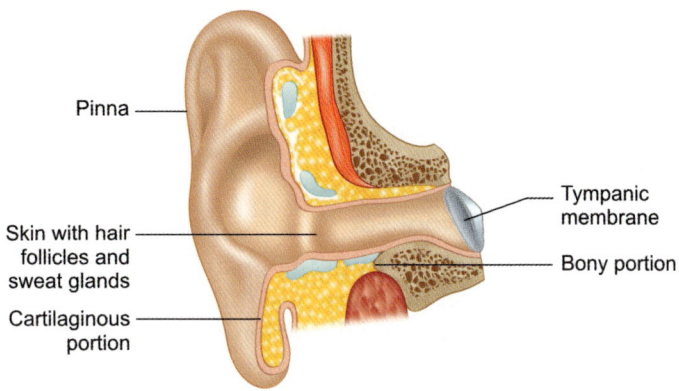

Pinna

Tympanic membrane

Skin with hair follicles and sweat glands

Bony portion

Cartilaginous portion

Fig. 1.4: Longitudinal section of the external auditory canal

cartilaginous part (8 mm), inwards and slightly downwards and forwards in the inner bony part (16 mm) (Fig. 1.4).

Therefore while examining the tympanic membrane, the pinna must be pulled backwards and upwards in order to straighten out the canal in adults. The junction between the cartilaginous and bony portions where foreign bodies are most likely to lodge is called the isthmus. The walls of the meatus are lined with skin, which in the bony portions gradually becomes thinner, loses its subcutaneous tissue and closely adheres to the periosteum. The skin covering the cartilaginous portion contains hair, sebaceous and ceruminous glands, which secrete the earwax or cerumen. The skin of the bony portion has neither hairs nor glands. The cartilaginous portion may have deficiencies other than incisura terminalis. The fissures of Santorini are amongst them providing potential paths of infection between the parotid gland and superficial mastoid regions. In children up to the age of about 4 years, and sometimes in the adult, the bony canal is deficient anteroinferiorly called foramen of Huschke. Through this gap infections may again pass between the adjacent parotid gland and the canal. The anterior wall is related to the articular head of the mandible, which explains why it is painful to open the mouth and chew in cases of inflammation of the anterior wall of the external auditory canal.

In the newborn, there is neither bony canal nor mastoid process. In place of the bony canal there is a bony ring or annulus, which is deficient in a small upper portion and is directly connected with the cartilaginous canal. The inner border of the annulus has a long furrow or sulcus into which the tympanic membrane is inserted. In the bone-free upper part, the tympanic membrane is directly attached to the squamous part of the temporal bone, the so-called notch of Rivinus. By the end of the third year, the external auditory canal is fully developed.

Physical Volume of Ear Canal

Normal volume is up to 1.0 ml in children and 2 ml in adults. In perforation of the tympanic membrane, the volume is more than 2 ml in children and more than 2.5 ml in adults as the middle ear volume is added with the volume of external ear canal.

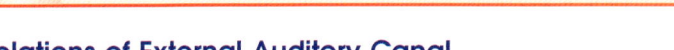

Relations of External Auditory Canal

The external auditory canal is related in front by the temporomandibular joint, behind by the mastoid air cells, above by the middle cranial fossa, and posteromedial and superomedial to the sloping squamous portion of the deep bony canal by the mastoid antrum.

Sensory Nerve-supply of External Ear

The great auricular nerve (C2,3) supplies the greater portion of the posterior or medial surface of the auricle and the more posterior portion of the lateral surface. Lesser occipital nerve (C2) supplies a small portion of the upper part of the posterior surface and overlaps with the great auricular nerve.

The auriculotemporal branch of the trigeminal nerve supplies the skin of the tragus, the anterior limb of the helix and a portion of the crus, the anterosuperior wall of the external auditory canal and the corresponding segment of the external surface of the tympanic membrane.

Auricular branch of the vagus nerve (Arnold's) joins the posterior auricular branch of the VIIth cranial nerve and supplies the concavity of the concha, posterior portion of the external auditory canal and the corresponding segment of the external surface of the tympanic membrane and a small area of the skin on the postero-medial aspect of the auricle and adjacent mastoid region. Thus mechanical irritation of the posterior wall of the canal, as in removal of wax, often causes reflex cough and even vasovagal attack owing to vagal irritation.

Blood Supply

The external ear is supplied with blood by branches of the external carotid artery, e.g. auriculotemporal branch of superficial temporal artery anteriorly and branches of posterior auricular artery posteriorly.

Lymphatic Drainage of the External Ear

The lymphatics of the tragus, anterior external portion of the auricle and anterior wall of the auditory canal drain into the superficial parotid lymph nodes (preauricular). The lymphatics of the posterior external and whole cranial aspect of the auricle and the posterior wall of the canal drain into the postauricular lymph nodes. From the lobule of the auricle and the floor of the canal lymphatics drain into the external jugular lymph nodes. Inflammations in the external auditory canal are often accompanied by swelling and pain in these lymph nodes.

Tympanic Membrane

The tympanic membrane or "drum head" is a thin, freely mobile, semitransparent, elliptical disc situated between the external and the middle ear. Functionally the tympanic membrane is a part of the tympanic cavity or "ear drum" and the tympanic membrane may be called 'drum head' (Fig. 1.5).

When seen under illumination it presents a pearly grey or mother-of-pearl appearance with a triangular cone of reflected light in its anteroinferior quadrant. The greater part of the tympanic membrane fitted into the bony sulcus of the

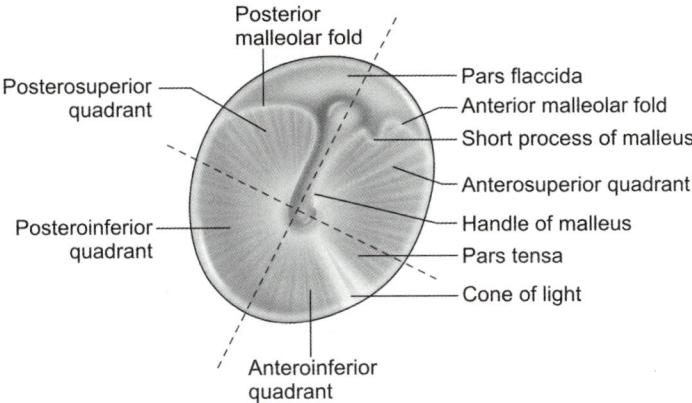

Fig. 1.5: Normal tympanic membrane (right)

tympanic ring is taut, and is called the pars tensa. The other smaller part which is directly attached to the notch of Rivinus is lax, and is called the pars flaccida or Shrapnell's membrane. The tympanic membrane consists of three layers: an outer layer or epidermal layer continuous with that of the auditory canal, a middle layer of radiating and circular connective tissue fibres, and an inner layer of mucosa continuous with the mucous membrane of the tympanic cavity. Shrapnell's membrane or pars flaccida consists only of two layers and lacks the middle layer of fibrous tissue.

In infancy the tympanic membrane is comparatively thick owing to the presence of a loose submucous layer. It grows compact with age and becomes quite thin in the elderly.

The tympanic membrane is set with an obliquity of about 55° to the floor of the meatus. The centre of it is retracted and is called the umbo. An ivory-coloured extension upwards from the umbo is the handle of the malleus. The handle of the malleus is embedded in the fibrous layer of the drumhead. It starts from the umbo and goes forward and upward to end above in a tiny knob of a pinhead size: the short process. From this process two folds stretch anteriorly and posteriorly, named accordingly the anterior and posterior malleolar folds. These two folds separate the upper lax membrane flaccida from the lower taut membrana tensa. Sometimes the veiled image of the long process of the incus and occasionally the stapedius tendon are visible when the posterior portion of the membrane is more transparent.

Artery Supply

The external surface of the tympanic membrane is supplied by deep auricular branch of the maxillary artery. After piercing the anterior bony wall of the external auditory canal, it sends small radial branches into the membrane from the whole circumference of the pars tensa and one or two manubrial branches that descend on the handle of malleus from the above.

The internal surface of the tympanic membrane is supplied by the stylomastoid branch of the posterior auricular artery from behind, and by the tympanic branch of the maxillary artery from the front.

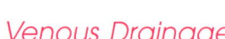
Venous Drainage

The superficial veins drain into the external jugular veins. Veins from the inner surface drain partly into the transverse sinus and veins of dura mater, and partly into the plexus of veins on the eustachian tube.

Nerve Supply

Posterior half of the external surface of the tympanic membrane is supplied by auricular branch of the vagus nerve and possibly filaments of glossopharyngeal and facial nerve, and the anterior half by the auriculotemporal branch of the trigeminal nerve. The inner surface of the membrane is supplied from the tympanic branch of the glossopharyngeal nerve.

Lymphatic Drainage

The lymph vessels pass to the parotid lymph nodes, post-auricular lymph nodes and cervical group of nodes.

MIDDLE EAR CLEFT

The middle ear cleft consists of:
1. Eustachian tube
2. Tympanic cavity
3. Aditus ad antrum
4. Mastoid antrum
5. Mastoid air cells

Eustachian Tube

It is about 3.5 cm in length and connects the middle ear cavity with the nasopharynx. The outer third of this, adjoining the middle ear, is bony. The inner two-thirds leading into the nasopharynx are made up of membrane and cartilage. The nasopharyngeal opening lies behind and on a level with the posterior end of the inferior turbinate. At rest, the tube remains closed, but it opens on yawning or swallowing movement by contraction of the soft palate muscles attached to it. In adults the tube lies obliquely with the inner end lowermost. In infants, the tube is more horizontal and relatively wide and short. Thus the middle ear infection in infants is more common than in adults.

Tympanic Cavity

It is a six-sided chamber. It lies between the external ear and the inner and is like a biconcave disc. Through the eustachian tube, it communicates with the nasopharynx in front. Through the aditus, it communicates with the mastoid antrum and the cells of the mastoid process. The tympanic cavity, similar to the cells of the mastoid process, contains air coming through the eustachian tube. It measures 15 mm from above downwards, 13 mm anteroposteriorly, and 2 mm (depth) in the middle (Fig. 1.6).

The tympanic cavity is divided into three parts: Mesotympanum—it is the middle ear proper and the biggest of the three; it corresponds with the pars tensa of the

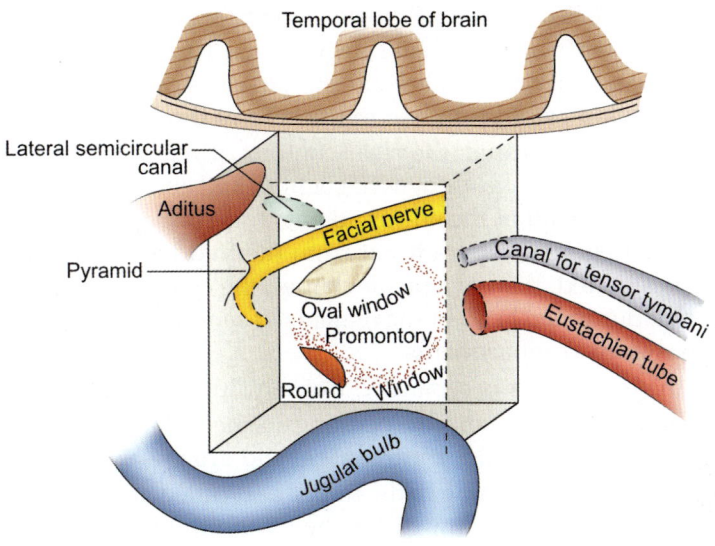

Fig. 1.6: Middle ear cavity, a six-sided area, with important relations

tympanic membrane; Epitympanum—the upper part, lying above the former and also known as the epitympanic recess or attic; Hypotympanum—the lower part, lying below the tympanic membrane level.

The outer wall of the tympanic cavity is formed mainly by the tympanic membrane, and above this—by the external bony wall of the epitympanum or attic.

The inner bony wall separates the middle ear from the inner ear. There is an eminence on this wall, corresponding to the basal turn of the cochlea, named promontory. Above and behind it is the oval window, which leads into the vestibule and is closed by the footplate of the stapes. Below and behind the promontory in a niche is the round window, which leads into the cochlea. The round window is closed by a thin membrane, the secondary tympanic membrane. The horizontal

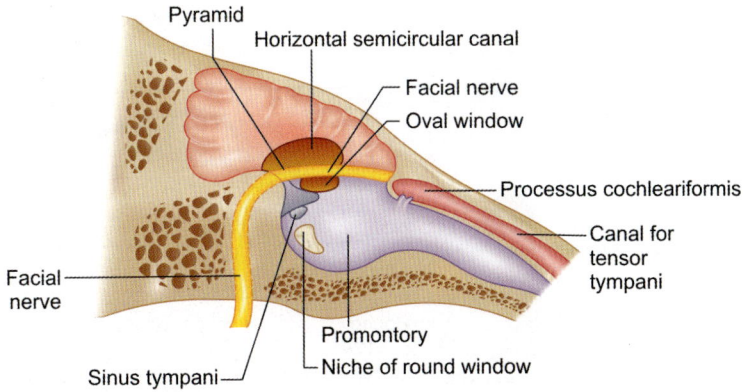

Fig. 1.7: Medial wall of middle ear

part of the facial nerve lies just above the oval window in a bony canal. On reaching the entrance to the antrum, the facial nerve canal turns downwards to form a descending knee, and then passes behind the posterior wall of the auditory canal and through the stylomastoid foramen to the base of the skull (Fig. 1.7).

Horizontal semicircular canal, the clear contour of which serves for orientation in operations of the mastoid, lies somewhat behind and above the facial nerve canal. This lies on the medial wall of the aditus ad antrum. The roof of the middle ear is a thin plate of bone (tegmen) separating it from the middle cranial fossa where the temporal lobe is situated. A bony spicule named the cog extends from the tegmen into the attic, anterior to the head of the malleus. It separates the epitympanum into anterior and posterior compartments.

The *floor* of the middle ear is separated from the jugular bulb by a bony plate.

The *eustachian tube* begins with an opening in the anterior wall separating the tympanic cavity from the canal for internal carotid artery.

The *posterior wall* has an opening in the upper part called aditus ad antrum, which leads to the mastoid antrum. Below this is the pyramid through the opening at the tip of which passes the tendon of the stapedius muscle, which is inserted into the neck of the stapes. The anterior wall has two openings:

i. Tympanic end of eustachian tube, below.

ii. Canal for tensor tympani muscle, above.

The tendon of the tensor tympani passes laterally around the processus cochleariformis and inserted into the handle of the malleus just below its neck.

The tympanic cavity contains three ossicles: the malleus, the incus and the stapes. They transmit sound waves from the surface of the tympanic membrane to the cochlear fluid.

The handle of the malleus is incorporated into the fibrous layer of the tympanic membrane. The footplate of the stapes is attached in the oval window by means of an annular ligament. The incus lies between the malleus and the stapes. This ossicular system is kept in place by ligaments fastening the malleus and incus to the walls of the tympanic cavity (Fig. 1.8).

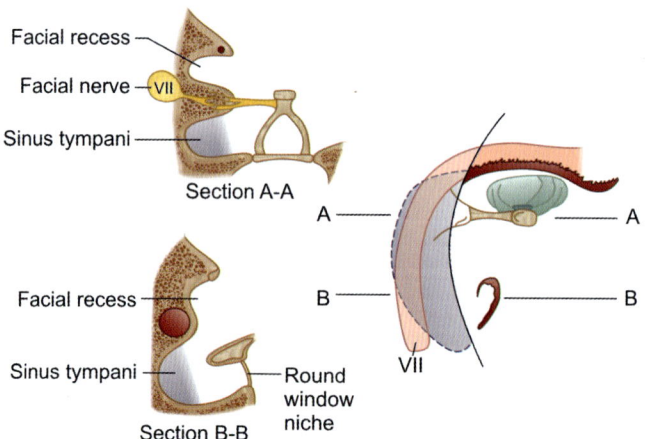

Fig. 1.8: The facial recess and sinus tympani of the right middle ear

There are two muscles in the tympanic cavity:
i. Tensor tympani, which keeps the tympanic membrane stretched. It is innervated by trigeminal nerve.
ii. Stapedius, which arises from the hollow pyramid and is attached to the neck of the stapes. It is innervated by facial nerve.

Aditus ad Antrum

It is a short channel connecting the epitympanum and the mastoid antrum. The bony prominence of the lateral semicircular canal lies between the medial wall and floor of the aditus. The short process of incus lies on its floor called fossa incudis. The facial nerve lies in a deeper plane in the floor of the aditus.

Mastoid Antrum

It is situated in the petrous temporal bone. Suprameatal triangle (Macewen's) forms its bony surface marking in the adult. It communicates with the mastoid air-cells by several openings.

Mastoid Air Cells

There is a considerable variation in distribution, number and size of mastoid air cells. There are three types of mastoid process,
1. Cellular or pneumatic, where air cells are large and numerous.
2. Diploeic, where cells are small and less numerous. Marrow spaces are present.
3. Acellular or sclerotic, where cells and marrow spaces are absent. The pneumatised mastoid is regarded as normal. 80 per cent of mastoids are pneumatised, and the rest 20 per cent is either diploic or acellular. The mastoid antrum is always present (Fig. 1.9).

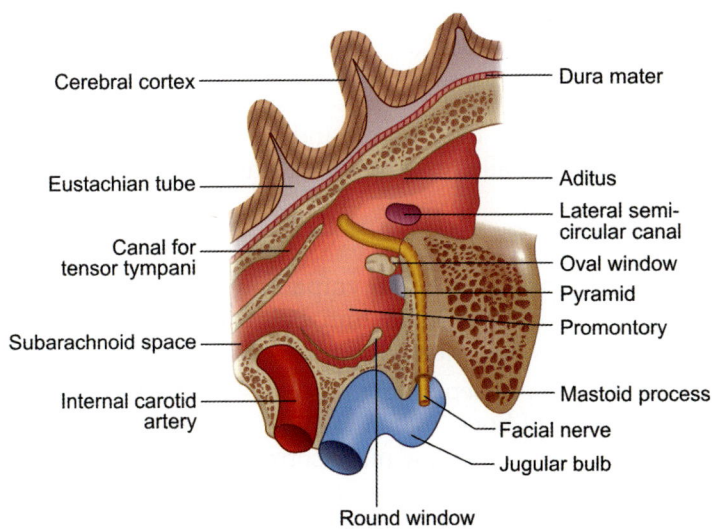

Fig. 1.9: Relations of the left tympanic cavity and facial nerve

Koerner's Septum

The remnant of the petrosquamous suture sometimes persists as a partition within the mastoid cells, extending upwards towards the antrum as Korner's septum. This septum produces a false floor of the mastoid antrum.

In searching for the mastoid antrum, which always lies just above and behind the posterosuperior bony meatal wall a few millimeters lateral to the annulus and sulcus tympanicus, one should be beware of:

1. Forward lying sigmoid sinus
2. Low middle fossa dura
3. Second genu (pyramidal segment) of facial nerve to begin its vertical course in the mastoid
4. A "false antrum" due to well-developed Korner's septum.

The landmarks for the vertical portion of the facial nerve are:

1. The posterior end of the bony horizontal semicircular canal
2. The digastric ridge and
3. The tympanomastoid suture in the posterior bony meatal wall.

Trautman's Triangle

The triangular area of the posterior fossa plate behind the antrum is the Trautman's triangle. It is bounded posteriorly by the sigmoid sinus, anteriorly by the solid angle of the bony labyrinth and superiorly by the superior petrosal sinus. Cerebellar abscess secondary to ear infection (otogenic brain abscess) can be drained through the Trautman's triangle.

Solid Angle

The solid bone medial to the antrum in the angle formed by the three semicircular canals is known as solid angle.

Sinodural Angle

The angle between the middle fossa above and the posterior fossa and the sigmoid sinus behind the antrum is called the sinodural angle.

Sinus Tympani

The medial wall of the posterior mesotympanum is divided into discrete bony pockets by the ponticulus and the subiculum. Below the ponticulus on the posterior aspect of the tympanum is the sinus tympani.

Ponticulus is a ridge of bone separating the oval window from the sinus tympani. The subiculum is a ridge of bone, which persists from the pyramidal eminence to the posterior lip of the round window niche separating the sinus tympani from the round window.

Facial nerve is normally located inferiorly and slightly medial to the horizontal semicircular canal and 1.72 to 0.92 mm from the tip of the short process of incus.

Facial Recess

The facial recess is a collection of air cells lying immediately lateral to the facial nerve at the external genu. This recess may serve as a route to the middle ear for extensive cholesteatoma. The landmarks used to expose the facial recess are the external genu of the facial nerve medially, the fossa incudis superiorly, the chorda tympani nerve laterally and the tympanic membrane anteriorly and laterally. Using a diamond burr (4 mm), the buttress of bone just inferior to the tip of incus is left intact and the bone over the facial recess is thinned, identifying the chorda tympani nerve and the posterior and posterolateral aspect of facial nerve at this point. A smaller burr (2 mm) is then used to open the confines of the facial recess. Opening the facial recess gives visualisation of the superior and posterior mesotympanum. The pyramidal process, the stapes superstructure, oval and round windows, the incus and malleus and the eustachian tube may be identified. After removing the bar of bone protecting the incus (incus buttress), the horizontal part of the facial nerve comes into clear view, as do the tensor tympani and cochleariform process.

Geniculate Ganglion

It is located in the anterior epitympanum. It can be found slightly superior and anterior to the cochleariform process as the nerve turns inward towards the internal auditory canal, bending around the cochlea.

Attic

The attic or "epitympanum" lies above the fallopian canal of the horizontal part of the facial nerve. It is bounded above by the thin bone (tegmen tympani) separating middle cranial fossa from the middle ear and posteriorly by the mastoid antrum. The aditus ad antrum is the opening from the epitympanum to the antrum. Anteriorly the attic is bounded by zygomatic air cells and below by an imaginary line at the level of anterior and posterior tympanic spine. The attic is the extension of the middle ear spaces and carries a continuation of the mucoperiosteum of the middle ear cavity.

Cog

It is a spine of bone that hangs inferiorly from the tegmen just above the cochleariform process. The facial nerve lies anterior to the cog just before it turns into the "First genu".

Cochleariform Process

The tensor tympani tendon comes out of its semicanal at the bony eminence known as the cochleariform process and inserts onto the malleus. Superior to the cochleariform process, the facial nerve takes a sharp bend towards the internal auditory canal named first genu of the facial nerve.

The tensor tympani muscle originates on the cartilaginous portion of the eustachian tube, passes across the cochleariform process as a tendon and inserts on the manubrium of the malleus.

Facial Ridge

The plate of bone just covering the facial nerve is called the facial ridge.

Cochlea

From apex to base the cochlea measures 5 mm and the diameter of the base is about 10 mm. The cochlea has two and three fourth turns.

Mike's Dot

It is a cribriform area of bone (macula cribrosa superior) that transmits the vestibular nerve to the ampulla of the lateral and superior semicircular canals. Mike's dot is a useful landmark for identifying the lateral end of the internal auditory canal located in the vestibule.

Mucosa, Folds and Compartments of the Middle Ear

The walls of the tympanic cavity, mastoid antrum and air cells are lined with continuous thin mucosa. The mucous membrane of the eustachian tube and of the adjoining part of the floor of the tympanic cavity is lined with pseudo stratified ciliated columnar epithelium. The mucosa of the cartilaginous part of the Eustachian tube contains mucous glands, which are absent in the mucosa of the other parts of the middle ear. The mucosa of the attic and antral region above the level of chorda tympani nerve is non-ciliated epithelium. It is a single-layered pavement or low columnar in type. The attic or epitympanum has no thoroughfare with mesotympanum except through two small ports of entry anteriorly and posteriorly, i.e. isthmus tympani anticus and isthmus tympani posticus respectively. The attic region is subdivided into anterior and posterior compartments by transversely placed superior malleolar fold. The posterior compartment is subdivided into lateral and medial incudal spaces by the superior incudal fold. The lateral incudal space is also called superior incudal space. Below the floor of the attic there are three compartments. The inferior incudal space bounded above by the lateral incudal fold, medially by the medial incudal fold, laterally by the posterior malleolar fold, and anteriorly by the interossicular fold, which lies between the long process of the incus and the upper two-thirds of the handle of malleus. Anterior and posterior pouch of von Troltsch lie anterior and posterior to the handle of malleus and between the anterior and posterior malleolar folds and the tympanic membrane respectively.

Prussak's space—a small space lying between the neck of the malleus and pars flaccida of the drumhead.

The mucosal folds limit infection to one or several of these compartments of the middle ear.

Internal Auditory Meatus

The internal auditory meatus is nearly 1 cm in length, which terminates in a perforated plate. It is divided into two portions by a transverse crest (the crista falciformis), which separates the nerves into upper and lower groups. The upper part is divided by a vertical ridge (Bill's bar) separating the superior vestibular nerve canal posteriorly and facial nerve canal anteriorly. The posterior part below

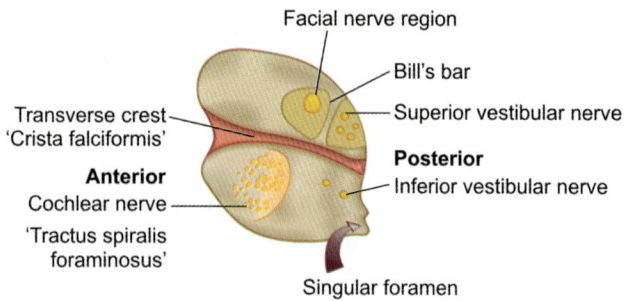

Facial nerve region

Bill's bar

Transverse crest—
'Crista falciformis'

Superior vestibular nerve

Anterior
Cochlear nerve

Posterior
Inferior vestibular nerve

'Tractus spiralis
foraminosus'

Singular foramen

Fig. 1.10: Right internal auditory meatus with its contents

the transverse crest is the inferior vestibular area, which transmits nerves to the saccule. The nerve to the posterior semicircular canal passes through the foramen singulare. The cochlea area is situated in the anterior part below the crista falciformis, named tractus spiralis foraminosus (Fig. 1.10).

Dissection of Internal Auditory Canal

After removing all the bone of the labyrinth and the bone between the jugular bulb inferiorly and the superior petrosal sinus superiorly the internal auditory canal is skeletonised by removing bone above (the roof) and below (the floor) as well as in the area near the posterior lip. Bone is removed so as to approach the posterior wall of the internal auditory canal. All of the dura is exposed first. A horizontal crest, the falciformis (transverse crest), separates the fibres of the superior vestibular nerve from the thin filaments of nerve to the saccule (inferior vestibular nerve). On the medial side of the superior vestibular nerve laterally in the canal, there is a vertical bony bar (Bill's bar). Anterior to Bill's bar is the facial nerve. The facial nerve enters the canal above the falciform crest and in front of the vertical crest. The superior vestibular nerve, which covers the vestibular nerve, is situated more superficially than the inferior vestibular nerve. The cochlear nerve can be seen only after resection of the inferior vestibular nerve.

The simple mastoidectomy and postauricular labyrinthectomy are the first two stages of the approach to the internal auditory canal. During labyrinthectomy in this procedure, the ampulla of the superior semicircular canal is preserved as a landmark to find the end of the superior vestibular nerve, Bill's bar and the facial canal. In approaching the internal auditory canal, one must remember that the medial wall of the vestibule represents the lateral wall of the internal auditory canal fundus where the nerves enter the inner ear structures. Minimal bone removal on the medial wall of the vestibule will expose the internal auditory canal. Posteriorly, at the posterior fossa dura, the route to the porus acousticus is much deeper because the internal auditory canal is slanting away from the dissector. The plane of the canal in an anterior-posterior direction is roughly from the external genu to the sinodural angle. The superior border of the internal auditory canal extends from the facial canal to the sinodural angle. The inferior border of the internal auditory canal is at a point approximating the junction of the external genu and descending portion of the facial nerve and parallel the superior border posteriorly to its junction with the posterior fossa.

Blood Supply

The middle ear is supplied with blood mainly by branches of the external carotid artery.

Venous Drainage

From the middle ear the veins of the duramater, the venous sinuses and the venous plexuses around the carotid artery maintain the venous drainage.

Lymphatic Drainage

Lymphatic drainage is carried out as follows:
1. Through peritubal lymphatics to the retropharyngeal nodes and further to the deep cervical glands.
2. Through the lymphatic vessels across the tympanic cavity to the lymphatic ducts of the external auditory meatus and pre- and post-auricular lymph nodes.

Nerve Supply

The nerve supply of the middle ear is from the tympanic plexus. It lies over the promontory and forms by branches of the glossopharyngeal, facial and sympathetic nerves.

Relations of the Middle Ear Cleft

Inflammatory and neoplastic diseases of the middle ear cleft may give rise to series of complications. It is important to know therefore the relations of the middle ear cleft (Fig. 1.6).
  i. The temporal lobe of brain with its meninges is separated from the tympanic cavity, aditus, and antrum by a thin plate of bone (tegmen tympani et antri).
  ii. The inner ear (labyrinth) lies in relation to the medial wall of the tympanic cavity, aditus and antrum.
  iii. The facial nerve, the horizontal and vertical portions of it is closely related to the medial and posterior wall of the tympanic cavity respectively.
  iv. The lateral sinus (sigmoid portion) is related to the posteromedial part of the mastoid process.
  v. The jugular bulb is separated by a thin plate of bone, i.e. floor of the tympanic cavity.
  vi. The cerebellum lies in the posterior cranial fossa, posteromedial to the lateral sinus.
  vii. The fifth and sixth cranial nerves are closely related to the petrous temporal bone.

ANATOMY OF INFRATEMPORAL FOSSA

It lies below the base of the skull deep to the ascending. ramus of the mandible, shaped rather like an inverted pyramid. It possesses roof, anterior, lateral and medial walls, a posterior edge and an apex inferiorly. It is filled with muscles, nerves and blood vessels and it communicates with adjacent anatomical spaces by fissures and openings.

The roof is formed by the infratemporal surface of the greater wing of the sphenoid bone and further back by a small part of the squamous temporal bone.

Inferiorly, the fossa is limited by the upper surface of the medial pterygoid and attachment of this muscle to the inner aspect of the lower part of the ascending ramus of the mandible. Behind the muscle, lies the hiatus, which communicates below with the parapharyngeal space.

The lateral pterygoid plate represents the anterior half of the medial wall of the infratemporal fossa with the tensor palati and superior constrictor forming the posterior half of the medial wall.

On the lateral side, the inner aspect of the zygomatic arch, the masseter and temporalis muscles, the ascending ramus of the mandible, the upper most part of the deep lobe of the parotid gland and styloid apparatus constitute the external boundary.

The anterior wall of the fossa is the rounded posterolateral wall of the maxillary antrum and the posterior margin of the innermost part of the tympanic plate.

The infratemporal fossa communicates with the pterygopalatine fossa through the pterygomaxillary fissure, which occupies the junction of anterior and medial walls.

The inferior orbital fissure similarly forms a connection with the orbit at the junction of the roof and the anterior walls. The gap between the anterior edge of the ascending ramus of the mandible and posterolateral wall of the maxilla represents a potential channel of communication between the infratemporal fossa and the oral cavity.

The muscles, which fill the infratemporal fossa, are the medial and lateral pterygoids and the temporalis. The maxillary artery crosses the fossa giving out its five named branches on the way to the infraorbital and pterygomaxillary fissures. The fossa contains thin-walled veins, some of which are grouped together within and overlying the pterygoid muscles as the pteroygoid venous plexus. The mandibular division of the fifth cranial nerve, its anterior and posterior subdivisions and their branches traverse the length of the fossa mainly in a downward and lateral direction between the pterygoid muscles.

INNER EAR OR LABYRINTH

The inner ear consists of bony and membranous labyrinth. The bony part, like a capsule, covers the membranous labyrinth, which is filled up with endolymph. Endolymph has high potassium and low sodium. The space between the bony and membranous labyrinth is filled up with perilymph, which contains high sodium and low potassium. The bony labyrinth has the following parts:

1. The vestibule
2. Three semicircular canals
3. The cochlea

The *vestibule* lies in the centre of the bony labyrinth. On its external wall, the oval window is situated. Within the bony vestibule a system of membranous sac is present. The saccule lies in front and communicates with the membranous cochlea. The utricle lies in rear and is connected with the three membranous semicircular canals by five separate openings. They represent three planes of spaces. The sacs of the vestibule contain the statokinetic receptors or maculae, the otoliths made up of specific neuroepithelium covered with a membrane containing granules of carbonate and phosphates of lime.

The *three semicircular canals*, horizontal, superior and posterior are set at right angles to one another. One end of each canal is dilated and is known as ampulla. The superior and posterior canals have a common even stem called crus commune.

The *ampulla* contains receptor organ called crista.

The receptors of the vestibule and semicircular canals are the peripheral nerve endings of the vestibular analyzer.

The *cochlea* is a bony tube of two-and-a-half turns around a central pillar called the modiolus and resembles a snail-shell in appearance.

An osseo-membranous lamina divides the tube lumen into two, i.e. the upper or scala vestibule and the lower or scala tympani. They communicate at the apex through a small opening known as the helicotrema. Both the channels are filled up with perilymph. The scala vestibule communicates with the vestibule, while the scala tympani borders the tympanic cavity through the round window covered by the secondary tympanic membrane.

The scala vestibule of the cochlea contains the thin Reissner's membrane which extends from the osseous spiral lamina to cut off a small membranous canal filled with endolymph and is known as the cochlear duct or ductus cochlearis.

The end organ of hearing is called the organ of corti. It rests on the basilar membrane. The basilar membrane is a structure of elastic fibres of different lengths strung from the edge of the bony spiral lamina to the outer wall of the cochlea.

The organ of Corti is a structure of complex histology containing hair cells and supporting cells. The cells are covered with a membrane called the tectorial membrane. The sensory hair cells are connected by a network of cochlear nerve branches leading to the spiral ganglion of the auditory nerve in the bony spiral lamina. The central ends of the bipolar cells of the spiral ganglion are connected with the superior temporal gyrus of the brain by intricate routes.

Organ of Corti

It consists of a series of neuroepithelial structures. Organ of Corti is divided into inner and outer portions by a triangular tunnel formed by the two rows of rods of Corti and the basilar membrane. On the inner side of the inner rod, there is a single row of hair cells, i.e. inner hair cells. These are bulbous in shape.

The hairs of each cell consist of 120 stereocilia arranged in two rows in the form of a double "V". On the outer side of the outer rod, there are three or four rows of hair cells, i.e. outer hair cells. These are columnar in shape, with 46–148 stereocilia arranged in three rows in the form of a triple "W". The outer hair cells cilia are 2 mm long in the basal turn and increase in length to 6 mm at the apex. The free surface of each hair cell is the cuticular plate, and the hair cells are separated by supporting cells. There are about 4,500 inner hair cells and 12,500 outer hair cells in each ear.

The tectorial membrane overhangs the organ of Corti. Outside the outer hair cells are the cells of Hensen. Lining the outer side of the scala media is the stria

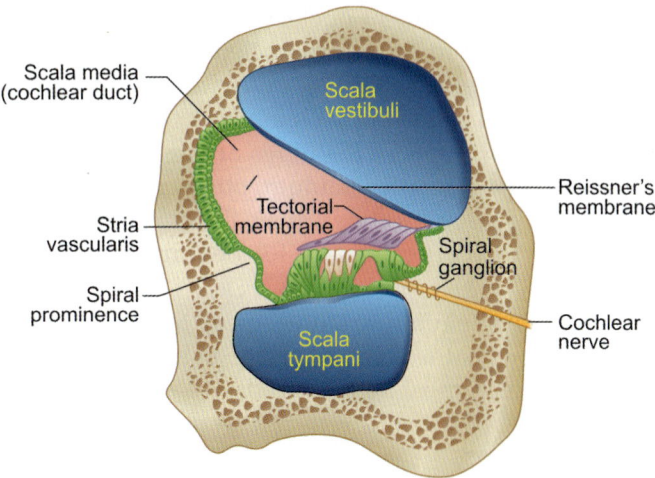

Fig. 1.11: A cross-section of the cochlea with organ of Corti

vascularis, which is important in regulating Na and K ions. The thickened endosteum lining the outer wall of the bony canal of the cochlea is called the spiral ligament.

The basilar membrane in the basal part of cochlea represents the high frequencies starting from 20,000 Hz. The most prominent part of the promontory lies at the region of basilar membrane representing 4000 Hz and the apical part of the basilar represents the low frequencies (Fig. 1.11).

Cochlear Division of VIIIth Cranial Nerve

The terminal fibres end in contact with the hair cells. These fibres are of two types: type I fibres are less granulated and probably afferent, and type II fibres are richly granulated and probably efferent. The fibres pass in the spiral lamina to the spiral ganglion in the modiolus, to become the auditory branch of the VIIIth cranial nerve.

Central Connections of the Cochlear Nerve

The cochlear nerve is composed of the central processes of the bipolar cell bodies of the spiral ganglion of the cochlea (the peripheral processes; connect with the organ of Corti). It lies on the lateral side of the vestibular nerve as it enters the brainstem. In the brainstem the cochlear fibres end in dorsal and ventral cochlear nuclei interposed by inferior cerebellar peduncle (restiform body) (Fig. 1.12).

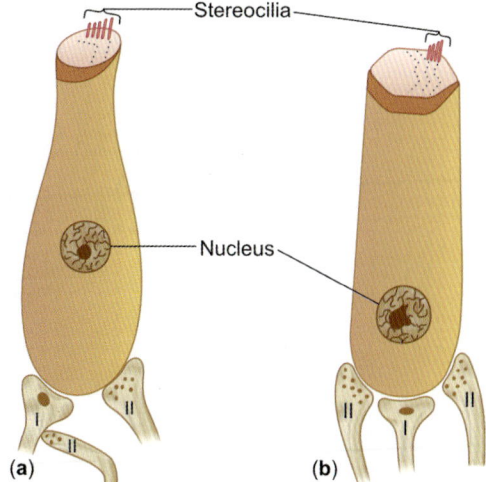

Fig. 1.12: Structure of cochlear hair cells. (a) Inner hair cell, (b) Outer hair cell

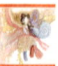

The axons of the cells of the cochlear nuclei (second neuron) pass across the floor of the fourth ventricle and end in the dorsal nucleus of the corpus trapezoideum of the same or of the opposite side. From the nuclei of the corpus trapezoideum a third neuron system ascends as the lateral lemniscus (Fig. 1.13).

On reaching the mid-brain some of the fibres of the lateral lemniscus end in the nucleus of the inferior corpus quadrigeminum, others reach the medial geniculate body. From the medial geniculate body new fibres (fourth neuron) carry the auditory impressions to the cortical centre for hearing in the superior temporal gyrus (Fig. 1.14).

Hearing is relayed almost equally from each ear to the acoustic cortex of both sides. This means that for deafness in either ear to arise from central causes the acoustic paths from both ears must be damaged.

Vestibular Receptor Organs

These are the ampullary cristae and the utricular maculae (otolith organ). Their epithelium is formed of cells surmounted by long hairlets. The vestibular cells are of two types: the type I cell which is rounded and flask-shaped and surrounded by a nerve chalice; and the type II cell which is cylindrical and has no nerve chalice. Hence the type I cell bears a morphological resemblance to the inner hair cells and the type II cell resembles the outer hair cell of the cochlea. The hairs jut into a mucus like substance, dome shaped in the ampulla (cupola), cylindrical in the utricle, where there are a number of calcareous particles (otoliths) embedded in it.

The bundle of sensory hairs protruding from the free surface of each sensory cell is composed of one kinocilium and 50–110 stereocilia. The kinocilium is the longest of the sensory hairs and each bundle of the stereocilia diminish in length with

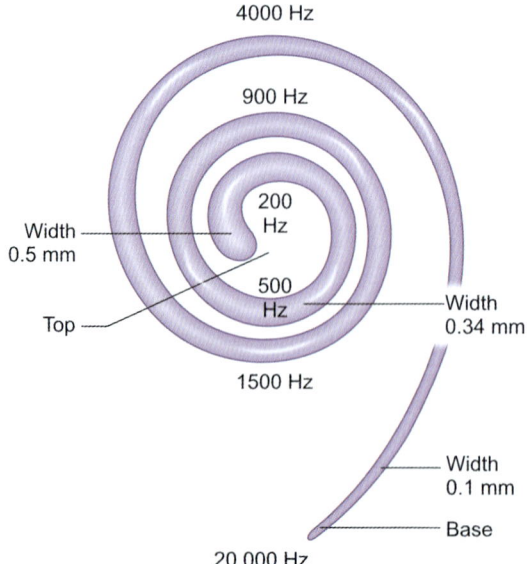

Fig. 1.13: The human basilar membrane showing the frequency dependent locations of sound receptors and analyzing receptors

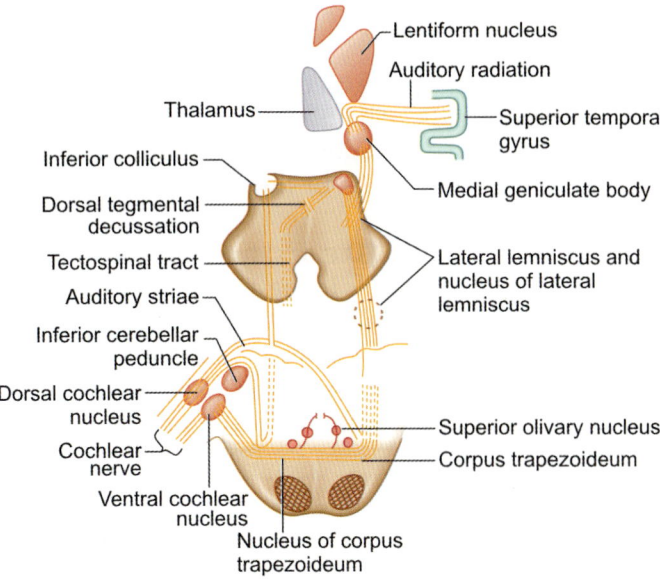

Fig. 1.14: Central connections of cochlear nerve

increase in distance from the kinocilium. Hence there is morphological (and functional) polarization of the vestibular cells, a displacement of the sensory hairs towards the kinocilium accompanied by depolarization of the cell and increased rate of discharge in the afferent nerve with a decreased discharge rate when the hairs are displaced in the opposite direction.

Central Connections of the Vestibular Nerve (Fig. 1.15)

The impulses from the different parts of the nonauditory labyrinth are conveyed by the vestibular branch of the VIIIth nerve to the superior, lateral, medial and

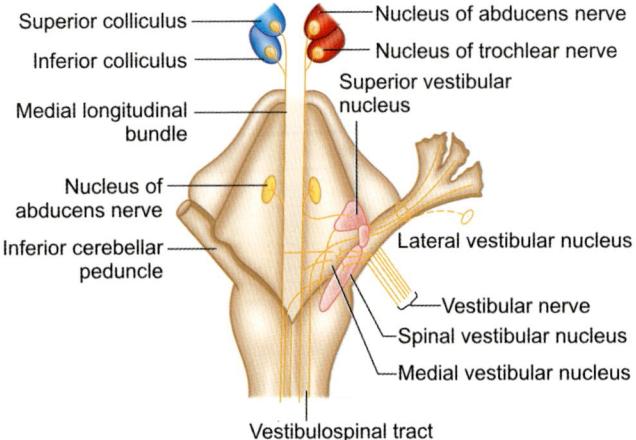

Fig. 1.15: Central connections of vestibular nerve

inferior vestibular nuclei in the medulla oblongata, from which relay fibres follow three pathways:

1. Ascending fibres from the superior, medial and inferior vestibular nuclei form the medial longitudinal bundle. The fibres from these nuclei terminate in the nuclei of the IIIrd, IVth and VIth cranial nerves and constitute the vestibulo-ocular tracts. The reflex movements of the eyes are brought about by these connections.

2. Descending fibres from the lateral (Dieter's) nucleus, constituting the vestibule-spinal tract end round the motor cells in the anterior horn of the spinal medulla. From the inferior vestibular nucleus descending fibres join the descending portion of the medial longitudinal bundle to establish connection with the skeletal system.

3. Some of the fibres of the vestibular nerve ascend in the inferior cerebellar peduncle to the flocullo-nodular lobe of the cerebellum on the same side. These constitute the vestibulo-cerebellar tract.

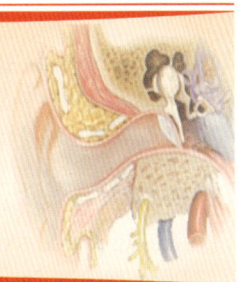

2

Physiology
of the Ear

The ear performs two functions. The main function is hearing and the other one is orientation in space and maintenance of equilibrium.

AUDITORY FUNCTION

The auditory function of the ear consists of the conduction of sounds through the external and middle ears or cranial bones and their reception by the organ of Corti. The auditory apparatus may be regarded as consisting of two main subdivisions: the sound conducting and the sound perceiving apparatus. In the former the external auditory meatus and the middle ear cleft, with the tympanic ossicles and labyrinthine fluids are included, while in the latter, the inner ear or labyrinth, with the auditory nerve termination, nerve trunk and ganglia are included. The auditory nerve and brainstem alone are not sufficient for hearing. It is a perceptive process. Sounds become meaningful only when they are detected and associated with the specific memory in the brain. Only the audiometry can determine the functions of the entire system.

The auricle in man, as it is almost completely immobile, is not of much importance in collection of sound waves.

The eustachian tube acts as a ventilating shaft for the middle ear. It opens up during each act of swallowing and maintains the air pressure in the middle ear at the same atmospheric pressure. If eustachian tube obstruction is, present, the tympanic membrane may be drawn in or even ruptured in a rapid aeroplane descent, owing to the inequality of pressure on the two sides of the tympanic membrane and the aviator may suffer from earache, deafness, nausea, and vertigo.

The external auditory canal conducts sound waves from the outer medium to the tympanic membrane. The atresia as well as its complete obstruction as occurs in earwax impaction, hinders the passage of sound waves and considerably impairs the hearing.

FUNCTION OF THE MIDDLE EAR

Ossicular Function

The malleus and incus rotate around a common fulcrum and transmit vibrations to the stapes in the oval window. The stapes moves mostly piston like motion up to 2.0 kHz. The motion becomes more complex at the higher frequencies. Above

2.0 kHz, anterior–posterior rocking motion rise logarithmically with frequency. Near 4 kHz level, the rocking and piston-like motions are almost equal.

A. Sound Pressure Transformation

1. *Ossicular leverage:* The difference in length between the handle of malleus and the long process of the incus constitutes the ratio of advantage gained by leverage. The leverage ratio in man is 1.31; not a very impressive figure of advantage.

2. *Hydraulic action:* The force of sound vibration exerted over the whole tympanic membrane is focused on to the footplate of the stapes with a gain in pressure per unit area. This gain in pressure may be expressed as the surface area of the larger divided by the smaller. The ratio varies between 15 and 26.6; the average lies at about 21.0. As only a central cone of the membrane, constituting two-thirds of the total area moves as a unit, in calculating therefore, the ratio between the tympanic membrane and the footplate, a reduction must be made to two-thirds. Thus if the anatomical ratio between the surface areas is about 21, the necessary reduction to two-thirds gives a physiological ratio of 14.

   The final figure of advantage for the sound pressure transformer system is $14 \times 1.31 = 18.34$.

B. Acoustic Separation

Sound protection of the round window: Eustachian tube function. The middle ear is essentially an air-containing space in bone lined by mucous membrane. The round window has this air-containing space as its immediate external relation. The oval window has the footplate of the stapes. The ossicular chain prevents the oval window from being directly influenced by the air space environment of the middle ear. The round window, on the other hand, is immediately susceptible to changes in this aerial environment, and the changes, which are most prone to influence it, are changes in atmospheric pressure. Changes in pressure adversely affect the mobility of the round window membrane and this increases the impedance of the inner ear to the propagation of sound waves. Variations in the middle ear pressure are essentially governed by the eustachian tube, which communicates with the atmosphere.

Thus occlusion of the eustachian tube causes negative pressure in the middle ear through absorption of air and therefore an increase in round window impedance owing to the negative "Pull" upon it. It also abolishes to some extent the sound protection effect.

The negative pressure in the middle ear impedes the mobility of the tympanic membrane and therefore of the ossicular chain. The net result of eustachian tube obstruction may therefore be an impairment of hearing of sufficient severity to exclude the reception of human voice sounds at normal speech intensity, i.e. a deafness exceeding 30–40 dB.

Sound Perception

The sound normally enters the cochlea through the oval window. It may enter the cochlea by round window and via the bones of the skull. Propagation of sound within the cochlea is controversial. Numerous theories have been advanced to explain how the energy of sound in all its complexities of frequency and intensity may be abstracted by the cochlea and transmitted to the auditory centers in the sensory cortex. The following are the three theoretical positions that form the basis of all the explanations:

a. The propagation depends exclusively upon the fluid (Resonance theory).
b. The propagation depends upon basilar membrane.
c. The propagation depends upon some interaction between the fluid and the basilar membrane (Wever's Volley theory) and combines both place and telephone principles, postulating that:
   1. High frequencies are perceived in the basal turn of cochlea (place).
   2. Low frequencies (below 1000 Hz) stimulate nerve action potentials at a rate equal to the stimulus frequency.
   3. Intermediate frequencies are represented in the auditory nerve by asynchronous discharges in groups of neurons whose combined activity represents the frequency of stimuli.

The second and third positions are variously assumed in the Standing Wave and Traveling Wave theories.

Theories of Hearing

Volley theory of Wever: It represents a combination of Place theory and Telephone theory, i.e. higher frequencies are perceived by place mechanism and lower frequencies are perceived by telephone mechanism.

Traveling wave theory of von Bekesy: It explains that sound waves travel along the basilar membrane. The higher frequencies stimulate the hair cells of the basilar membrane at the basal turn of cochlea and the lower frequencies at the apical turn.

The two best-known names in connection with the resonance theories are Helmholtz (1863) and Rutherford. Helmholtz also held the place theory, that is, the movement of the fluid is distinctive for every tone and the movement travels a particular tonal pathway through the basilar membrane from window to window. There is thus a "Place" on the basilar membrane specifically activated by a particular tone. "Place" theory of cochlear action postulates that perception of pitch of a sound depends upon the selective vibratory action of the basilar membrane. Rutherford, on the other hand, considered that the whole fluid and whole basilar membrane were stimulated by every sound, the telephone theory, and pitch perception is based upon the rate of firing in individual nerve fibres.

Anomalies of Auditory Perception

Conversation in a quiet environment is conducted around 40 dB hearing level, a doorbell output is, on an average, 60 dB and conversation on the telephone between 40 and 70 dB, within limited frequency band of 200–1200 Hz. The ability of a person with sensorineural deafness to discriminate speech is not necessarily helped when the speaker raises the intensity of the voice. Indeed the listener may say, 'don't shout, I'm not deaf.

Recruitment of loudness is characteristic of a cochlear hearing loss. A relatively small increase in the intensity of the auditory stimulus may cause frank discomfort to the listener. Poor speech discrimination without recruitment, especially if unilateral, suggests an auditory nerve lesion.

Autophony is the abnormal perception of one's own breath and voice sounds and is often associated with a permanently open, or patulous eustachian tube.

Fluctuant hearing loss may result from disease causing either conductive or sensorineural pathology. The fluctuant nature of the hearing loss associated with upper respiratory tract infections, eustachian tube dysfunction and otitis media with effusion is well known.

VESTIBULAR FUNCTION

Many receptors are responsible for the orientation of the body and its individual parts in space. In addition to the eyesight, the location of body and its parts is identified through the nerve endings lying in the skin, muscles, joints and tendons. These are called proprioceptors.

Stimulation of the receptors of the vestibular analyzer produces a number of reflex reactions, which cause a change in the tones of some muscle bundles of extremities, neck and eyes. This causes the whole body to change position and maintain balance.

Nystagmus is one of the unconditional reflexes observed in stimulation of the semicircular canals.

3

Examination of the Ear

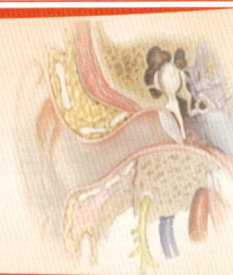

HISTORY TAKING AND CLINICAL METHODS

Careful and methodical history taking and clinical examinations with investigations are essential for accurate diagnosis and adequate treatment. For examination of patients a good set up is required. An examination chair for the comfortable sitting of the patient, a revolving stool for the examiner, a light source (Bull's eye lamp with plano-convex lens), one head mirror, a sterilizer, one X-ray view box, a suction and irrigation machine and one set of examination instruments are essential.

Light source is (a Bull's eye lamp) placed on the left-hand side of the patient on a level of patient's head or shoulder. The bulb should be of 100 W and milky white type. Otherwise, the reflected light becomes shattered.

It is preferable to use fibre optic headlight, the illumination of which is brighter than any other light source, if one can afford to do so. An ENT OPD unit provides fibre optic light, suction, cautery, endoscopy, etc (Fig. 3.1).

Head Mirror

The forehead mirror is usually 9 cm in diameter with 0.9 cm central hole. The focal length of the mirror is about 23 cm.

The examination of the ear includes collection of data about the case, inspection of the ear, palpation of the pinna and the mastoid process and functional examination of hearing and vestibular function.

The symptoms with duration as described by the patient should be noted in chronological order. Attention should be focused on the following:

a. Pain in the ear and its character

b. Discharge—its amount, colour, smell, nature (purulent or mucopurulent)

c. Impairment of hearing or total loss of it

d. Tinnitus or extra sound in ear.

e. Dizziness

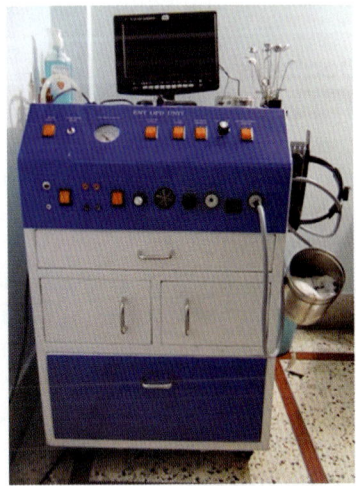

Fig. 3.1: ENT OPD unit displaying the facilities for fibreoptic headlight, endoscopy with display in the monitor, suction, cautery, etc.

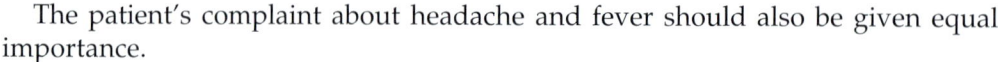
The patient's complaint about headache and fever should also be given equal importance.

It is important to know if the ear disease in question was preceded by common colds, influenza, etc. because one of the most important etiological factors producing acute otitis media is inflammation in the nose and throat.

The history of past illness, infectious diseases in particular, personal and family history specially regarding deafness and allergy should be noted.

Otalgia, discharge, deafness, tinnitus, vertigo and headache are the symptoms of ear disease. Otalgia or pain in the ear may be due to local causes such as otitis externa of bacterial, fungal or viral origin, myringitis bullosa hemorrhagic, acute otitis media, otitis media with effusion (glue ear), eustachian tube dysfunction when the middle ear pressure is markedly reduced with retraction of the tympanic membrane.

Sudden relief of pain in cases of acute otitis media indicates perforation of the tympanic membrane. Pain is not present in chronic suppurative otitis media unless it is associated with otitis externa or intracranial complication like meningitis. Pain in the ear may be a presenting symptom of diseases in other areas supplied by, the fifth, ninth and tenth cranial nerves. The common causes of referred pain in the ear are dental disease, lesions of the posterior one third of tongue, pharynx and larynx.

Ear Discharge (Otorrhoea)

The causes are otitis externa, CSF otorrhoea, acute and chronic otitis media. In chronic otitis media, the discharge is often long-standing and foetid due to saprophytic organisms, cholesteatoma and otitis externa. The onset of bleeding in chronic otitis media may be due to granulation tissue or due to neoplastic change. Bleeding from the ear may also be due to trauma, glomus tumours or vascular anomalies in the middle ear or external ear canal.

Deafness

This may be conductive or sensorineural. In conductive deafness the defect is in the conducting apparatus of the ear, i.e. from pinna up to the medial wall of the middle ear. If it is bilateral, the patients speak in low voice. Patients may hear better in the noisy environment which is known as paracusis willisii and is usually associated with Otosclerosis.

In sensorineural deafness there is poor speech discrimination, particularly in noisy surroundings and the patients speak loudly. When the speaker raises the intensity of the voice, the person with sensorineural deafness hear the sound but cannot understand due to poor discrimination of speech.

Recruitment is a characteristic phenomenon of a cochlear disease. A relatively small increase in the intensity of the auditory stimulus may cause frank discomfort to the listener. Poor speech discrimination without recruitment, especially if unilateral, suggests acoustic neuroma of auditory nerve damage. Diplacusis is a symptom of endolymphatic hydrops or Meniere's disease, which is the apparent difference in the pitch of a tone between the two ears.

Autophony is usually associated with serous otitis media or a permanently open or patulous eustachian tube.

Sudden deafness: In majority of the cases of sudden deafness the cause is unknown, though many are assumed to be due to vascular disease and/or viral infection. In 10% of acoustic neuroma, sudden deafness may be the presenting symptom. In perilymph fistula resulting from increased venous pressure due to straining or weight lifting, there may also be sudden deafness, commonly after stapedectomy.

Family history of deafness may reveal a hereditary cause.

Occupational history of noise exposure and army service are important. Pop music, rifle shooting and motor racing are the social noise trauma, which may lead to sensorineural deafness.

Past history—Receiving aminoglycoside antibiotics used for life threatening infections, diuretics like Fursemide are potentially ototoxic. Other drugs such as Salicylates, Quinine and cytotoxic therapy in oncology have been implicated as a cause of hearing loss.

Tinnitus—Means perception of extra sound.

A rhythmic beating or pounding tinnitus synchronized with the pulse is suggestive of a vascular lesion, e.g. glomus tumour. A dull, continuous tinnitus is sometimes found in association with a conductive deafness.

Body sounds transmitted via an abnormally patent eustachian tube may be reported as tinnitus.

The history of rushing, hissing or ringing sound in the ear or head is usually due to the diseases in the cochlea, auditory nerve or cerebral cortex. Tinnitus in general may be caused by all of those agents, which produce deafness.

It may be in the form of voice, music and bells in psychological patients as in Schizophrenia.

Vertigo: It may be defined as a "hallucination of movement", that is the patients feel that they or their environments are moving. Peripheral lesions usually produce vertigo of sudden onset. In Meniere's disease, the attacks are recurrent and usually associated with fluctuating deafness and tinnitus. Movement tends to make vertigo of peripheral origin worse. Vertigo associated with coughing or straining suggests the presence of a perilymph fistula, Tullio' phenomenon is the vertigo caused by loud sounds, in endolymphatic hydrops, or in labyrinthine fistula.

Central lesions tend to produce less intense vertigo. It is usually associated with disturbance of gait. Vertebrobasilar ischaemia, diabetes mellitus or atherosclerosis, ototoxic antibiotics particularly gentamycin may damage the vestibular system and cause vertigo. Vertebrobasilar ischaemia can cause sudden onset of vertigo and drop attacks, without loss of consciousness.

It is important to ask the patient about the first attack of vertigo. The onset, whether sudden or gradual, precipitating factors, duration of attack and associated symptoms are noted. The frequency and severity of attacks should be enquired about.

Clinical Examination

Note any congenital abnormality of the pinna and ear canal in the form of anotia or microtia. Presence of the tragus is considered a good prognostic feature for middle ear reconstruction.

Acquired conditions on the pinna include gouty tophi, squamous carcinoma, basal cell carcinoma and the painful nodules of chondrodermatitis helicis.

It is important to look in the postaural region for any surgical scar, fistula or any other pathology. Endaural incision can usually be noted in the area between the tragus and helix.

The external auditory canal is examined using an aural speculum and headlight or an otoscope. Pulling the pinna upwards and backwards helps to straighten the canal and facilitates vision in adult. Anterior sulcus of the canal cannot be seen in patients with prominent anterior meatal wall.

OTOSCOPY

The inspection of the external auditory canal and the tympanic membrane is called otoscopy.

Good illumination is essential for the examination of the ear. The best source of illumination is preferably a 100 W gas-filled, frosted-glass bulb, enclosed in a lantern fitted with a bull's eye condensor so as to concentrate the rays. These rays are then reflected on to the area under inspection by a forehead mirror. The lamp is placed close to the left side of the patient on a level with the patient's head.

The forehead mirror, provided with a central aperture, should have a focal length of about 20 cm. The examination is made in a sitting posture. The examiner adjusts the forehead mirror, with the aperture opposite his right eye. He should sit on a stool slightly lower than the patient's chair. The patient should sit in a chair facing the examiner.

Both eyes are used when making an otoscopic examination, the right eye necessarily peering through the mirror hole. One should see the diameter of the meatal opening to use an ear speculum of a suitable diameter, before inserting it. Children are examined with the aid of an assistant. The assistant keeps the child's head fixed to her chest with the left hand and holds her arms with the other. The legs of the child are pressed in between the legs of the assistant (Fig. 3.2).

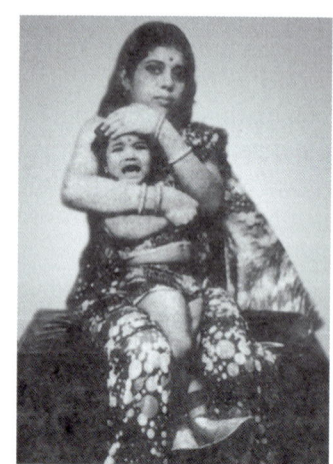

Fig. 3.2: Technique of holding the child during ENT examination

The ear speculum with its dilated part is held between the thumb and forefinger. It is then carefully introduced into the meatal opening to a depth of about 8 mm without touching the bony part. At the same time the pinna is pulled upwards and backwards in adults and downwards and backwards in children with the help of middle and ring finger to straighten out the meatus. In cases of swellings, fissures

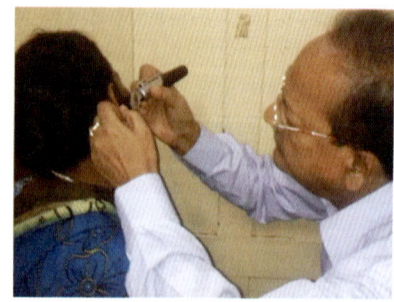

Fig. 3.3: Method of holding the otoscope during ear examination

and eczema, the speculum should be introduced with particular caution to avoid pain.

The normal tympanic membrane may be identified by the following features:

1. Distance—In adults after introducing the speculum up to about 8 mm, the tympanic membrane is seen to lie at a depth of about 16 mm from the tip of the speculum.
2. Colour—Pearly grey
3. Certain landmarks:
   i. Short process of the malleus.
   ii. Anterior and posterior malleolar folds.
   iii. Handle of the malleus.
   iv. Umbo.
   v. Cone of light with the tip pointed to the centre (umbo) and the base facing the antero inferior edge of the tympanic membrane.

Pneumatic Massage

The response of the tympanic membrane to the use of a Siegle's or pneumatic speculum is invaluable. The normal mobility can be recognised with experience; as can the immobility of an effusion in the middle ear. Some middle ear effusions are associated with a characteristic snap back of the displaced membrane as the pressure is released. A very thin excessively flaccid tympanic membrane can be recognised and often a thin tympanic membrane that has been sucked into the middle ear can be sucked out again from its subjacent mucosa, allowing identification of a retraction pocket and distinction between that and a perforation. The dusky red colour of a glomus tumour may become pale under raised pressure with the pneumatic speculum.

Patency of Eustachian Tube

Patency of Eustachian tube can be determined by the following methods:

1. Valsalva's autoinflation—The production of a high pressure in the nasopharynx by blowing out against closed lips and nose, normally results in an increase in middle ear pressure with the tympanic membrane bulging outwards. This can be observed by auriscope in place.
2. Toynbee's maneuver—When a swallow is made with the lips and nose closed the tympanic membrane moves outwards. This should return to its normal position with swallowing again with an open nose.
3. Frenzel maneuver (nasopharyngeal pressure test)—This test is more effective than the Valsalva or Toynbee test. The air in the nasopharynx is compressed by the contraction of the muscles of the floor of the mouth and tongue. This is done with the closure of the nostrils and glottis. It facilitates opening of the eustachian tube.
4. Politzerization.
5. Eustachian catheterization.
6. Impedance audiometry.
7. By passing out air through the external auditory meatus during swallowing in the presence of a TM perforation.

EXAMINATION OF THE AUDITORY FUNCTION

The functional examination of hearing is made by means of the following:
   i. Voice tests
      a. Whispered voice (WV)
      b. Conversational voice (CV)
   ii. Tuning fork tests
  iii. Audiometric tests

Voice Tests

These are of limited value because under differing acoustic conditions, the intensity of voice varies considerably. If a patient can hear the spoken word clearly at a distance of 12 ft. in each ear separately and together, it is unlikely that any gross hearing defect is present.

The results of voice tests are noted as follows: CV as the symbol for conversational voice and WV as the symbol for whispered voice. In a sound treated room WV from a distance of 5 ft and CV from a distance of 30 ft indicate normal hearing. A patient of bilateral conductive deafness speaks in a low tone and perceptive deafness in a high tone.

Tuning Fork Tests

These tests are helpful in knowing only the quality of deafness. They are as follows:

Rinne's Test

Essentially this test consists of comparing the auditory acuity of each ear to bone and air conduction. The tuning fork is struck gently so as not to produce overtones and dysharmonics. The fork is then placed firmly on the mastoid with observer's hand steadying the head (Fig. 3.4). The patient is asked to indicate when the sound disappears and the fork is then immediately placed erect and in the line with the external auditory meatus. If the patient still hears the sound, the patient is termed 'Rinne positive' (air conduction being better than bone conduction); 'Rinne negative' if the patient does not still hear it (bone conduction better than air conduction).

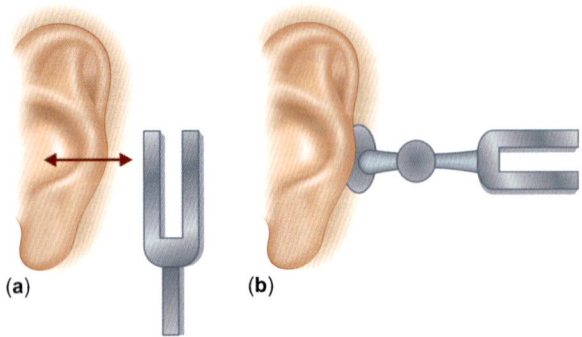

(a)   (b)

Fig. 3.4: Rinne's test. (a) Air conduction, (b) Bone conduction

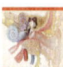

In conductive deafness Rinne's test will be negative (–ve), if the hearing loss is greater than 15–20 dB. The tuning fork is placed 2.5 cm lateral to the pinna in line with the external auditory canal.

Alternatively, and more usually, in routine clinical practice, the patient is asked to compare the sound intensity of the fork in the mastoid position (bone conduction) with that in the meatal position (air conduction). If there is a considerable sensory-neural deafness, the fork will not be heard by bone conduction at all, and obviously in the severe cases not by air conduction either. A conductive deafness of greater than 25 dB usually gives a negative Rinne test with a 512 Hz fork. However, with 256 or 128 Hz fork; this may be reduced to 10–15 dB and with the higher frequency forks 1024, 2048 and 4096 Hz, the conductive deafness needs to be greater than 25, 30 and 35 dB, respectively.

A Rinne test result, that is equal or negative for 256 but positive for 512 and 1024 indicates a mild conductive loss with air-bone gap of 20–30 dB. A Rinne test result, that is negative for 256 and 512, but positive for 1024, indicates a moderate conductive loss with a 30–45 dB air-bone gap. A negative Rinne test result for all three forks (256, 512 and 1024) indicates a maximum conductive loss with an air-bone gap of 45–60 dB.

False negative Rinne: If the patient has no hearing in the test ear, the bone conduction stimulus may be perceived by the contralateral (non-test) ear, although the patient often says that he/she hears it in the test ear. As there is no hearing by air conduction, the test result is labeled Rinne negative suggesting that the deafness is conductive in nature. This mistaken impression of function in a non-functioning ear is called a false negative Rinne. This phenomenon occurs because the interaural attenuation for bone conduction is less than 5 dB, that is sound passes freely across the skull stimulating both ears equally, regardless of where the tuning fork is placed.

Weber Test

This is valuable in unilateral deafness.

Principle: In comparison to the bone conduction, this consists of both ears simultaneously.

Technique: A vibrating tuning fork is placed on the vertex in the midline. It is heard equally on both sides in normal persons and in bilateral hearing loss of equal quantity (Fig. 3.5).

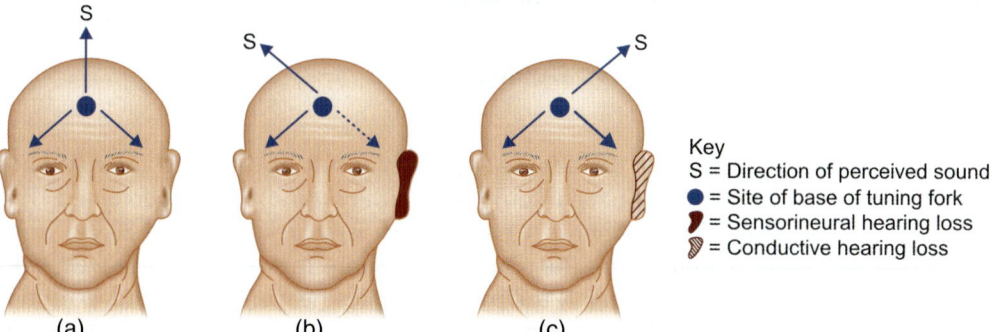

Key
S = Direction of perceived sound
● = Site of base of tuning fork
🎜 = Sensorineural hearing loss
🎝 = Conductive hearing loss

(a)   (b)   (c)

Fig. 3.5: Weber test. (a) Normal; (b) Sensorineural hearing loss; (c) Conductive hearing loss

Interpretation: It is expressed as "lateralized" or not.

In conductive deafness it is lateralized in the deaf or the deafer ear. In neurosensory deafness it is lateralized to the healthy or better ear.

It is important to remember that the word of the patient is often unreliable in this test. During this test they often state that the fork is heard better in the good ear, because they think that this must necessarily be so. Hence, this test is fallacious.

Schwabach Test

In this test the bone conduction of the patient is compared with that of the examiner (taking the examiner having normal hearing) without occluding the external auditory meatus. The test is not a reliable test; hence not recommended nowadays.

In sensorineural hearing loss the bone conduction is reduced, same as ABC test, whereas bone conduction is lengthened in conductive deafness.

Absolute Bone Conduction (ABC) Test

This is a modification of Schwabach's test and is a test for knowing the presence or absence of neurosensory deafness.

Principle: This consists in comparing the duration of bone conduction of the deaf person with that of an individual with normal hearing, keeping the ear canal blocked by finger.

Technique: The examiner and the patient, each block his external auditory meatus with the finger.

The examiner places the base of a vibrating tuning fork on his own mastoid (presuming that his hearing is normal) and waits till he no longer hears the fork sounding. He then transfers the fork to the patient's mastoid process and asks him if he hears it.

Interpretation: The test is interpreted as whether the duration of hearing by the patient is shortened or not. In perceptive deafness it is shortened.

Bing's Test

Bone conduction of the patient is tested with occlusion of the external auditory meatus. In normal hearing patients and in patients with neurosensory type of hearing loss, the bone conduction is lengthened (positive), whereas there will be no change in patients having conductive deafness (negative).

Tuning Fork Tests in Nonorganic Deafness

Stenger Test

Principle: Normally if sounds of identical frequency but of different intensity are presented simultaneously to each ear, only the louder sound will be perceived. The examiner stands behind the patient. A tuning fork is struck and held 20 cm from the 'good ear'—the patient hears the sound. The same fork is then removed, and placed 5 cm from the `feigned ear'—the patient denies hearing the sound. Another fork is simultaneously held 15 cm from the good ear without the patient noticing. If there is a genuine hearing loss, the patient will hear the fork in the good ear, but if

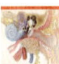

there is a non-organic hearing loss, the patient will not be able to hear the fork in the good ear because the fork which is closer, and of louder intensity, is being heard in the so-called bad ear.

Chimani-Moos Test

This is a modification of the Weber test. When the vibrating tuning fork is placed on the vertex, the patient indicates that he hears it in the good ear and not in the feigned deaf ear. The meatus of the good ear is then occluded. A genuinely deaf patient will still lateralise the sound to the good ear, but the malingerer will usually deny hearing the sound at all.

Audiometric Tests

The audiometer is an electronic instrument, which provides an uniform standard of measurement of hearing. Audiometry may be subjective or objective.

In subjective audiometry the measurement of hearing depends on the voluntary response of the patient. These are:
1. Pure-tone audiometry
2. Speech audiometry
3. Bekesy self-recording audiometry

In objective audiometry the measurement of hearing does not require the active cooperation of the subject. These are:
1. Impedance audiometry,
2. Electric (Evoked) response audiometry (ERA):
    i. Cortical ERA (CERA)
    ii. Crossed acoustic response (CAR)
    iii. Electrocochleography (E Coch G) which may be:
        a. Transtympanic E Coch G.
        b. External E Coch G (brainstem response),
3. Psychogalvanic skin resistance (PGSR) audiometry, which is not much used.

Both quality and quantity of hearing loss can be measured by audiometric tests.

Pure Tone Audiometry

The audiometer, an electronic machine, delivers pure tone sounds to the ear at a desired frequency ranging from 125 Hz to 8000 Hz and intensity ranging from 0 to 100 dB. It consists of an *oscillator*, which produces the frequencies, a frequency selector, an *attenuator* to control the intensity and a *receiver* to deliver the pure tones to the ear.

At a particular frequency if the sound is just heard by a person with normal hearing, it is designated 0-dB and this is 0 threshold. A person with normal hearing therefore should have an audiogram showing straight lines across the graph at 0 to 15 dB both by air and bone conductions. The testing tone may be delivered both by air and bone conduction (Fig. 3.6). The untested ear may be masked by using filtered whitenoise (FWN), which is fed by an insert-type earphone. A pure tone audiometer may also be used to do the loudness recruitment test in distinguishing the cochlear

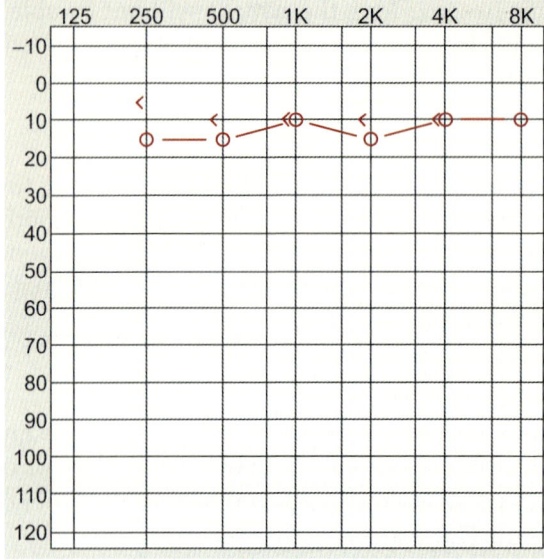

Fig. 3.6: Normal air conduction audiogram, right ear

and retrocochlear lesions in neurosensory type of deafness. The threshold of hearing by air and bone conduction is plotted against each frequency on the audiogram with symbols "O" for the right ear, and "X" for the left. The symbols are joined together by interrupted lines in the case of bone conduction and by continuous lines in the case of air. The colour of the symbols and the line is drawn in red for the right ear and in blue for the left.

Bone Conduction

Measurement of sensitivity of cochlea is rather problematic. It is almost universally adopted that a vibration stimulus to the mastoid process travels directly through the bones of the skull to the cochlear fluids independent of the outer and middle ear. This is thought to be an incorrect assumption nowadays.

The bone conduction is carried into the cochlea by three routes. These are:

1. The direct bony route.
2. The route passing from the bone to the middle ear and then to the cochlea via the ossicles and the air of the middle ear cavity. The inertial component (arises from the inertia of the mass of the ossicles) is a part of this mechanism.
3. The route passing from the skull to the ear canal and middle ear. The audiogram thus shows hearing as a curve or line. From the curve patterns the type and degree of deafness may be ascertained.

In pure conductive deafness bone conduction curve lies in the range of 0 to 15 dB level, whereas the air conduction curve lies lower down (for example, at 30 dB or 40 dB level) with a distinct bone-air gap (Fig. 3.7). On the other hand, in pure neurosensory deafness both bone and air curve will be together or inter-weave with increase in hearing threshold (for example, at the level of 30 dB or more) depending on the degree of hearing loss (Fig. 3.8). An audiogram may be interpreted as mixed

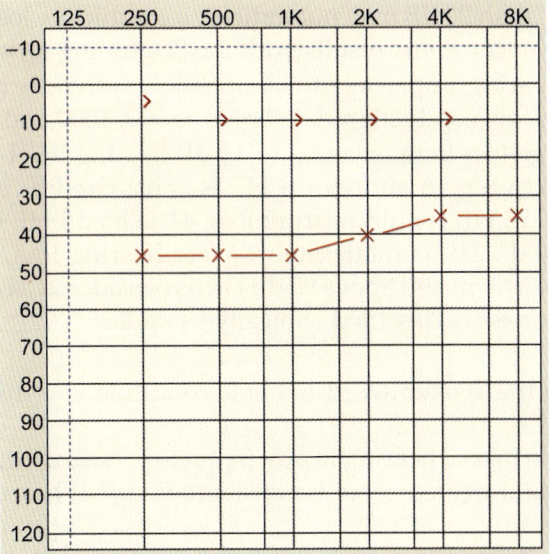

Fig. 3.7: Air conduction and bone conduction audiograms in conductive deafness, left ear

deafness, if the bone conduction curve lies below the 0 dB level (for example, at 30 dB) with a clear bone-air gap, as the bone conduction curve is a measure of the perceptive mechanism of the ear.

An air-bone gap of 20–30 dB indicates a mild or very early conduction loss; 30–45 dB, moderate conduction loss; 45–60 dB, a maximum conduction loss. Because of a possible 10 dB variation inherent in air and bone conduction audiometry, an

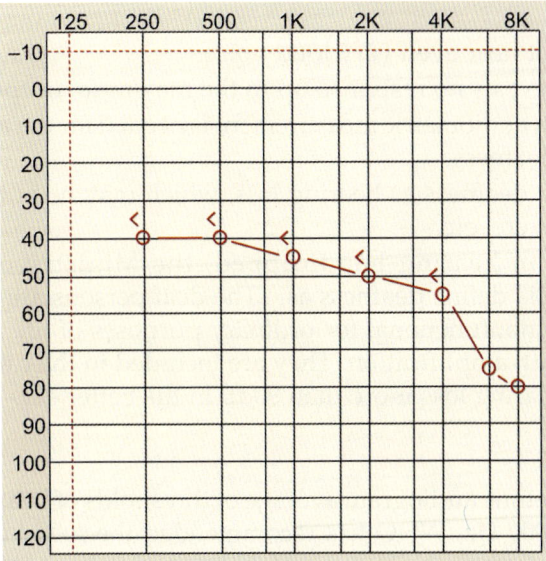

Fig. 3.8: Air conduction and bone conduction audiograms in sensorineural deafness, right ear

air-bone gap of less than 20 dB may not indicate a conductive loss unless confirmed by equal or negative Rinne test results with the 256 tuning fork.

Magnitude of hearing impairment classification system is based on the pure-tone average for the air-conduction thresholds at 500, 1000 and 2000 Hz.

Pure tone average less than or equal to 15 dB hearing level (HL) is considered normal hearing, between 16 and 25 dB HL is considered as slight hearing loss, between 26 and 40 dB HL is mild hearing loss, 41 to 55 dB HL is moderate degree hearing loss; 56–70 dB HL is moderately severe hearing loss, 71 to 90 dB HL is severe hearing impairment and above 90 dB HL, is considered as profound deafness. The severity of deafness is classified clinically as under:

1. Normal

   Voice test: Hears the spoken word in clinic condition at a distance of 18 feet or more.

   PT Audiogram: No loss of hearing in any frequency. Loss up to 15 dB when tested in a properly sound treated room is considered normal hearing.

2. Mild deafness

   Voice test: May not hear the conversational voice in the clinic condition beyond 12 feet distance.

   PT audiogram: Shows a loss of hearing between 15 and 30 dB in the speech frequencies.

3. Moderate deafness

   Voice test: Not being able to hear spoken voice in the clinic beyond 3 feet.

   PT audiogram: Shows a speech frequency loss of up to 60 dB.

4. Severe deafness

   Voice test: Conversational voice is not heard at all. May understand amplified speech. In the clinic he will hear nothing less than a raised voice at the meatus.

   PT audiogram: Reveals a loss over 60 dB in speech frequencies.

5. Total deafness

   Voice test: Cannot hear even very loud voice.

   PT audiogram: Reveals no response up to the maximum output of the machine.

   However, speech audiometric measurement is needed for the accurate assessment of the severity of deafness.

We use the term deafness as hearing loss, which may be of any degree such as mild, moderate, severe, etc.

For assistance in hearing handicapped, the Ministry of Social Welfare, Government of India define deafness as: "The deaf persons are those in whom the sense of hearing is nonfunctional for ordinary purposes of life." They do not hear any sound even with amplification. They are included in the category of profound deafness having hearing loss more than 90dB in the better ear.

WHO Classification of Degree of Hearing Loss

On the basis of puretone audiogram average of thresholds of hearing for frequencies of 500, 1000 and 2000 Hz, WHO has recommended the following classification in 1980:

1. Mild: 26–40 dB

2. Moderate: 41–55 dB
3. Moderately severe: 56–70 dB
4. Severe: 71–91dB
5. Profound: >91 dB
6. Total deafness
   0–25 dB is considered as normal hearing or no apparent impairment of hearing.

Percentage of Hearing Impairment

The percentage of hearing impairment is calculated as per recommendations of the Personal Department of the Government of India. It depends on pure tone audiometry and speech audiometry.

Pure-tone averages in speech frequencies (500, 1000 and 2000 Hz) by air conduction and discrimination score in speech audiometry are taken into account for categorization of hearing loss. In conductive type of hearing loss, no change occurs in speech discrimination score (SDS), hence they are not considered for the calculation of the percentage of impairment.

The recommended classification by the Personal Department, Government of India is as under:

Category I: Less than 40% impairment, i.e. mild hearing impairment; 26–40 dB in better ear and SDS is 80 to 100%.

Category II: 40 to 50% impairment, i.e. moderate hearing impairment; 41–55 dB in better ear and SDS is 50 to 80% in better ear.

Category III: 50 to 75% impairment, i.e. severe hearing impairment; 56–70 dB in better ear and SDS is 40 to 50%.

Category IV: 75 to 100% impairment, i.e. profound hearing impairment; 71–90 dB in better ear and SDS is less than 40%.

Category V: Near total or total deafness: 100% impairment, i.e. 91 dB and above in better ear or no hearing and no SDS.

Facilities for the Hearing Handicapped

Category I: No special benefits given.

Category II: Given hearing aids (free or concessional rates).

Category III: Hearing aids, job reservations, scholarship at school. Single language formula.

Category IV: Same as Category III. Three language formula (to study in the recommended single language); also for consideration of admission under special category in IIT (Indian Institute of Technology) and ITI (Industrial Training Institute).

Speech Audiometry

Uses of speech audiometry:

1. To find out Speech Reception Threshold (SRT), i.e. average of speech frequencies of pure-tone audiogram which is usually within 10 dB of the pure-tone average.
2. SRT more than 10 dB of pure-tone average suggests a functional deafness.

3. Speech discrimination score (SDS) helps in fitting a hearing aid. The volume of hearing aid may be adjusted with the intensity at which the SDS is the best.
4. It helps to determine the sensory form of neural type of neurosensory deafness.

Speech Reception Threshold (SRT)

When 50% of spondee words (two syllabic words such as baseball, sunlight, doorbell etc.) are heard properly and repeated when produced through the headphone of the audiometer in the minimum intensity of sound, it is called Speech Reception Threshold (SRT).

Normally SRT is within 10 dB of the average pure tone threshold of the speech frequencies (500, 1000, 2000 and 4000 Hz).

Speech Discrimination Score (SDS)

The ability to understand the spoken speech is called Speech Discrimination Score. Single syllabic phonetically balanced (PB) words (like pin, sin, sit, hit, etc.) are delivered 30 dB above his SRT in each ear. The percentage of words heard properly by the patient is recorded. The normal persons and patients with conductive deafness score 90 to 100%, whereas in NSHL the scores are less than 90%. In acoustic neuroma the SDS becomes very low, < 40%.

Bekesey Audiometry

It is similar to a conventional pure-tone audiometer but in this case the frequencies are automatically raised in a continuous manner. The intensity is also controlled automatically, which increases until the patient presses a button to signify that it is heard. The patient keeps the button pressed as long as the signal continues to be heard. When the button is released the signal intensity again increases, at a slightly higher frequency until the patient again pushes the button. This appears as a tracing on the audiograph by a pen-recorder attached to the audiometer. It helps in establishing the pure tone threshold and in localisation of a lesion in neurosensory deafness.

Impedance Audiometry

By means of an impedance audiometer two tests such as tympanometry, and acoustic reflex threshold may be performed. These tests help in diagnosing different causes of conductive deafness, differentiation between conductive and neurosensory deafness, measurement of middle ear pressure and of eustachian tube function, information on the presence of recruitment, and the site of the lesion in facial paralysis. The peculiarity of impedance audiometry is that here the sound reflected from the tympanic membrane is measured, whereas in all other forms of audiometry the sound energy which is absorbed by the ear and converted into nerve impulses is measured.

In tympanometry, variance in air pressure introduced into a sealed air-canal provides information regarding the amount of air-pressure in the middle ear cavity as well as the mobility (compliance) of the tympanic membrane and ossicular chain. The graphic recording of this information is called the tympanogram and it is usually

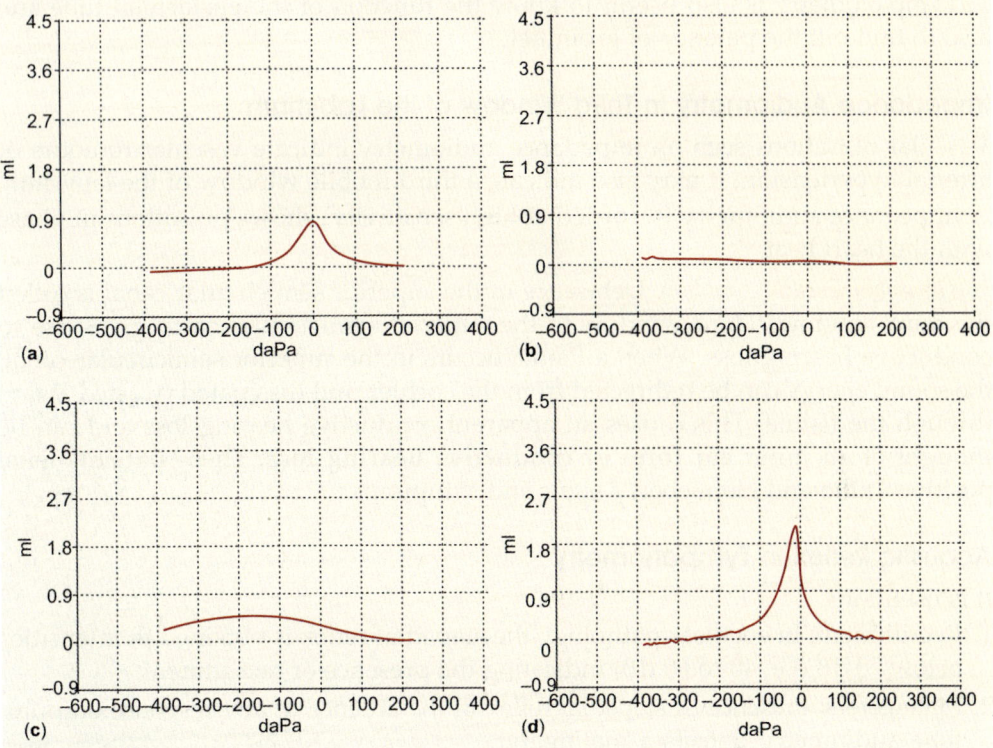

Fig. 3.9: Tympanograms. The horizontal axis is the pressure in the external auditory canal, which can be varied by the pump. The vertical axis is compliance, which is measured in millimeters and is the reciprocal of stiffness. This gives a measure of the elasticity of the drums and ossicles. (a) Normal response, (b) Fluid in the middle ear, (c) Reduced middle ear pressure (due to eustachian tube dysfunction), (d) Discontinuity of the ossicular chain (e.g. disarticulation of incudostapedial joint)

classified into five basic types. As for example, type A, type A_S, type A_D, type B and type C (Fig. 3.9).

Type A: Normal pressure (± 100 mm of H_2O) and normal static compliance (0.25 to 1.6 cc)

Type A_S: Normal pressure (± 100 mm of H_2O) and reduced static compliance (Less than 0.25 cc)

Type A_D: Normal pressure (± 100 mm of H_2O) and high compliance (greater than 1.6 cc)

Type B extreme negative pressure (greater than –250 mm of H_2O) and low static compliance (.10 to .25 cc)

Type C negative pressure (–100 to –250 mm of H_2O) and normal compliance (0.25 to 1.6 cc)

Acoustic reflex measurements: It is the observation of changes in compliance caused by contraction of the middle ear muscles in response to auditory stimuli. In normal persons, the acoustic reflex is elicited at approximately 85 dB hearing level.

Tympanometry is also useful to know the function of the eustachian tube and also to find out the patency of grommet.

Impedance Audiometry in Third Window of the Labyrinth

Vascular pulsations seen on impedance audiometry indicate vascular tumours or arterial hypertension. It may also indicate a third mobile window of the labyrinth.

Impedance audiometry (recorded at high sensitivity) shows pulsations in phase with the heart beat.

Third labyrinthine window: Dehisence in the superior semicircular canal is called the third window. Third window in the superior semicircular canal gives rise to conductive hearing loss. When a fistula occurs in the superior semicircular canal, the sound energy can be redirected from the cochlea and dissipated (wasted away) through the fistula. This causes an apparent conductive hearing loss and can be thought of an **inner ear form of conductive hearing loss**. These patients have positive Tullio and Hennebert's signs and symptoms.

Acoustic Reflex in Tympanometry

It is useful in:
1. Recruitment: In cochlear pathology the stapedial reflex is obtained in intensities below 70 dB (i.e. 40 to 60 dB) indicating the presence of recruitment.
2. Malingerers: Presence of stapedial reflex in the absence of any response on pure-tone audiometry detects a malingerer.
3. Objective method of testing the hearing in infants and younger children
4. Stapedial reflex decay indicates VIII cranial nerve lesions. If a continuous tone of 1000 Hz is delivered 10 dB above the acoustic reflex threshold for 10 seconds, it brings down the reflex amplitude to 50%, which is called stapedius reflex decay.
5. In normal hearing persons if the stapedius reflex is absent, it indicates VII cranial nerve lesion proximal to the nerve to stapedius.
6. *Brainstem lesion:* If ipsilateral stapedial reflex is present but contralateral reflex is absent, it indicates brainstem lesion.

Eustachian Tube Function Tests by Tympanometry

A negative or a positive pressure ($-$ 200 to $+$ 200 mm of H_2O) is created in the middle ear and the person is asked to swallow 5 times in 20 seconds. The ability to equalize the pressure indicates normal eustachian tube function.

Stapedius Reflex Threshold (SRT)

The minimum intensity of sound required to evoke reflex is termed the stapedius reflex threshold. A very high intensity of sound > 70 dB causes contraction of stapedius muscles of both sides. The speech frequencies (500 to 4000 Hz) are used for testing SRT.

In normal hearing persons the SRT for pure tones occurs with 70 to 100 dB sounds. The SRT for noise stimuli (wideband sound) occur at lower intensities, i.e. below 70 dB.

In conductive deafness the reflex is absent. Reflex may be obtained if the sounds of 70 to 110 dB above threshold are given.

In recruiting type of deafness (cochlear) the reflex occurs below 70 dB of subjective threshold.

In neural deafness (retrocochlear) the reflex is obtained if more than 70 dB above subjective threshold is used.

Hearing aquity may be predicted if SRT for pure-tones and for wideband noise are known by using a formula as under:

$$PTT = SRT_1 - 2.5 \times (SRT_1 - SRT_2)$$

PTT – Pure-tone threshold

SRT_1 – Average of speech frequencies i.e. 500 to 4000 Hz of pure tones.

SRT_2 – Threshold for wideband noise which is always lower than the pure-tone threshold.

SRT is important for screening the young children and for malingerers. In malingerers who claim to have no hearing and does not respond in pure-tone audiometry will have stapedius reflex. Stapedius reflex decay (SRD) will be present in neural deafness. It will not be present in normal hearing persons. The absence of stapedial reflex in a normal hearing person indicates that facial nerve paralysis is above the level of stapedius muscle.

HEARING TESTS IN CHILDREN

To overcome a hearing handicap and integrate a deaf child into normal society, an auditory defect should be diagnosed as early as possible. If a parent suspects a child to be deaf, that child is deaf until proved otherwise.

a. Reflex tests:
    i. At birth—Moro or Startle reflex causes crying.
    ii. At 3 months—Smiling, blinking and frowning.
    iii. At 5 months—Turns eyes to a sound source.
    iv. At 6 months—Turns head to a sound source.

b. Behavioural tests: At 7 to 18 months—distraction tests are used.

c. Performance tests: Between 18 months and 5 years—"Go" and "Show me" game.

d. Subjective tests:
    i. Peepshow audiometry.
    ii. Conditioned audiometry.

e. Objective tests: ART, CERA, CAR, ECochG are used.

These help only to test. the integrity of the auditory pathway and do not show that the child understands sounds.

Blinking reaction to loud sounds is probably the most frequent reaction of newborn infants. Children as young as one month can be tested for hearing. Four groups of tests are well known:

1. Voice and speech.
2. Percussion toys such as bells and drums.
3. A range of pitch pipes (120–1700 cycles).
4. "Meaningful sounds" such as the chink of a feeding bottle or a knock at the door.

The "Peepshow" apparatus is based on a conditioned response to a light sound signal, and is useful between the ages of three and six years. The action of a child in response to the sound offered may be involuntary or voluntary. In case of involuntary reactions the techniques are described as distraction techniques used for the child below the age of $2^1/_2$ years. The startle reflex and head turning response are the most valuable tests to determine whether the sound has been heard.

In the case of voluntary reactions the techniques are described as conditioned techniques used from about the age of $2^1/_2$ years. "Go" and "Show Me" game are the two well-known conditioning techniques. By conditioning the child who has reached the mental age of 4, a pure-tone audiogram may be obtained.

Brainstem Auditory Evoked Response (BAER)

These are a series of neurogenic potentials that can be recorded using surface electrodes in response to click stimuli in 10 milliseconds immediately after the stimulus. The patient may be awake or asleep but should be relaxed to reduce myogenic activity, which tends to mask these tiny potentials. The active and reference electrodes are placed at the vertex and ear lobules, or mastoid processes with a ground electrode on the forehead.

The latency of each of the waves decreases with increasing intensity but the interwave relationship remains constant.

The main value of auditory evoked potentials is primarily in detecting lesions involving the auditory nervous system particularly the vestibular schwannoma and neurological conditions. With decreasing intensity of stimulus, wave V is the most resistant and persists to a level that relates closely to psycho-acoustic thresholds. Comparison of wave-V latency after stimulation of each ear separately is of value in distinguishing cochlear from retrocochlear pathology. In cochlear lesions with loudness recruitment, there is a progressive disappearance at high intensities of stimulation of interaural difference in the latency of wave-V, which may be observed consistently at low frequencies. In contrast, the patients with retrocochlear hearing loss exhibit a consistent interaural difference in the latency of wave-V.

The value of interwave latency measurement, particularly the wave I to V interval, in evaluating disorders of VIIIth cranial nerve has been established.

Wave-I is developed by the auditory nerve. Wave-II is from the cochlear nuclei in the pons. Wave-III is formed by superior olivary complex in the pons. Wave-IV is formed by lateral lemniscus in the pons. Wave-V is formed by inferior colliculus in mid-brain. Wave-VI is formed by the medial geniculate body in thalamus. Wave-VII is formed by auditory radiations (thalamocortical).

Otoacoustic Emissions (OAEs)

OAEs are sounds reflected in the external auditory canal that originate from physiologically vital and vulnerable activity inside the cochlea. It happens that OAEs are generated only when the organ of Corti is in near normal condition, and, of course, they can emerge (or at least can be detected) only when the middle ear system is operating normally as well. The sounds generated by the cochlea are small but potentially audible; sometimes amounting to as much as 30 dB speech level. They can emerge spontaneously, as sound already in the cochlea perpetually recirculates but more commonly OAEs follow acoustic stimulations. To observe OAEs, no electrodes are required. They are not electrical in nature, rather they are vibratory responses. In fact, a microphone is used to detect them and it is converted to an electrical analogue, which can be easily processed.

The sounds or ear canal pressure fluctuations, called OAEs, are actually created by motion of tympanic membrane driven by the cochlea through the middle ear ossicular chain. Consequently, to record OAEs we need a healthy middle ear with good sound conduction. The cochlea itself does not significantly radiate sound through the air of the middle ear. At frequencies below 3000 cps (3 kHz), the OAE vibrations transmitted through the middle ear is undetectable without physically closing the ear canal during measurement.

Healthy cochlea contains a mechanism capable of returning sound to the middle ear and significantly impaired cochlea normally does not. This makes OAEs a uniquely valuable clinical tool.

FUNCTIONAL EXAMINATION OF THE VESTIBULE

The function of the vestibular labyrinth can be assessed by the following ways:

Caloric Test

If water at 30°C and 44°C (i.e. 7°C below and above normal body temperature) is run into the ear, nystagmus is produced in the normal persons with a healthy labyrinth. The nystagmus lasts for about 2 minutes from the beginning of stimulation. If the time of nystagmic-reaction lasts for less than average, it is termed canal paresis. Directional preponderance of nystagmus either to right or to left is another important finding of this test as shown in Fig. 3.10. Each ear can be tested separately.

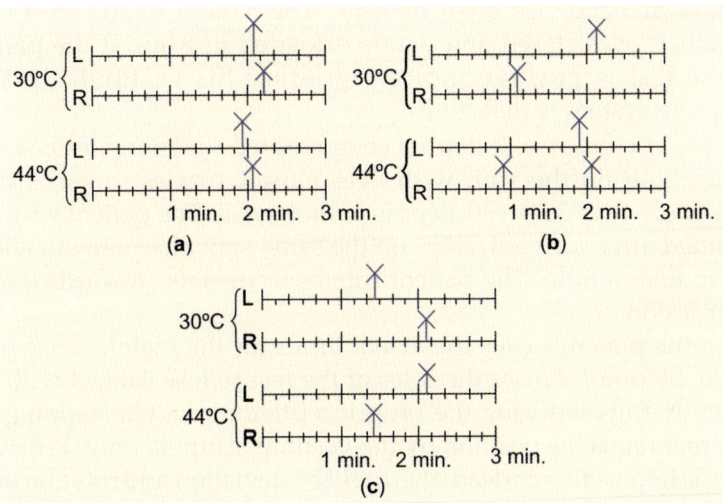

Fig. 3.10: Calorigrams. (a) Normal caloric responses; (b) Right canal paresis; (c) Directional preponderance to the left

Both canal paresis and directional preponderance may occur either singly or in combination. Canal paresis will be present in majority of patients with Meniere's disease, vestibular neuronitis and acoustic tumours. In the lesions of the posterior part of the temporal lobe, directional preponderance will be demonstrated towards the side of the lesion.

Dundas Grant Test (Cold Air Caloric Test)

If there is perforation in the tympanic membrane this test will be convenient. If cold air is blown into the ear and there is an active labyrinth, nystagmus is induced after 15–30 seconds. Other tests used for vestibular function estimation are:

- *Rotation test:* The patient sits on a special chair and rotates with eyes closed 10 times in 20 seconds. The after nystagmus is measured with a stopwatch, which varies from 15 to 30 seconds in a normal individual. In active labyrinth the nystagmus will be on the opposite side of the rotation.
- *Fistula test:* A fistula in the bony wall of the horizontal semi-circular canal may result from erosion by cholesteatoma or from the fenestration operation for otosclerosis. In either case, compression of air in the external auditory canal either by pushing the tragus with a finger or by compression of the bulb of Seigle's speculum, will produce movement of endolymph in the duct, hence vertigo and nystagmus, as long as the vestibular labyrinth is functioning. This is interpreted as fistula test positive (+ve). The fistula test may be negative (−ve) in the presence of fistula if the labyrinth is dead or if there is no fistula.
- *Hennebert's sign:* It occurs when there is a positive fistula test with an intact tympanic membrane and no evidence of middle ear disease. It is seen most commonly in congenital or late tertiary syphilis, but is sometimes found in Meniere's disease. It is also thought to be due to either adhesion in the vestibule or to the presence of a third window somewhere in the labyrinth caused by osteitis.
- *Romberg's test:* Eye closure results in a dramatic loss of balance in cases of either unilateral or bilateral vestibular damage. The patient stands erect with his feet close together, eyes closed and hands extended in front. If the patient grossly sways, the test is positive indicating either his vestibular system or his propioceptive system is defective.
- *Unterberger's stepping test:* It detects compensated unilateral lesions. The patient while marching on the spot with eyes closed rotates towards the weakest labyrinth. More than 30° in 30 steps is pathological. The patient with eyes closed and extended arms forward, steps on the same spot alternatively with each foot 90 times in one minute. The patient rotates or deviates towards the side of the vestibular lesion.

  By closing the patient's eyes the visual input for the maintenance of balance is eliminated. Stepping causes the soles of the feet to lose contact with the ground intermittently thus reducing the proprioceptive input. On stepping the patient therefore maintains his position by the vestibular inputs only. Where one of the vestibules is hypoactive or dead, there will be deviation and rotation of the patient towards the affected or weaker side. If the patient is ataxic due to a central lesion, it causes swaying movement from side to side to maintain his balance during stepping.

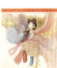
- *Electronystagmography (ENG):* This test helps in detecting nystagmus, which may not be visible to the naked eye. It is a means by which the nystagmus can be permanently recorded. This is possible due to the presence of an electrical potential in between the cornea and retina, which can be picked up by placing electrodes close to the eyes. The movement of the eyes can be accurately recorded as because the electrical axis of the eye corresponds to the optical axis. The nystagmus can be recorded during caloric or rotation tests even if the tests are done in darkness or with the eyes closed.
- *Craniocorpography (CCG):* Craniocorpography is a quick, non-invasive and simple test of the vestibulospinal system. It helps to differentiate between the peripheral and central vestibular disorders without stimulation of the vestibular apparatus either by caloric or rotation tests. In this test (CCG) the angular deviation and rotation of the patient is measured which indicate the peripheral disorders. The side to side swaying is also recorded and measured which indicates the central pathology.

Technique

The CCG is performed by CF. Claussen's technique. One helmet fitted with two small bulbs in the Saggital axis, the anterior bulb placed on the forehead and the posterior one on the occiput, is made to wear by the patient. Over each shoulder of the patient, one small bulb is fitted representing the coronal plane. On the roof of the testing room, a convex mirror is fitted. One Polaroid camera is placed on an adjustable stand with its lens directed upward towards the convex mirror. This camera is placed in between the head of the patient and the convex mirror.

The blindfolded patient is asked to perform the stepping on a spot 9 times in one minute (approx) like Unterberger's test when the room is darkened. The patient's movement is monitored by the lights on his helmet and shoulders, which are reflected on to the convex mirror and from there to the film in the Polaroid camera. The camera is set in the 'B' position (i.e. constant exposure) and records the movement of the patient during stepping.

Interpretation

i. *Angular deviation:* Some amount of deviation from the spot of stepping is common in all individuals. It is considered as normal if the deviation is 70° to the right and 50° to the left of the midline. Any deviation beyond this range is taken as the vestibular hypoactivity or inactivity on the side of the deviation.

ii. *Angular rotation:* Rotation around his own vertical axis may be there during stepping test. It is considered as normal if the rotation is 100° to the right and 70° to the left of the midline. Rotation beyond this range suggests vestibular hypoactivity or inactivity on the side of the rotation.

iii. *Lateral sway:* The swaying movement from side to side with each step is recorded. The breadth of this sway is considered as normal if it ranges from 3 to 20 cm. The sway greater than 20 cm occurs in central pathology.

The forward and backward displacements of the patient are not considered as significant.

REFERRED PAIN IN THE EAR

Causes: These are best considered on an anatomical basis.

1. Via the 5th Cranial Nerve

a. *Lesion of the teeth and jaws*
  i. Impacted wisdom tooth—particularly in the lower jaw.
  ii. Caries tooth.
  iii. Apical abscess.
  iv. Malocclusion, over closure of jaws (Costen's syndrome).
b. *Lesions of the nasopharynx*
  i. Ulceration or neoplasm.
  ii. Acute nasopharyngitis.
  iii. After adenoidectomy.
c. *Lesions of the nose and paranasal sinuses*
  i. Sinusitis
  ii. High deviation of the septum causing pressure on the middle turbinate.
d. *Lesions of salivary glands and ducts*
  i. Acute infection.
  ii. Calculus.
e. *Sphenopalatine neuralgia*

2. Via the Ninth and Tenth Cranial Nerves

a. *Lesions of the oropharynx*
  i. Acute tonsillitis and pharyngitis.
  ii. Peritonsillar abscess (quinsy).
  iii. Retropharyngeal and parapharyngeal abscesses.
  iv. After tonsillectomy.
  v. Tuberculous ulceration.
  vi. Neoplasms.
b. *Lesions of the laryngopharynx*
  i. Tuberculous ulceration.
  ii. Neoplasms.
c. *Lesions of the tongue*
  i. Ulceration.
  ii. Neoplasms.
d. *Elongated styloid process* (Eagle's syndrome)
e. *Glossopharyngeal neuralgia*

3. Via the Second and Third Cervical Spinal Nerves

  i. Cervical disc lesions.
  ii. Arthritis of the cervical spine.
  iii. Fibrositis of the upper part of the sternomastoid muscle.
  iv. Herpetic lesions.

4. Via the Seventh Cranial Nerve

Herpes zoster oticus including the Ramsay Hunt syndrome.

4

Deafness, Tinnitus and Vertigo

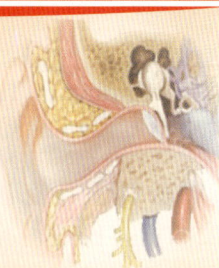

Deafness may be congenital or acquired. "Congenital deafness" may be defined as a more or less pronounced loss of hearing present at birth; leading to mutism, and transmitted by hereditary or acquired by chemical, physical or mechanical influences in the prenatal period. However, certain forms of hereditary deafness develop later in life. Thus these are excluded from the terms congenital according to the above definition. It will perhaps be simpler if the causation of deafness is considered under two headings as follows:

a. Prenatal, and

b. Postnatal.

Causes of Congenital Deafness

 i. Hereditary group ("Bad Seed"): It causes defective development of the cochlea, middle ear including otosclerosis, and external ear.

 ii. Pregnancy group ("Damaged Embryo")
Rubella: Rh-incompatibility, other infections, drugs, toxemia, threatened abortion, major surgery under general anaesthesia.

iii. Birth group ("Hazardous Birth")
- Prolonged or difficult labour
- Premature birth
- Anoxia
- Convulsions
- Cerebral palsy
- Jaundice

Causes of Postnatal Deafness

I. Conductive Deafness

Due to any lesion of the conductive apparatus of the ear. This may be:

1. *Traumatic:* Acquired atresia of the external auditory canal, rupture of tympanic membrane either from explosive blast or from trauma by matchstick, pencil end or hairgrip, fractured base of the skull, foreign bodies or unskilful attempts at their removal, haematoma middle ear, ossicular disruption and barotrauma.

2. *Inflammatory:* Eustachian salpingitis, acute and chronic otitis media, furunculosis of external ear, adhesive otitis media and secretory otitis media.

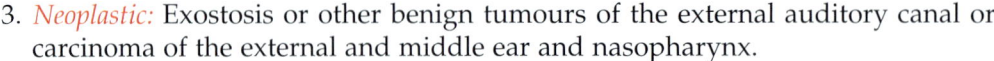

3. *Neoplastic:* Exostosis or other benign tumours of the external auditory canal or carcinoma of the external and middle ear and nasopharynx.
4. *Miscellaneous:* Otosclerosis, cerumen.

II. Perceptive Deafness

This may be caused by any lesion affecting the perceiving apparatus of the ear. This may be:
1. *Traumatic:* Fractured base of the skull involving the labyrinth. Explosive blast and 'acoustic trauma', and noise-induced hearing loss.
2. *Inflammatory:* Infective labyrinthitis.
   Drug toxicity: For example, dihydro-streptomycin, quinine, aspirin, kanamycin, neomycin, framycetin, polymyxin-B, chloromycetin (rarely), tobacco, alcohol, arsenic. Aniline dyes (in hair and fur works) also may affect the inner ear.
3. *Neoplastic:* VIIIth nerve tumour in internal auditory canal, and cerebellopontine angle tumors.
4. *Miscellaneous:* Senility (presbycusis), Meniere's disease.

III. Psychogenic Deafness

Malingering, hysteria.

NOISE AND DEAFNESS

Basically noise may produce deafness in four ways:
1. Acoustic trauma
2. Noise-induced hearing loss
3. Acoustic accident
4. Otitic blast/injury.
1. Acoustic trauma—Very brief exposure to very loud sound, such as gunfire, magazine explosions, causes aural damage resulting in sensorineural hearing loss permanently. Audiogram shows a severe and abrupt loss for higher frequencies, such as 5500 frequency level.
2. Noise-induced hearing loss—Prolonged exposure to loud sound in certain industrial workers causes inner ear damage. Cochlea is affected. Vestibule remains normal. The hearing loss is characteristically greatest at 4000 frequency level.
3. Acoustic accident—Brief exposure to a loud noise in a bent forward position causes sudden severe unilateral deafness. Audiogram shows a characteristic U-shaped curve with maximum loss at 500–1000 frequencies.
4. Otitic blast/injury—Sudden blast from bursting shells, bomb explosions, etc. causes injury to external, middle and inner ear. Positive wave causes injury to the middle ear and the negative wave to the inner ear.

Tinnitus

Tinnitus is a subjective sensation of noises in the ear or head. Occasionally it may be objective in the form of clicks or buzzing sounds due to clonic contractions of the intra tympanic or palatal muscles.

It may occur in two clinical forms:

1. **Tinnitus with hearing loss:** In this type the pitch of the tinnitus nearly always corresponds with the frequency of maximal hearing loss. Tinnitus may be present in any type of deafness. It is very troublesome particularly in Meniere's disease and senile deafness. In drug toxicity and noise trauma it is often the warning symptom. If it is unilateral, acoustic neuroma should be suspected.
2. **Tinnitus without hearing loss:** It may be found in focal sepsis, carious or impacted wisdom teeth, anaemia, atherosclerosis, cerebrovascular disease, intracranial vascular tumours, hypertension and hypotension. In great majority of patients no cause may be found out.

Treatment

Usually tinnitus disappears with the cure of causative aural conditions. Sometimes it persists. In persistent tinnitus the patient should be explained about the symptom and reassured about its harmless nature and advice the patient to ignore the sound. Sedatives in the form of phenobarbitone may be prescribed if the tinnitus interferes with sleep. Tranquillizers may sometimes help.

Vertigo

Vertigo could be defined as a "false sense of orientation of the patient with respect to his environment". The patient feels that he is moving or that the surroundings are moving.

Dizziness is a sensation of imbalance with a tendency to fall.

Causes

A. Vertigo with deafness
1. Meniere's disease.
2. Labyrinthitis: Viral, bacterial
3. Acoustic neuroma
4. Labyrinthine trauma: Following fracture of the temporal bone, following operation, e.g. stapedectomy and mastoidectomy.
5. Miscellaneous: Wax occluding the external auditory canal, serous otitis media, eustachian tube obstruction and labyrinthine haemorrhage due to blood dyscracia.

B. Vertigo without deafness
1. Vestibular neuronitis (epidemic vertigo).
2. Benign paroxysmal positional vertigo (BPPV) (fatigable).
3. Dysequilibrium of aging—Due to degenerative changes in the maculae and the cristae. Cervical spondylosis may be associated in some patients.
4. Drugs, e.g. aminoglycosides (streptomycin, kanamycin, gentamycin, etc.) are well known ototoxic drugs and may cause both vestibular and cochlear damage.
5. Miscellaneous, e.g. anaemia, hypotension, diabetes mellitus, migraine, psychogenic, acute vertiginous aura in epilepsy.

C. Vertigo with signs of intracranial disease
   1. Central (malignant) positional nystagmus (non-fatigable), e.g. tumours of the posterior cranial fossa, mid-brain, disseminated sclerosis and vascular lesions. Posterior-inferior cerebellar artery thrombosis (lateral medullary syndrome).

Vertebrobasilar Insufficiency

This affects elderly people with atherosclerosis and often precedes a stroke due to microemboli originating from plaques of atherosclerosis in the major arteries.

Investigations

History of vertigo with or without deafness, earache, discharge and tinnitus should be noted. Patient should be asked for about fluid and salt intake, smoking habits, overwork, head injuries and emotional upsets which act as contributory factors.

Examinations

1. General examination: To exclude CSOM with attic cholesteatoma.
2. Special examinations of ears and labyrinth in the absence of chronic otitis media
   i. Examination of the eyes for nystagmus
   ii. Audiogram to assess hearing. Tone decay test, SISI and loudness balance test for recruitment
   iii. X-ray of each internal auditory canal (Towne's, Stenver's and transorbital views)
   iv. Caloric test (Gold standard)
   v. Labyrinthine function tests, e.g. positional test, positioning test, caloric test, Romberg test, unterberger test, ENG and CCG (Fig. 4.1)
   vi. Neurologist's opinion to exclude diseases of the central nervous system
   vii. Contrast study of the internal auditory meati
   viii. Computerized tomography (CT)
   ix. MRI (Magnetic resonance imaging).

Nystagmus

It may be defined as an involuntary, rhythmical, oscillatory movement of the eye. The slow component is labyrinthine, while the quick component is cerebral. In clinical practice nystagmus is named after the direction of the quick component.

Types

i. *Physiological (optokinetic nystagmus); "Railway nystagmus"*: Unlike pathological nystagmus quick phase is towards the centre or rest-point.
ii. *Pathological*: Congenital bilateral blindness (ocular). The two phases of nystagmus are of the same speed and amplitude (pendular).
   Vestibular nystagmus: Two phases are in the opposite direction
   Brainstem lesions: Produce nystagmus in the vertical direction

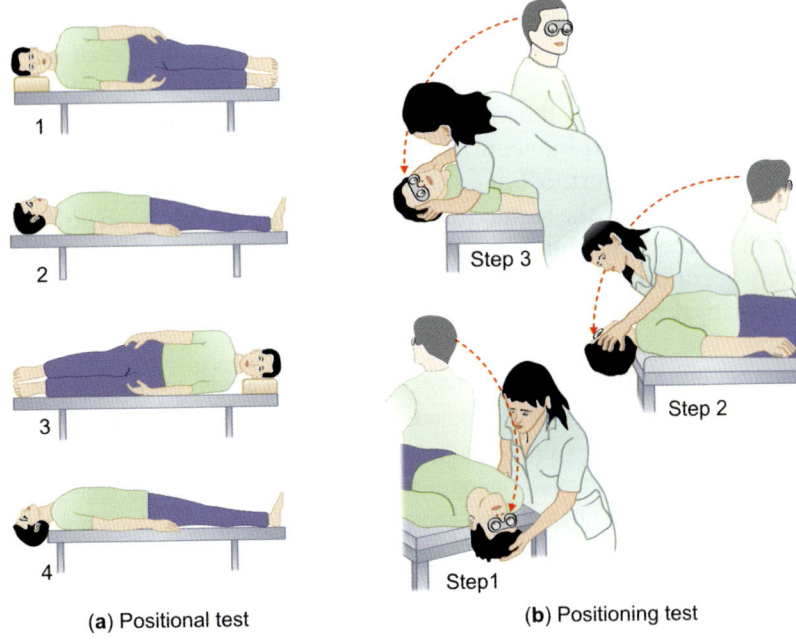

(a) Positional test　　　　**(b)** Positioning test

Fig. 4.1: (a) Positional test; (b) Positioning test

Cerebellar lesions: Produce horizontal nystagmus, usually more marked to the side of the lesion.

Toxic nystagmus: It is a horizontal nystagmus usually due to excess of alcohol, sedatives, anticonvulsants, etc.

Rotatory nystagmus: It is seen in labyrinthine or brainstem lesions.

Ataxic nystagmus: It is a horizontal nystagmus and is seen in lesions of the medial longitudinal bundle. Multiple sclerosis is a common cause.

Degrees of Nystagmus

1. *First degree:* Only if the eyes are directed away from the rest point, i.e. peripherally in the direction of fast component
2. *Second degree:* Nystagmus on looking straight ahead.
3. *Third degree:* There is so violent nystagmus to one side that it does not stop if the gaze is to the opposite side, i.e. when the patient looks in the direction of the slow component.

Vestibular end organ or vestibular nerve will produce nystagmus with its quick phase towards the opposite side.

In unilateral cerebellar lesions the quick phase of the nystagmus is to the same side.

Nystagmus due to peripheral cause is fatigable and in central pathology it is nonfatigable.

Positioning Nystagmus (Dix-Hallpike Test)

The patient is seated up on a examination table. Head of the patient will project over the table when he lies down. The patient is instructed to keep his eyes open and to look at the centre of the examiner's forehead. The patient's head is held with both hands and is slowly turned to one or other side at an angle of 45° from the sagittal plane, and he is laid swiftly backwards into the supine position until the head of the patient overhangs the table edge. After a latent period of about 20 seconds a rotatory nystagmus will be seen in positive cases in BPPV. The nystagmus is directed towards the undermost ear and lasts for a few seconds. The nystagmus is associated with vertigo of the same quality that the patient has been suffering from. On repetition of the test, the nystagmus fatigues. A nystagmus on the reverse direction may occur on sitting the patient up. This suggests that in unilateral disease the abnormal labyrinth is that of the undermost ear.

Differentiation between peripheral and central causes of nystagmus		
	Peripheral nystagmus	Central nystagmus
Onset	Delayed (0 to 20 seconds)	Immediate
Distress	Distressed during nystagmus	No distress
Nystagmus	Fatigues on repetition of the test	Does not fatigue

BPPV

BPPV is treated by canalolith repositioning procedure, i.e. Epley maneuver.

Epley Maneuver

The principle of this maneuver is to bring back the otoconial debris from the posterior semicircular canal to their original position in the ampula. Like Dix-Hallpike's maneuver, the patient is made to lie down supine with his head over the edge of the examination table. The head is turned 45° towards the affected side. This will result in vertigo and nystagmus. Wait till the signs stop. The head is then turned bringing the affected ear up. The patient is then rotated towards the normal ear with the face positioning downwards. After that the patient is brought to the sitting position keeping the head turned by 45°. The head is then turned forwards with chin down to 20°. Each position should be maintained till the nystagmus stops, the change of each position should be performed very rapidly.

After completion of the maneuver the patient should maintain an upright position for 48 hours. If required the maneuver may be repeated. The majority of the patients are cured by one maneuver. Success rate is nearly 90%.

a. *Positional test (stalic):* This test starts in the supine position. The patient rolls on to the right side and then rolls back in the supine position. Then rolls back to the left side. After, that the patient adopts a head hanging position.

b. *Positioning test (dynamic)* i.e. Dix-Hallpike maneuver.

Semont Maneuver

One hour after Dix-Hallpike test (DHT), the patients underwent Semont's maneuver as follows:

- After identification of the affected ear by DHT, the patient is seated on an examination table. The patient's head is turned 45° towards the unaffected side and the patient is suddenly laid down on the affected side and kept in this position for 4 minutes. Maintaining the head in the same position relative to the trunk, the patient is suddenly turned 180° to the unaffected side and kept in this position for another 4 minutes and then the patient is slowly raised into a sitting position. If symptoms disappear, DHT becomes negative. Single Semont maneuver effectively resolves about 75% of all cases of unilateral BPPV affecting the posterior semicircular canal. Orthographic nystagmus in the second position of Semont maneuver (nystagmus of the same direction observed in the first position of Semont maneuver) is a sign of good prognosis. Orthotropic nystagmus is more common in patients with shorter latency periods (related to cupulolithiasis).

The labyrinthine reflexes are normally connected with others, e.g. visual and proprioceptive in the maintenance of posture. Postural reflexes are of two types:

1. *"Static reflex" (Utricular reflex):* These are the postural reactions of the body when at rest. Static reflexes are of two types:
   a. Tonic labyrinthine reflex—with effects on the limbs, neck, trunk and eyes.
   b. Labyrinthine righting reflexes—restore the body to its normal position when it is brought to rest in an abnormal position.
2. *Kinetic reflexes:* This is the postural reaction of the body when in movement. The kinetic reflexes bring the body into its normal stance while pose is maintained by the static reflexes.

5

Diseases of the Ear

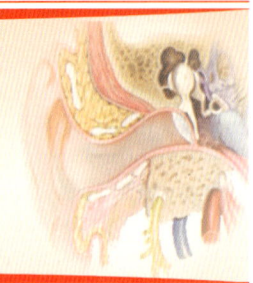

DISEASES OF THE EXTERNAL EAR

Congenital

Types

1. Complete or partial absence of auricle
2. Pre-auricular sinus
3. Accessory auricles
4. Atresia of external auditory canal
5. Changes in size and shape of auricle.

Treatment

In auricular defects of minor type plastic surgery improves the appearance. Prosthesis is suitable in major defects of auricle. If the pre-auricular sinus is repeatedly infected and gives rise to discharge, complete excision is the treatment of choice. Deafness of congenital malformations may be corrected by surgery.

Traumatic

Lacerations

All degrees are encountered including complete severance of auricle.
   Treatment: Immediate dressing, repair of injuries and antibiotics.

Blows

Haematoma auris occur usually on the external surface of the auricle. Sometimes haematoma may arise spontaneously in the elderly. Organisation of the blood may cause permanent thickening of the auricle called 'Cauliflower ear'.

Treatment
   i. Aspiration
   ii. Pressure bandage.

Burns and Frostbite of the Auricle

Frostbites of the auricle are more frequent than burns. Light frost/bites cause intense redness and slight swelling of the skin followed by severe burning sensation and pain. More severe frostbites cause blebs on the skin, and very severe freezing produces necrosis of the skin and cartilage.

Treatment: Burns are treated by common surgical methods.

Frostbites

In the early stages—gradual rewarming (thawing), by rubbing with snow.
In the later stages—should be treated in the line of the treatment of gangrene.

Traumatic Rupture of Tympanic Membrane

Causes

1. By foreign bodies, or unskilled instrumentation.
2. Blows, slap, blast, rapid descent in nonpressurized aircraft may cause rupture of the tympanic membrane by sudden air compression.
3. Forceful inflation of the eustachian tube.
4. Fractured base of the skull.

Clinical Features

Pain, deafness, tinnitus and vertigo. Perforation shows red and irregular margin. Blood in the meatus.

Treatment

1. Systemic antibiotic is to be given to prevent infection.
2. Blood clot should not be disturbed for about 10 days or more.
3. Never syringe or put any eardrop. No local treatment should be carried out except cleaning with sterile swab.
4. Ask the patient to abstain from getting water into the ear during bathing and not to swim or dive.
5. Myringoplasty should be done if the perforation fails to heal.

Inflammatory

Perichondritis

It is the infection of perichondrium and auricular cartilage. This may cause necrosis of the auricle. Perichondritis may follow haematoma auris or operations involving the auricular cartilage.

Treatment: Systemic suitable antibiotics in adequate doses.

Otitis Externa

Causes

1. Local—bacterial, fungal or viral.
2. General—allergy, systemic infection by bacteria or viruses.

Clinical Types

Infective
1. Bacterial

a. Furuncle
b. Erysipelas
c. Diffuse otitis externa
d. Malignant otitis externa
2. Fungal: Otomycosis
3. Viral: Herpes simplex, Herpes zoster, Myringitis bullosa.

Reactive
1. Eczematous otitis externa
2. Seborrhoeic otitis externa

Furuncle of External Auditory Canal

It is a staphylococcal infection of hair follicle or sebaceous gland in the cartilaginous portion of the external auditory canal. It commonly recurs. Diabetics are especially susceptible.

Clinical Features

i. Pain in the ear and tenderness in the region of the meatus. It is aggravated by movements of the pinna. If situated in the anterior wall, it causes pain on opening the mouth, yawning, and chewing. In extreme stages it may cause trismus (inability to open the mouth).
ii. Swelling and redness of the meatal walls.
iii. Deafness—if the canal is occluded by swelling, it may cause deafness of conductive type.
iv. Involvement of regional lymph glands.

Pus from the furuncle may spread
1. Backwards—over the mastoid with obliteration of the postauricular sulcus.
2. Forwards—into the parotid region through the fissures of Santorini.
3. Inwards—rarely infect the tympanic cavity through the notch of Rivinus.

Differential Diagnosis

Diagnosis between furunculosis and mastoiditis may sometime be difficult.

Furuncle with post-auricular cellulitis	Mastoiditis with subperiosteal abscess
No preceding history of otitis media	Preceding history of otitis media
Deafness not present unless the canal is occluded	Deafness present
Tympanic membrane is normal if visualized	Tympanic membrane shows signs of middle ear infection
Movement of the auricle is painful	No pain on moving the auricle
Obliteration of post auricular groove	Post auricular groove remains
Swelling forms in the cartilaginous portion of the canal	Swelling forms in the bony portion of the canal
Auricle pushed outwards and becomes prominent	Auricle pushed outwards, forwards and downwards
X-ray mastoids show no change	X-ray mastoids show changes

Treatment

Local treatment:

1. Before rupture—tight packing with a wick of cotton wool or ribbon gauze soaked in 10% ichthyol in glycerine or with steroid antibiotic ointment like betamethasone with neomycin cream. This helps by:
   a. Lessening pain by counter pressure and prevention of the movement of the cartilaginous external ear canal during chewing and yawning (splinting action);
   b. Constant medication.
2. Dry hot fomentation.
3. Rarely it may require incision and drainage. Damage to the cartilage during this procedure should be avoided to prevent infection and necrosis. This at times may give rise to deformity of the ear canal and auricle.
4. Following rupture of the furuncle aural toilet should be done.

General treatment:

1. Analgesics for pain.
2. Suitable antibiotics or chemotherapeutics should be given in adequate dosage.
3. A course of autovaccine may be tried in recurrent furunculosis.

Diffuse Infective Otitis Externa

Predisposing causes are scratching, unskilled instrumentation and the discharge of acute or chronic suppurative otitis media usually due to streptococcal infection.

Clinical Features

Itching is the first symptom followed by pain. Inflammatory swelling and oozing are seen in the canal wall. Crusting, desquamation and discharge are present in varying degrees. In chronic forms scaling, fissuring and stenosis are seen.

Treatment

Local—wicks of ribbon gauze soaked in 8 per cent aluminium acetate (mild astringent) may be introduced. Aural toilet and instillation of Chloramphenicol or Gentamycin drops help.

General—systemic antibiotic is required in severe cases.

Malignant Otitis Externa

In diabetic elderly patients, sometimes pseudomonas infection in external ear may be fatal due to spread of infection in the surrounding bone causing osteitis or osteomyelitis. It may cause paralysis of the V, VI, VII, IX, X, XI and XII cranial nerves. Meningitis and sigmoid sinus thrombosis are not uncommon leading to a fatal outcome. It may also occur in non-diabetic patients.

Clinical Features

Pain in the ear, discharge, granulation tissue, and cranial nerve paralysis are present. A Gradenigo's syndrome may result.

Treatment

1. Control of diabetes.
2. Antibiotics—preferably gentamycin or cephalosporins and quinolones.
3. Removal of granulation and radical mastoidectomy.

Erysipelas

It is the cuticular lymphangitis of the ear canal, which often follows a scratch. The causative organism is a streptococcus. Cellulitis is common.

Large swelling and erysipelatous redness in the ear canal are preceded by fever, malaise and headache. The disease lasts for 3 to 4 days if correctly treated. The local reaction of the skin on the mastoid process on the first day may be mistaken for mastoiditis.

Treatment

1. Systemic disinfections by suitable antibiotics.
2. Ultraviolet light in an erythematic dose.
3. Painting the skin with neutral ointments.

Otomycosis

Fungal infection of the ear canal is frequently seen in damp and rainy seasons. Varieties of fungi are found but aspergilli (especially *Aspergillus niger*) and *Candida albicans* are the commonest.

Clinical Features

Itching and deafness may be present.

A grayish or brownish-black mass is seen in the meatus resembling "wet newspaper". On magnification by otoscope or microscopic examination spores with stalks are seen in certain cases.

Treatment

1. Removal of mass by syringing and thorough cleaning.
2. The canal wall may be painted with keratolytic agents (2 per cent salicylic acid in alcohol) for 2 or 3 days.
3. Mercuric perchloride in alcohol 1:4000 (fungicide) or multifungin solution may be applied with good results.
4. Nystatin is effective in candida infection.
5. Clotrimoxazole 1% in the form of ointment or lotion acts well in all types of fungi.
6. Batrafen cream.

Myringitis

This is seen during certain epidemics of influenza. Severe pain in the ear and tinnitus are the associated symptoms. On examination blisters of a reddish-brown or purple colour may be seen. This condition is called myringitis bullosa or hemorrhagic otitis externa. The causative organism is β-hemolytic streptococcus combined with virus.

Treatment
- Systemic antibiotics
- Local instillation of drops of 10% icthyol in glycerine
- Bullae may require incision and drainage under general anaesthesia when severe pain is present.

Herpetic Lesions of External Ear

Probably caused by neurotrophic viruses. There are three varieties:
1. Herpes simplex—may occur as elsewhere
2. Otitis externa haemorrhagica (myringitis bullosa)—*see* above.
3. Herpes zoster oticus.

It usually causes severe pain. Sometimes pain may persist (postherpetic neuralgia). Vessication occurs but disappears early. Cranial nerve involvement may cause other symptoms:
a. Deafness—perceptive variety
b. Vertigo
c. Facial nerve palsy. The **Ramsay Hunt syndrome** includes all the above features.

This may be treated early with acyclovir, which is highly sensitive against herpes virus. Analgesics should be used sparingly.

Eczematous Otitis Externa

It is an allergic dermatitis of the external ear. The allergen may be extrinsic or intrinsic. Analgesics should be used sparingly.

Clinical Features

Irritation, redness and edema of the skin of the external ear. These are followed by vessication, weeping and crust formation. The picture may be changed by secondary infection. In chronic state scaling and fissuring occur. This may end in stenosis of the ear canal.

Treatment

Acute stage: Hydrocortisone acetate ointment gives dramatic improvement. Antihistaminics should be given systemically. Aluminium acetate 8% or resorcin 5% may be applied.

Chronic stage: Silver nitrate 10% solution is applied. In stenosis plastic surgery may be required.

Seborrhoeic Otitis Externa

It is a greasy scaling and crusting condition of the skin of external ear canal. Mostly results from the scalp condition.

Treatment: Shampooing of the scalp once or twice a week with soft soap or spirit shampoo.

Aural toilet: Ointment containing antibacterial, antifungal and steroids should be used.

Neoplasms of External Ear

Benign—papilloma, angioma, chondroma, osteoma, adenoma, ceruminoma and neurofibroma are the common benign tumours of the external ear.

The commonest benign tumours are the **exostosis** of the bony canal.

Malignant—squamous cell carcinoma and rodent ulcer (basal cell carcinoma). Rodent ulcer occurs more commonly on the auricle than in the external canal.

Sarcomas are very rare; may be in the form of osteosarcoma or chondrosarcoma.

Miscellaneous Group

Foreign Body

Various types of foreign bodies are found in the ear. These are found commonly in children.

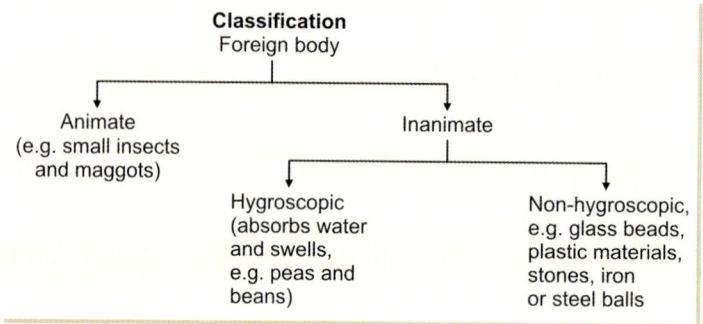

Classification
Foreign body

Animate (e.g. small insects and maggots)

Inanimate

Hygroscopic (absorbs water and swells, e.g. peas and beans)

Non-hygroscopic, e.g. glass beads, plastic materials, stones, iron or steel balls

Treatment

Treatment is removal of foreign body. In case of animate foreign bodies, such as insects and maggots, pour any bland oil into the ear canal. By this the foreign body will be killed by suffocation. Maggots are initially paralysed by inhaling ether or chloroform soaked in a cotton ball before removal. Turpentine oil may also be used for removal of maggots. Then the foreign body may be removed either by syringing or by forceps.

Inanimate foreign bodies which are not impacted and non-hygroscopic should be removed by syringing the ear.

Hygroscopic foreign body of small size, which has not been interfered with, should be removed by syringing in the first attempt.

If the foreign body is swollen by absorbing water, advise for instilling absolute alcohol into the ear for 24 hours. Then syringe the ear.

If the foreign body is impacted and the patient is a child, its removal should be done under general anaesthesia with the help of aural hook. When diffuse inflammation of the meatus has been set up by unskilled attempts at removal, wait till the inflammation subsides and treat for the inflammation. Then take steps to remove the foreign body.

Rarely the foreign body may be driven into the middle ear. In such cases an external operation is required for its removal.

Wax

Wax (cerumen) is a mixture of the secretions of the ceruminous and sebaceous glands. These are situated in the cartilaginous part of the ear canal. Normally it comes out from the canal in flakes, aided by movements of the jaws. It forms plug in the ear canal if there is excessive formation and its retention owing to stenosing conditions in the canal.

Clinical Features

Deafness—only when there is complete occlusion of the canal. There may be sudden onset of it after swimming or taking bath if water enters into the ear canal.

Tinnitus, pain, and vertigo may accompany the deafness.

On examination with aural speculum, a dark-brown or blackish mass is seen to obstruct the view of the tympanic membrane.

Treatment

Treatment is removal either by ring probe and scoop or by syringing with water at body temperature after softening by repeated instillation of a saturated solution of sodium bicarbonate or any oily drop such as liquid paraffin and olive oil. Suction clearance under operating microscope is also helpful and comfortable for the patient.

Keratosis Obturans

The external auditory canal is filled up with a plug of desquamated epithelium. It behaves like a cholesteatoma of the middle ear and mastoid. It produces symptoms like wax. But it usually does not soften by saturated solution of sodium bicarbonate. Sometimes it needs general anaesthesia for removal. Formation of keratosis may be prevented by regular use of keratolytic agents (2% salicylic acid in alcohol).

DISEASES OF THE MIDDLE EAR

Congenital Malformations

Developmental defects of various degrees of the tympanic cavity and ossicles are sometimes found. Middle ear defects are usually associated with deformities of the external ear.

Traumatic

a. *Fractured base of skull:* It may be longitudinal and transverse type. Longitudinal type is the more common of the two and the fracture line is in the long axis of the petrous bone. In this type there may be conductive deafness, bleeding from the ear and cerebrospinal otorrhoea

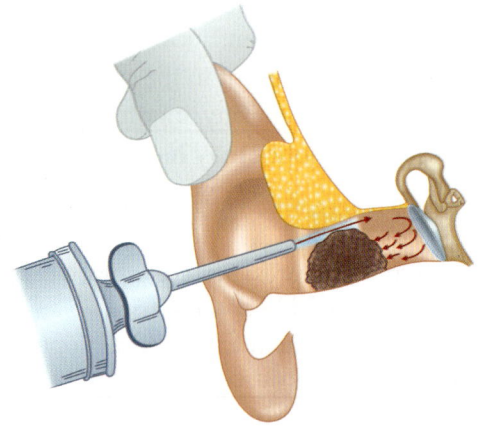

Fig. 5.1: While syringing the ear, the jet of water should be directed along the roof of the canal

of short duration. In transverse type labyrinth is commonly involved causing perceptive deafness, vertigo, nystagmus and occasionally facial paralysis.

The treatment of longitudinal type of fracture is the same as that of the ruptured tympanic membrane. There is practically no treatment in the transverse type.

b. *Barotraumatic otitis media:* This is also called otitic barotrauma. It occurs during rapid descent in non-pressurized aircraft, or during compression in a caisson. Rapid descent produces "Locking" of the eustachian tube resulting in retraction of the tympanic membrane owing to relative lowering of pressure in the middle ear. "Locking" occurs when the pressure difference between the middle ear air and surrounding atmosphere becomes 80 mm water. The decrease of pressure occurs because of absorption of oxygen by the tissue.

Reaction of the Middle Ear to Negative Pressure

When a negative pressure develops in the middle ear, the pars flaccida retracts first because of its elasticity. When the negative pressure reaches 50–90 mm of water a transudate from the blood vessels lying in the middle ear fills the cavity. This transudate by itself diminishes the middle ear volume and prevents a further decrease in its pressure. These changes constitute barotrauma.

Clinical Features

Increasing discomfort and pain are the first symptoms. They usually disappear in a few hours. Deafness may persist for a few days. Tinnitus is a common symptom. Sometimes may complain of vertigo.

On examination—the tympanic membrane becomes red soon after the onset. If fluid is present, a hairline may be seen between the air and fluid level. Foam-like bubbles also may be seen sometimes.

Treatment

- "Unlocking" may be done by frequent autoinflation. This technique usually fails if the tube has been "locked" for more than an hour.
- If no fluid is present in the middle ear, eustachian catheterization usually helps.
- If fluid is present, myringotomy may be necessary.
- Use of antibiotics may have to be considered in case of threatened infection.

Prevention of Otitic Barotrauma

Flying in a non-pressurized aircraft, especially in the presence of upper respiratory infection, should be avoided.

As the eustachian tubes are not opened by swallowing during sleep, one should not sleep during descent of an aircraft.

In the presence of minor nasal congestion one should instill decongestive drops during descent of an aircraft.

During descent, autoinflation by valsalva technique should be performed.

Otitis Media

Otitis media is an inflammation of the lining of the middle ear. So long as the process remains confined to the lining mucosa, the disease does not produce complications. Complications arise only when the disease involves any part of the bony walls or spreads beyond these walls to adjacent structures. A fairly common complication is mastoiditis.

Classification of Otitis Media

Otitis media may be classified as follows:
1. Non-suppurative
     i. Acute
     ii. Chronic
2. Suppurative
     i. Acute
     ii. Chronic
3. Specific
     i. Tuberculosis
     ii. Syphilitic
4. Adhesive

Secretory Otitis Media (SOM)

Synonyms—non-suppurative otitis media; serous otitis media; mucinous otitis media; glue ear; exudative otitis media; catarrhal otitis media; otitis media with effusion (OME), etc.

Aetiology

Aetiology is still uncertain. The factors responsible for such a condition are as follows:
1. *Anatomical:* DNS, cleft palate and other abnormalities of the hard and soft palate and nasopharynx that cause poor eustachian tubal ventilation.
2. *Physiological:* Allergy plays the dominant role. Neurovascular and neuroendocrine factors also cause hypersecretions.
3. *Pathological:* Adenoid hypertrophy, polypoid degeneration of the posterior ends of turbinates, nasopharyngeal tumours, chronic paranasal sinusitis and rhinitis, nasopharyngitis, etc. These lesions may develop tubal obstruction with defective middle ear ventilation.
4. *Iatrogenic:* Undue reliance upon antibiotic therapy neglecting the necessity of surgical drainage in acute suppurative otitis media is responsible for this condition in large proportion of cases.
5. *Geographical factors:* Geography and climate play a great role upon an infection or an allergic cause. In a tropical country, like ours, this disease is not so common. In Western countries, like the USA and the UK, this condition is very prevalent. Twenty-five percent of children entering school have 6-OME, in the UK.

Clinical Features

1. Deafness: Conductive in type. In children it is commonly bilateral. The onset may be sudden or gradual. Changes of head position may cause changes in degree of deafness if the fluid is thin and serous. Patient hears better in bed when supine but the hearing gets worse in erect position.

   Audiogram shows conductive deafness with a low frequency loss in the early stage and a high frequency loss in later stage. Impedance audiometry shows negative middle ear pressure with reduction in compliance.

2. Tinnitus and autophonia.

3. Otoscopic examination reveals dull and retracted tympanic membrane. Partial filling up of the middle ear with fluid may show a horizontally placed crescentic hairline and bubbles. The colour of the tympanic membrane may be near normal but may be pale yellow, gray or even blue. On siegalization there is characteristic snapback of the tympanic membrane due to the surface tension of the fluid during release of suction.

   The fluid may be serous, seromucoid, seropurulent, mucoid, mucopurulent or purulent with glue like consistency.

   The colour of the fluid may be clear or opaque; yellow or dark brown. The fluid is generally sterile. In allergic cases eosinophils may be present in the effusion.

Gradation of the Retracted Pars Tensa

Grade I: A slight retraction of the tympanic membrane over the annulus.

Grade II: The tympanic membrane touches the long process of the incus.

Grade III: The tympanic membrane touches the promontory.

Grade IV: The tympanic membrane is adherent to the promontory (Fig. 5.2).

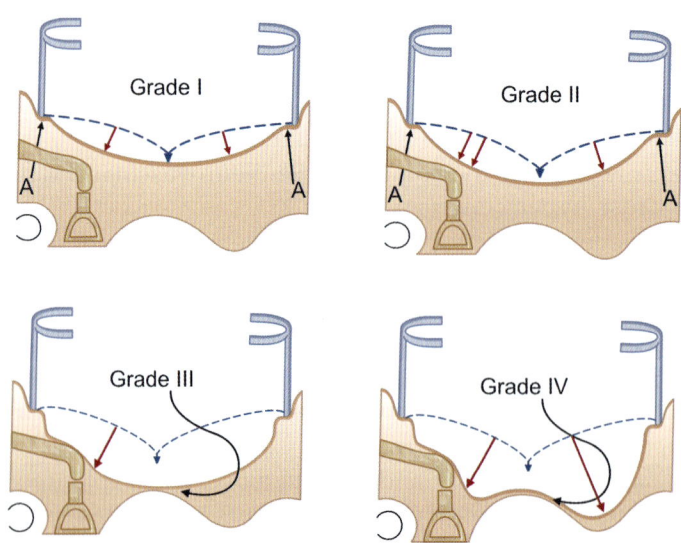

Fig. 5.2: Grades of pars tensa retraction

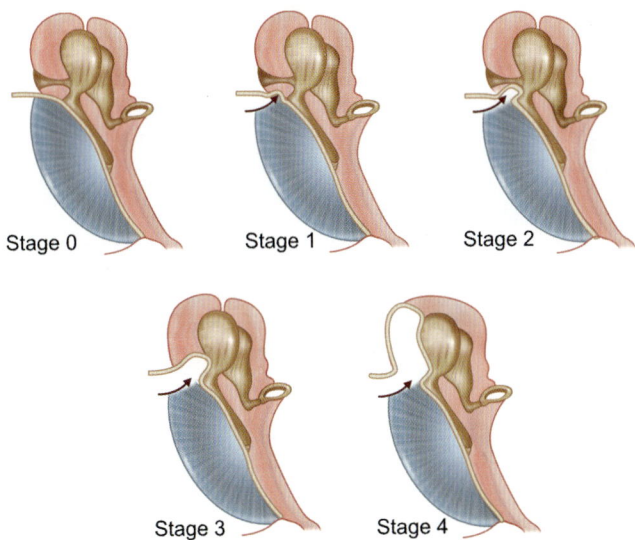

Stage 0 Stage 1 Stage 2

Stage 3 Stage 4

Fig. 5.3: Stages of pars flaccida retraction

Staging of the Retracted Pars Flaccida

Stage 1: A slight dimple.

Stage 2: Pars flaccida is retracted maximally and is draped over the neck of the malleus.

Stage 3: As stage-II, but with erosions of the outer attic wall (the scutum).

Stage 4: The retraction is deep and accumulated keratin cannot be cleaned by suction clearance. The last stage is a full-blown attic retraction pocket (Fig. 5.3).

Treatment

Elimination of etiological factors, as far as possible, should be done.

1. Medical treatment: It should be tried in all acute cases at least for 2 to 3 weeks in the form of:
    i. Decongestive nose drop, e.g. ephedrine hydrochloride solution 1/2 to 2% should be instilled in nose thrice a day. Xylometasoline HCl or oxymetazoline HCl aqueous solution (0.05%) may be used as nasal drops or spray.
    ii. Oral nasal decongestive drugs like phenylephrine present in coriminic, pseudoephedrine in actifed and phenylephrine, etc. should be used for a prolonged period.
    iii. Politzerisation in children, autoinflation and eustachian catheterization in adults help in dispersing and reabsorption or evacuation of the effusion, by raising the pressure in the middle ear.
    iv. Mucolytic drugs like chymotrypsin, alfatrypsin, bromhexine, ambrodil, etc. also help in liquefying and evacuation of the middle ear effusion.
2. Surgery
    i. Myringotomy and evacuation of fluid.
    ii. Grommets or indwelling teflon tubes inserted through the tympanic membrane act as a ventilating tube of the middle ear (Fig. 5.4).

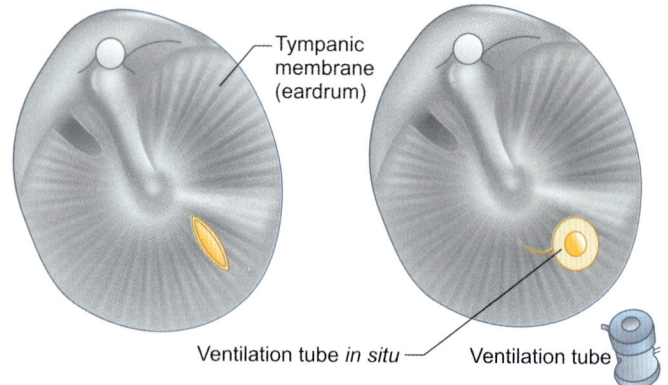

Fig. 5.4: Myringotomy and insertion of ventilation tube (grommet)

iii. Urea solution injection into the middle ear helps evacuation of thick 'glue'.
iv. Cortical mastoidectomy though recommended is of a little value.

Acute Suppurative Otitis Media (ASOM)

This is an infection of the lining membrane of the middle ear cleft by pyogenic organisms. It is commonly a disease of childhood. The most common organisms responsible for this disease are *Streptococcus haemolyticus, Staphylococcus aureus* and the *Pneumococcus.* Less common organisms are *H. influenzae, E. coli,* non-haemotytic *Streptococcus, B. proteus, P. pyocyaneus* and *H. influenzae.* The classification of ASOM may be based on duration of the disease.

• Up to 3 weeks duration is considered as acute.
• From 3rd week to 3 months duration as subacute.
• More than 3 months in duration as chronic.

Routes of Infection

1. Via the eustachian tube from the nasopharyngeal infection.
2. Via the external auditory meatus where the membrane is already perforated.
3. Rarely by blood-borne infection.

   The type of inflammation and its progress depend not only on the violence of the infecting organisms and the resistance and age of the patient but also on drainage and therapy, particularly with antibiotics.

   The clinical course is influenced by the degree of pneumatisation of the mastoid. A high degree of pneumatisation provides a large surface area and produces a large amount of inflammatory exudate. The clinical picture is severe in high degree of pneumatisation and mild in the acellular type.

Aetiology

It is common in childhood. Males are more commonly affected than females.

Predisposing Factors

The common predisposing factors are:

1. Rhinitis–usually the common colds, less often the allergic type, with secondary infection later.
2. Sinusitis.
3. Tonsillitis and adenoids.
4. Influenza and other infectious fevers.
5. Nasopharyngeal tumours, ulcerations and pack if kept for more than 24 hours.
6. Swimming and diving can cause forceful entrance of infected water into the middle ear through the eustachian tube.

Exciting Factors

Various organisms are found. The commonest of them are

1. *Streptococcus haemolyticus*.
2. *Pneumococcus*.
3. *Staphylococcus aureus*.
   Rarely *H. influenzae* and *B. friedlander* are found.

Pathology

Hyperemia and oedema of mucosa of the middle ear and the eustachian tube cause tubal obstruction. This is followed by exudation, which is serous at first and later becomes purulent. Bulging of tympanic membrane follows owing to excessive collection of exudate. By pressure necrosis rupture of the tympanic membrane occurs with discharge of pus.

Clinical Features

- *Stage-I:* Stage of hyperemia
  In this stage there is congestion and oedema of the middle ear mucosa causing:
  - Acute tubal obstruction
  - Sensation of fullness in the ear
  - Deafness of conductive type
  - Autophony
  - Retraction of tympanic membrane.
  There is injection of the vessels along the handle of malleus and between the umbo and the periphery resembling the spokes of a cartwheel.
- *Stage-II:* Stage of exudation
  In this stage there is exudation in the middle ear and generalized congestion and bulging of the tympanic membrane with loss of landmarks. Deafness increases with progressive discomfort. Bubbling sounds occur followed by pain in the ear of stabbing or boring character.
  In children these may be associated with malaise and fever.
- *Stage-III:* Stage of perforation
  Discharge from the ear (otorrhoea) follows rupture of the tympanic membrane.

The nature of discharge depends on the degree of infection. If the perforation of the tympanic membrane is very small, pulsating discharge is visible during otoscopy with intermittent reflection of light synchronizing with the heartbeat. This is due to inadequate drainage of pentup pus. Pain will be immediately relieved after drainage of pus.

Tuning-fork test: In the early stage Rinne's test may be positive which later becomes negative with progress of the disease. Weber's test will be lateralised to the worst ear.

Tenderness of bone: Mastoid process is tender in every case of acute suppurative otitis media. This is known as mastoidism and not a clinical mastoiditis. Mastoidism is due to the extension of inflammatory changes from middle ear mucosa to that of mastoid antrum and the mastoid air cells.

- *Stage-IV:* Stage of coalescent mastoiditis. In acute mastoiditis there is coalescence of air cells due to hyperemic decalcification and pressure necrosis of the bony cell walls with formation of pus.
- *Stage-V:* Stage of complication

  In this stage infection from the middle ear and mastoid extends to an adjacent structure with the manifestation of post-aural subperiosteal abscess, facial nerve paralysis, labyrinthitis, perisinus or extradural abscess, sigmoid sinus thrombophlebitis, brain abscess, or meningitis.
- *Stage-VI:* Stage of resolution

  If the patient of acute suppurative otitis media is treated properly and adequately, there is a complete resolution of infection with healing and return of normal hearing.

Differential Diagnosis

1. Furuncle or diffuse otitis externa.
2. Reflex otalgia—usually with normal tympanic membrane and normal hearing.
3. Herpetic lesions of the ear—difficult to diagnose especially after rupture of the vesicles.
4. Post-aural lymphadenitis—usually present with infection of the scalp. It is not accompanied by deafness and changes in the tympanic membrane.

Treatment

Local treatment

1. *Before rupture:* Sedative drops to relieve pain, i.e. guttae glycerin et acid carbolic (two drachm of acid carbolic in an ounce of glycerin).
   Myringotomy:
   i. When the patient passes more than one sleepless night owing to intense pain.
   ii. In the bulging stage.
   iii. Threatened intracranial complications.
2. After rupture or myringotomy—the treatment is primarily meant for helping better drainage and drying up of the discharge.

Aural toilet: Cleaning the ear as frequently as necessary followed by antiseptic eardrop instillation as follows: Guttae phenol or guttae boro spirit or otogesic, etc.

This may be followed by insufflation of an antibiotic, boric acid or iodine in boric acid powder (0.75 per cent iodine in boric acid). Myringotomy is also needed in cases with pulsating discharge indicating inadequate drainage in pinhole, perforation.

Nose drop: One to two per cent ephedrine in normal saline should be instilled into the nose three to four times daily. Oxymetazolin hydrocloride or xylometasoline solution of 0.05% may be used as nasal drop or spray.

Inflation of the ear either by autoinflation or by eustachian catheterization and politzerization helps restoration of the normal hearing.

Systemic Treatment

Adequate dosage of either oral sulfonamides and antibiotics like amoxycillin alone or with clavelunic acid, cephalosporin or intramuscular injection of antibiotics should be given in all stages of the infection for 5–10 days depending on the severity of the case.

Symptomatic Treatment

1. Rest in bed
2. Analgesics and sedatives
3. Local application of heat.

If the discharge from the ear continues, search should be made for other sources of infection. The common sources are the nasopharyngeal diseases, sinusitis and inadequate nasal airway. The treatment of these conditions is necessary for a cure.

Sequelae

1. The infection may be checked at any stage.
2. Healing may be complete with return of normal hearing.
3. The perforation may be closed either by scar or by a thin veil like membrane.
4. A perforation may remain open, which may be dry or moist. It is central in type.
5. A certain amount of deafness may persist in the presence of perforation or secretory otitis media due to unresolved ASOM.
6. "Chalk patches", otherwise called tympanosclerosis, may result.

Certain authors do not agree that the "chalk patches" are invariably connected with past infection.

Criterion of cure: Return of normal hearing is the only criterion of cure.

Myringotomy (Paracentesis Tympani)

Definition: Incision of the tympanic membrane (Fig. 5.5).

Indications

1. In acute suppurative otitis media—if the patient passes more than one sleepless night owing to severe pain in the ear.

2. In the bulging stage of acute suppurative otitis media.

3. In acute suppurative otitis media with threatening intracranial complication.

4. In acute suppurative otitis media with small perforation where the drainage is inadequate.

5. In secretory otitis media with non-purulent middle ear effusion for drainage and for application of grommet.

Complications

1. Injury to incudo-stapedial joint and other ossicles, laceration of the tympanic membrane and intratympanic muscles.

2. Injury to chorda tympani nerve.

3. Injury to jugular bulb in the floor of middle ear.

Anaesthesia: General anaesthesia. In secretory otitis media with uninflamed tympanic membrane no anaesthesia is required.

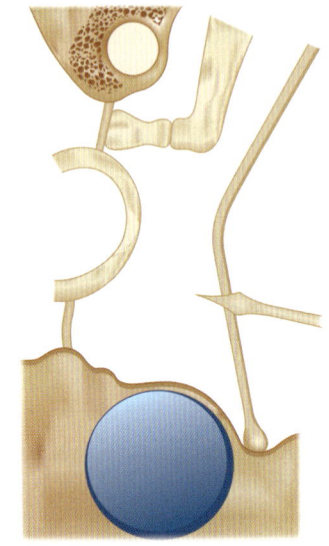

Fig. 5.5: Position of the myringotome during myringotomy

Technique

Preparation of the Patient

Preferably performed under an operating microscope. In every case full theatre facility should be available. A good light is essential for the performance of this operation. After anaesthesia and draping the patient is placed in a suitable position with the same ear upward. The external canal is cleaned either by wiping out with spirit or by suction after instillation of antiseptic solution.

The operation is done under general anaesthesia with the help of an aural speculum and angled myringotome, a radial incision is made in the postero-inferior quadrant (Fig. 5.6). Maximum

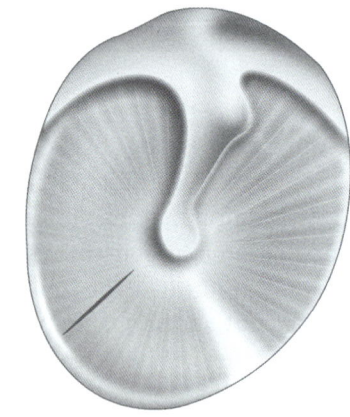

Fig. 5.6: Position of radial incision in ASOM

bulging occurs in the posterior part of tympanic membrane in ASOM. This inferior incision avoids the risk of damaging the ossicular chain, chorda tympani and facial nerve. Pus under pressure then gushes out. Residual pus is gently sucked out. The incision should be about 3–4 mm. in length from the umbo to the annulus.

In otitis media with effusion (OME) the radial incision is preferably taken in the anteroinferior quadrant.

Aftercare

In acute suppurative otitis media drainage is maintained by daily cleaning. There should be no interference in secretory otitis media. The patient is warned against getting water in the ear for about a week.

Before declaring a patient cured, careful examination of the hearing must be made. If required, the eustachian tube must be inflated. This is one of the important parts of the treatment. If one fails to effect inflation of the eustachian tube, the patient may develop permanent partial deafness.

Perforation of the Tympanic Membrane

Three types of perforation of the tympanic membrane are found (Fig. 5.8). These are as follows:

1. Central
2. Marginal
3. Attic

Central Perforation

In this type a margin of tympanic membrane remains all round the perforation. It is found in pars tensa. The underlying infection is limited up to the mucosa only. Bone is not involved.

Marginal Perforation

In this type the tympanic annulus is involved and disease of the underlying bone is present. This type is very often associated with cholesteatoma formation and presents in the posterosuperior quadrant of the tympanic membrane (pars tensa).

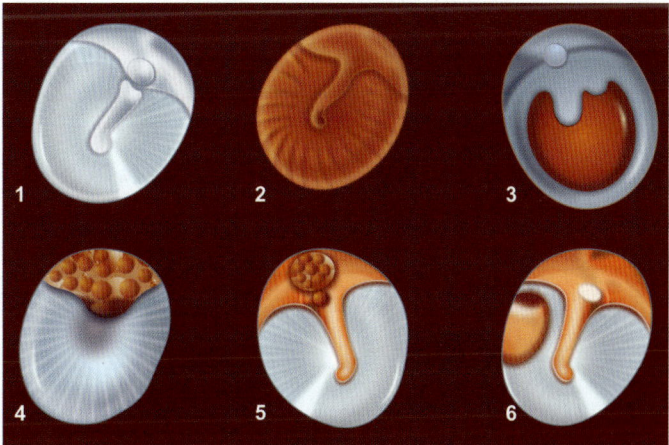

Fig. 5.7: Different types of tympanic membrane conditions. (1) Normal tympanic membrane (right), (2) Cartwheel appearance with generalized congestion of right tympanic membrane in acute otitis media, (3) Chronic suppurative otitis media with a large central perforation of the left tympanic membrane, (4) Chronic suppurative otitis media with granulation covering pars flaccida and part of posterosuperior quadrant (right), (5) Attic perforation with granulation (left tympanic membrane), (6) Posterior marginal perforation (right tympanic membrane) showing incudostapedial joint.

Attic Perforation

This type is situated in the membrana flaccida. This perforation is characterized by lack of symptoms and may cause serious complications due to extension of disease by erosion of neighbouring bone and cholesteatoma formation.

Prognosis

Prognosis is good in central perforation and bad in marginal and worse in attic perforations.

Special forms of Acute Infection of Middle Ear Cleft

1. Infection in Infants

The wide, short and almost horizontal eustachian tube predisposes to infection in infants. During bottle-feeding in supine position the contaminated milk may enter the eustachian tube. In infants acute upper respiratory infection is a common etiological factor in acute otitis media. Vomiting and teething with associated rhinitis are also the causes of otitis media in infants.

In babies with poor nutrition otitis media may be associated with gastroenteritis. In this type of otitis media diarrhoea is the prevalent symptom.

2. Infection Associated with Non-pneumatised Mastoid

In this type the symptoms are relatively mild. The patient complains of mere discomfort and heaviness of the ears. The perforation of the membrane is often marginal or attic type. The condition assumes a chronic character from its inception.

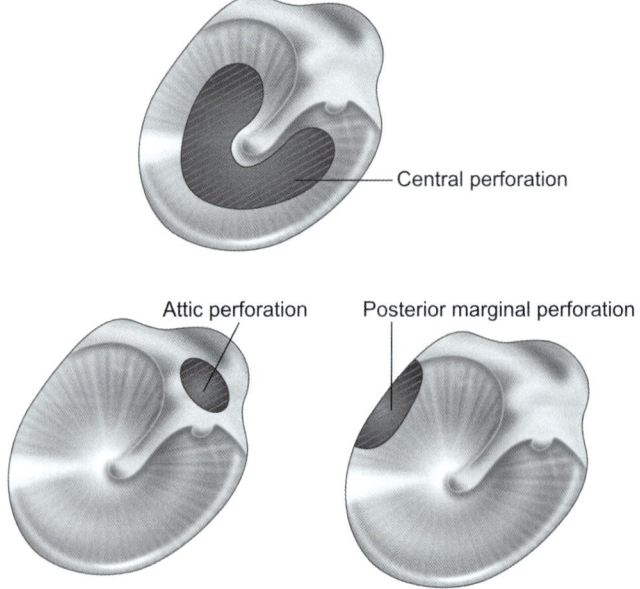

Fig. 5.8: Three types of tympanic membrane perforation

3. *Petrositis or Apisitis*

This is due to the extension of infection to the pneumatised petrous apex. Rarely there may be formation of abscess.

Suppuration in the petrous temporal bone is usually accompanied by serous meningitis, which may be either in the middle or in the posterior cranial fossa. A septic meningitis may follow the perforation of the bone with the formation of extradural abscess. A parapharyngeal abscess may rarely be formed following tracking of pus along the internal carotid artery.

Clinical Features

Petrositis is always associated with an established mastoiditis.
 i. Owing to irritation of the fifth cranial nerve there will be deep temporal or retro-orbital pain.
 ii. Persistent otorrhoea.
 iii. Due to compression of the sixth cranial nerve, there will be paralysis of the external rectus muscle. This results in internal squint and diplopia.

Unilateral headache, sixth cranial nerve paralysis, and mastoid infection together constitute **Gradenigo's Triad**.

Diagnosis is confirmed by radiographic demonstration of the petrous abscess.

Treatment

a. Mastoidectomy—appropriate to the mastoid disease, i.e. cortical or modified radical is to be performed.
b. Large doses of suitable antibiotics should be administered systemically.

Drainage of the abscess in the petrous apex may be established by following the track from the base of the petrous pyramid.

The route of infection to the petrous apex, i.e. posterosuperior (around the semicircular canals) or anteroinferior (around the cochlea), should be defined.

Exploration of the posterior cell track is generally undertaken first,
 a. Above the horizontal and behind the superior vertical canal,
 b. Through the arch of the superior semicircular canal (Frencknes's approach),
 c. Beneath the posterior canal and behind the vertical portion of the facial nerve.

If no diseased cell tracks are found in the posterior region, the anterior tracks should be explored.

The **Ramadier-Lempert approach** excavates between the carotid artery and the cochlea.

The **Thornval approach** exposes dura over the superior aspect of the petrous pyramid. The dura is elevated inwards until the apex is reached and opened.

4. *Acute Necrotic Otitis Media*

It is the infection of the middle ear complicating an acute infectious disease. Measles, scarlet fever, and rarely diphtheria and typhoid are the infectious fevers responsible for this type of otitis media. The organism known for the rapid necrosis of the tympanic membrane is a **β-haemolytic streptococcus**. Almost complete destruction of the tympanic membrane results in a large kidney-shaped perforation. Squamous epithelium from the external auditory meatus migrates in the middle ear cavity with formation of cholesteatoma and chronic suppuration. This causes severe deafness.

5. Pneumococcus (Type III infection)

This type deserves special mention.

The clinical triad of acute pain in the ear, fever and inflamed membrane in a typical case of simple acute otitis media is modified in this type. The onset is insidious leading to **quiet necrosis**. Pain in the ear and complications are slight. An unexpected complication with sudden onset may arise in exactly the same way as from a mastoiditis masked by antibiotics.

6. Haemorrhagic Otitis Media

It is a primary otitis media seen in influenza epidemics. It may be associated with myringitis bullosa and is principally established by the presence of a sanguinous middle ear effusion. Culture of discharge generally reveals a haemolytic streptococcus. Pain in the ear is severe and mastoid tenderness develops early.

Chronic Suppurative Otitis Media (CSOM)

The word "Chronic" carries an implication of time. The long-standing suppuration of the middle ear is called chronic suppurative otitis media or chronic otorrhoea.

There are two main clinical types:
1. Safe or benign or tubo-tympanic type.
2. Unsafe or dangerous or atticoantral type.

The second type is called dangerous for the following reasons:
   i. Owing to anatomical relationship of attic and antrum with middle and posterior cranial fossa, lateral sinus, lateral semicircular canal and facial canal.
   ii. The mucosa of the attico antral region is of pavement type. It cannot regenerate if it is damaged by infection. Hence osteitic erosion occurs.
   iii. Cholesteatoma formation is common in this type of CSOM, which erodes the surrounding bone by exerting pressure and by some enzymatic reaction.

Chronic suppurative otitis media may be
a. Active with discharge of pus.
b. Quiescent with an intermission of discharge of a period of less than six months.
c. Inactive with cessation of discharge for six months without probability of resumption in the near future. But it may be active by reinfection of the middle ear through the perforation of the tympanic membrane.
d. Healed otitis media implies total extinction of disease and healing of perforation of the tympanic membrane.

Aetiology

Exciting factors: These are pus-producing organisms. The predominant organisms are gram-negative bacilli, e.g. *B. proteus* and *Pseudomonas pyocyaneus.*

Predisposing Factors

i. Poor socioeconomic condition and lack of hygiene
ii. Non-pneumatised mastoid
iii. Diseases in the nose, paranasal sinuses and pharynx
iv. Lowering of local or general resistance of the patient
v. Hereditary disposition to catarrhal, and suppurative affections of the upper respiratory tract, including the middle ear cleft.

Pathology

In the safe or benign type the perforation can be of any size or shape and central in type. This may be anterior or posterior to handle malleus and inferior to umbo. It may be large kidney shaped or subtotal perforation. The mucosa of the middle ear is velvety and pink, and may be oedematous. Occasionally a polypus is seen arising from the medial wall of the middle ear. Mastoids are usually cellular. Mastoiditis is a common complication in this type.

In the dangerous type the infection invades the bony walls of the middle ear. The perforation of the tympanic membrane is either marginal or attic. It may be associated with cholesteatoma, granulations and polypus. The mastoids are sclerotic. Intracranial complications are common in this type.

Histopathology of chronic otitis media reveals healing accompanied by fibrosis. Inflammatory oedema in the cells causes hypertrophy and permanent swelling.

A polypus is formed by extrusion of the swollen middle ear mucosa through a perforation in the tympanic membrane. Thus a polypus appears in the external auditory meatus.

Granulation tissue replaces other cells. It is a vascular tissue composed of numerous newly formed blood vessels, histiocytes and fibroblasts. The tissue may show infiltration of polymorphs and other leucocytes.

A so-called granuloma which is nothing but a tuft of granulation tissue may appear in the areas of osteitis. Posterior tympanic ring margin is the commonly affected area.

Clinical Features

Deafness, discharge from the ear and perforation of the tympanic membrane are the chief symptoms and signs of chronic middle ear suppuration. Tinnitus may be present. Vertigo may be present sometimes. In an uncomplicated case of CSOM, no pain is present. If a case of CSOM complains of pain, it is nearly always due to some grave complications and should be seriously dealt with if it is not due to defective drainage or diffuse otitis externa.

A summary of symptoms and signs of the safe type and dangerous type of chronic suppurative otitis media is given:

	Safe type	Unsafe type
Disease site	Tubotympanic	Attico-antral
Type of perforation	Central	Attic or marginal
Character of discharge	Mucoid or odourless	Purulent, thick and foul
Amount of pus	Profuse	Scanty
Granulations	Not common	Common
Polypus	If present usually pale and edematous	If present usually hyperemic and fleshy
Deafness	Conductive, slight to moderate	Conductive or mixed, moderate to severe
X-ray mastoids	Pneumatic mastoid	Sclerotic mastoid
Cholesteatoma	Very rare	Very common

Headache, rise in temperature with chill and rigor with sudden fall of it (Hectic type), vertigo and facial twitchings in case of CSOM indicate involvement of duramater, lateral sinus, labyrinth and facial nerve respectively.

Investigation of Chronic Suppurative Otitis Media

Investigation of chronic suppurative otitis media must include the tools to confirm or eliminate the involvement of important neighbouring structures especially in unsafe or dangerous type of the disease.

1. *Hearing:* By voice test the hearing of the patient is assessed. If required, adequate masking sound should be used in the better ear while testing the diseased ear.
2. *Tuning fork test:* There will be conductive type of deafness. Adequate masking sound should be used in severe hearing loss.
3. *Fistula test:* The test will indicate presence or absence of fistulous connection between the middle and the inner ear and also the living or dead inner ear (labyrinth).

   The symptoms of vestibular irritation (fistula test) may be elicited either by sudden pressure on the tragus, by Siegle's pneumatic speculum or by politzerization.

   In case of aural polyp—this test may be performed by its manipulation with an aural probe.
4. *Cold air caloric or dunda grant test:* The test is carried out in the presence of perforation of tympanic membrane to know the function of the vestibular labyrinth.
5. Tests to exclude facial nerve paralysis.
6. *Radiological examination:* This is important to know the presence or absence of cholesteatoma, bony erosion in the attic or antral region.
7. *Audiometric test of hearing:* Pure-tone audiometry is more commonly used than any other audiometry.
8. Aural discharge should be tested for the growth of the bacteria and their sensitivity to different antibiotics.
9. Nose and pharynx should be examined and investigated in a routine manner to exclude the septic foci.

Treatment

There are two main objectives of the treatment of chronic suppurative otitis media.

1. Arrest of the disease
2. Preservation and/or restoration of function

These objectives may be secured by medical and/or surgical treatment. In the chronic otitis media surgical treatment gives best results. The degeneration, destruction, fibrosis, granulations and polyp formation are the features responsible for the failure of medical treatment either by topical or by parenteral medication.

Two factors should be always kept in mind in treating such a case such as safety of the patient and preservation of auditory function. Safety of the patient should of course get the priority. The restoration of hearing may be possible by plastic reconstructive surgery (tympanoplasty).

Treatment (tubotympanic disease)

- Topical antibiotics—when active. Avoid ototoxic antibiotics.
- Aural toilet—should be meticulously done under direct vision. It should be done as frequently as necessary.
- Elimination of septic foci if present in tonsils, adenoids and sinuses.
- Mastoidectomy—is not usually required in safe type. If fails to improve with the presence of a profuse discharge with haziness of the mastoid air cells on radiography, then cortical mastoidectomy may be required to eradicate a reservoir of infection in the cells.
- Myringoplasty or type I tympanoplasty may be performed for a dry perforation.
- Ossiculoplasty may be performed along with tympanoplasty if the ossicles are found damaged.

Repair of TM Perforations Using Epidermal Growth Factor (EGF)

For EGF efficacy for the repair of TM perforations, the excision of the epithelial margin of the perforation is not required. There is no necessity for placement of the paper patch over the perforation to act as a scaffold-because the action of the EGF requires continuous contact with the target issue for at least 5 hours. Gelfoam or some other sponge like substance is probably necessary for EGF efficacy.

This is based on experimental study on animals.

Treatment (attico-antral disease)

1. *Conservative:* If the cholesteatoma is small and accessible, a trial with conservative procedures as follows may be given:
   - Removal of cholesteatoma by fine crocodile forceps and suction-irrigation under operative microscope.
   - Removal of polypi and/or granulation tissue with cup forceps under magnification.
   - Permanent periodical inspection.
2. *Surgical:* If conservative treatment fails or when complications are present or threatening.

Surgical Treatment

Primary objectives of operative treatment are the following:

1. To render the patient safe. For this the diseased bone, disorganized mucosa, granulations, polyp and cholesteatoma should be removed.
2. To prevent further deterioration of function.
3. To stop discharge permanently.
4. To treat complications such as extradural abscess, brain abscess, facial nerve palsy and labyrinthitis.

　The surgical treatment may be:

1. Cortical mastoidectomy (simple or Schwartze operation).
2. Classical radical mastoidectomy.
3. Modified radical mastoidectomy.

　The choice of treatment will depend on the type of pathology.

In the Safe or Tubotympanic Type

With active stage, treatment should be in the form of topical application, removal of polypus if present and weekly check-up. Even if the discharge persists, investigation and treatment of upper respiratory tract and mastoid air cells are necessary. If mastoid infection is present simple mastoidectomy should be done.

　With quiescent stage the patient should be under monthly observation for a period of 6 months. If the perforation persists permanent precaution should be taken.

　With inactive stage—myringoplasty or Type I tympanoplasty should be performed. In case of the recurrence of perforation a repeat, myringoplasty is advisable or permanent precautions should be taken.

In Unsafe or Attico-antral Disease

Active Stage

　i. With cholesteatoma—modified radical mastoidectomy and tympanoplasty.
　ii. With polypus—removal of polypus.
　iii. With granulations—remove or reduce granulation.
　iv. With pus alone—local medical treatment and bi-weekly observation should be made. If medical treatment fails, mastoidectomy and tympanoplasty should be performed.

Quiescent Stage

The patient should be kept under monthly observation for 6 months. If there is recurrence of discharge, mastoidectomy with tympanoplasty should be performed.

Inactive Stage

With persistent perforation one should take permanent precautions and hearing aid may be prescribed.

　If associated with complications like facial nerve palsy, labyrinthitis, and intracranial extension—mastoidectomy is the choice of treatment.

Differential Diagnosis of Otitis Media

The knowledge about the pathology of different types of otitis media is essential for their better management.

The salient features of each type are indicated below:

1. Acute suppurative otitis media—this is an acute infection of the mucoperiosteum of the middle ear cleft. The tympanic membrane perforation is always small and always in the pars tensa. The disease is self-limiting and responsive to anti-bacterial therapy.

2. Tubercular otitis media—this is comparatively rare. The perforations are multiple. The hearing loss is conductive in type and disproportionate to the extent of the disease. It may be associated with pulmonary tuberculosis. The condition is painless. It may lead to facial nerve paralysis and a cold subperiosteal abscess.

3. Syphilitic otitis media—it is a rare disease nowadays. It can occur in both early and late forms of congenital syphilis, and tertiary stage of acquired syphilis. The middle ear is affected by a gummatous osteoperiostitis though otolabyrinthitis is common in syphilis involving both middle and inner ears with neurosensory deafness.

   Gummatous change produces foul smelling, painless discharge with mastoid bone destruction. Serological tests for syphilis (STS) are confirmatory. Antisyphilitic treatment cures the patient. Sometimes mastoidectomy may be required.

4. Allergic otitis media—it is much more common, characterized by its stubborn chronicity and resistance to therapy. The discharge is mucoid in nature.

5. Acute necrotic otitis media—it occurs in debilitating children suffering from acute infectious fever. The tympanic membrane perforation is invariably large due to necrotic sloughing of tissue.

   Three types of chronic otorrhoea result from an acute necrotic otitis media, which depends on the extent of the original necrosis of tissue:

   i. A benign type of chronic suppurative otitis media with a central perforation.

   ii. A bone-invading secondary acquired cholesteatoma with a marginal perforation. The discharge is scanty, foul smelling and non-mucoid in nature.

   iii. A bone-invading chronic osteitis, chronic osteomyelitis or sequestrum. The discharge is foul and purulent in this type.

   Of these three, the benign type of chronic otorrhoea is the most common, the secondary acquired cholesteatoma being next in frequency. Chronic osteitis, without cholesteatoma is comparatively rare.

   There is another bone-invading variety of chronic suppurative otitis media. That is, primary acquired cholesteatoma, which arises insidiously as a result of the indrawing of pars flaccida of the tympanic membrane.

6. Adhesive otitis media—it is a chronic adhesive process and is often bilateral. It usually follows secretory otitis media or unresolved acute suppurative otitis media.

Clinical Features

   i. Deafness

   ii. Tinnitus

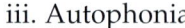

iii. Autophonia

iv. Tympanic membrane is dull lusterless and adherent to the medial wall of the middle ear. Mobility is absent. Audiometry shows conductive deafness. Tympanometry reveals negative pressure in the middle ear with flat curve (no compliance).

Treatment is usually unsatisfactory. Tympanotomy and placement of teflon or silastic sheet after severing the adhesive bands and removal of the sheet after a few months may cure the patient.

Cholesteatoma

Cholesteatoma or "epidermosis" or cholesteatosis occurs in two forms as described below which can be diagnosed histologically.

Cholesteatoma is a misnomer, because it is neither a tumour nor does it necessarily contain cholesterol crystals. The term cholesteatoma has still been retained as it has a firmly established place in the literature.

Classification

Cholesteatoma are of two types histologically:

1. *Epidermoid cholesteatoma (epidermosis):* It is a bag-like cystic structure lined by keratinizing stratified squamous epithelium resting on a fibrous stroma. Desquamation of epithelium produces pearly laminae and form the bulk of the cholesteatoma. This variety is the commonest one tackled by ENT surgeons.

2. *Cholesterol granuloma:* It is a granulomatous structure formed by variable numbers of cholesterol crystals, foreign body giant cells and granulation tissue. Cholesterol granuloma develops at a site of suppuration or haemorrhage.

Cholesteatoma may be **congenital** or **acquired**. The acquired variety may be again primary, secondary or tertiary.

The useful classification of cholesteatoma is based on the anatomical site of the disease with reference to tympanic membrane pathology. This classification is valuable, because different types of cholesteatoma are often distinct from pathological, clinical and therapeutic standpoints. Three types of cholesteatoma are recognised: Pars tensa cholesteatoma, pars flaccida cholesteatoma and occult cholesteatoma.

Occult cholesteatoma occurs deep to an intact tympanic membrane and is often congenital. Four main theories have been used to explain the development of cholesteatoma—the presence of congenital cell rest, metaplasia of middle ear epithelium, papillary ingrowth through the intact tympanic membrane and migration of epithelium into a pre-existing retraction pocket or through a perforation of the tympanic membrane.

Papillary Ingrowth

Papillary ingrowth refers to the development of cholesteatoma arising from the pars flaccida. Cholesteatoma could be generated by the application of foreign material onto the medial aspect of the pars flaccida, with the active proliferation of basal cells (papillary ingrowth of the epithelium) breaking through the basement membrane. Cholesteatoma could be generated by an inflammatory reaction in Prussack's space usually due to poor ventilation in this area.

Congenital Cholesteatoma

It arises in an embryonic cell rest in any of the cranial bones. It is etiologically not connected with chronic suppurative otitis media and is typically located in the anterior middle ear (Fig. 5.9).

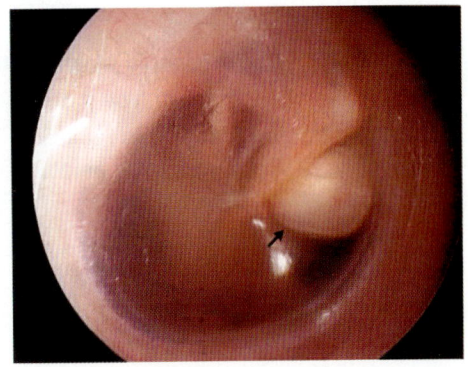

Fig. 5.9: Congenital cholesteatoma seen through the intact tympanic membrane at the anterosuperior part of middle ear

Diagnosis

1. Development behind an intact tympanic membrane.
2. No previous history of ear infection.
3. Origin from embryonic inclusion of squamous epithelium within the developing temporal bone.

Primary Acquired Cholesteatoma

The genesis of acquired cholesteatoma is debatable. In the primary acquired type, there is no history of otitis media. The explanations in favour of its formation are as follows:

1. Ingrowth of active prickle cells in the region of membrana flaccida. This is caused by repeated inflammatory episodes.
2. Indrawing of the pars flaccida due to negative pressure in the middle ear and formation of a pouch. There is desquamation of epithelium in the pouch with the formation of cholesteatoma.
3. Epithelial metaplasia. Due to subclinical infection, the normal pavement epithelium changes to keratinizing squamous epithelium. Subsequent desquamation from squamous epithelium forms cholesteatoma.

Secondary Acquired Cholesteatoma

This is secondary to chronic infection and is due to migration of squamous epithelium from the external auditory meatus into the middle ear through a perforation especially in the marginal type. It may also be due to metaplasia from pavement to squamous epithelium by the stimulus of infection.

Tertiary Acquired Cholesteatoma

This type has been included recently in the classification of cholesteatoma. After tympanoplasty operation especially with "onlay" graft, cholesteatoma may be developed sometime if bits of squamous epithelium during the process of de-epithelialization are inadvertently left behind underneath the graft. It is named graft cholesteatoma and one of the rare complications of onlay tympanoplasty (tertiary acquired cholesteatoma).

Black Cholesteatoma

It is generally found in children. On opening the diseased mastoid air cells, dark-coloured secretion is found. The mucosa stains black. The tympanic membrane appears blue.

Tos otoscopic classification of cholesteatoma (modified)			
Attic	*Tensa type 1*	*Tensa type 2*	*Intact TM*
Arising in retraction pocket of pars flaccida	Arising in retraction pocket of post ½ of pars tensa	Arising in retraction pocket of centre of tympanic membrane	Arising behind intact tympanic membrane

6

Complications of Otitis Media

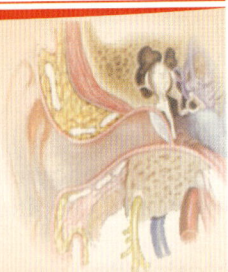

Spread of infection from the middle ear may occur through the tegmen to the middle cranial fossa causing subdural abscess, meningitis or temporal lobe abscess. Spread posteriorly into the posterior cranial fossa causes meningitis or cerebellar abscess. This may cause intratemporal spread resulting labyrinthitis, facial palsy, petrositis, sigmoid sinus thrombophlebitis. Spread into the subperiosteal area due to destruction of mastoid cortex develops infratemporal abscess of Berzld, zygomatic abscess, Citellis abscess and Lue's abscess (Fig. 6.1).

The complications of otitis media may be divided into two groups as follows

1. Meningeal.
2. Non-meningeal.

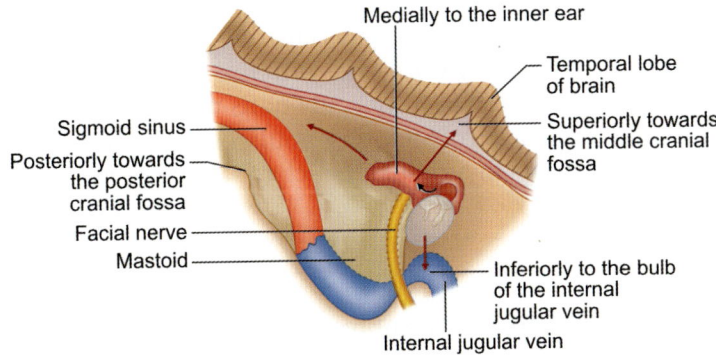

Fig. 6.1: Routes of infection from the middle ear and mastoid antrum

Meningeal complications are of the following

1. Extradural abscess
2. Subdural abscess
3. Venous sinus thrombophlebitis
4. Otitic hydrocephalus
5. Meningitis

Non-meningeal complications are of the following

1. Mastoiditis
2. Petrositis

3. Facial nerve paralysis
4. Labyrinthitis
5. Brain abscess

The complications of otitis media may also be classified by rearranging the above-mentioned conditions as extracranial and intracranial.

Mastoiditis

It can occur in two main forms, acute and chronic. A very common complication of acute suppurative otitis media is an acute mastoiditis. It frequently occurs in primary acute otitis media but may also be seen due to an acute exacerbation of a chronic otitis media. Acute mastoiditis occurs in a cellular type of mastoid bone.

The mastoid air cells are distributed in groups. These include:

1. Tip cells
2. Perisinus cells—overlying the lateral sinus
3. Petrosal angle cells—in the angle between the dura and the lateral wall
4. Subdural cells—between the roof of the mastoid antrum and the dural plate
5. Zygomatic cells—into the zygoma
6. Facial cells—under the posterior meatal wall surrounding the facial nerve canal
7. Perilabyrinthine cells—surrounding the semicircular canals
8. Peritubal cells—surrounding the bony part of the eustachian tube
9. Apical cells—around the petrous apex.

Acute mastoiditis is a coalescence of air cells due to hyperemic decalcification and pressure necrosis of the bony cell walls, with the formation of an empyema. It is derived by extension of infection from acute otitis media.

Chronic mastoiditis is invasion of bone by granulation tissue arising from a chronic otitis media. It always occurs in a cellular or sclerotic type of mastoids.

Acute Mastoiditis

Aetiology and Pathology

Extension of inflammation from acute otitis media in the mastoid air cells through the aditus is one of the common etiological factors. If the virulence of the organisms is great, resistance of the patient is low and the drainage of the cleft via the eustachian tube and/or perforation of the tympanic membrane are poor, more pus will be produced with increased intra air-cell tension. This increased tension if not relieved will result in pressure necrosis of the bony cell walls. The bone destruction will be enhanced by hyperemic decalcification.

This process results in the formation of an empyema. Ultimately the cortex of the bone will be destroyed and a subperiosteal abscess is produced. If the production of pus and drainage is not properly balanced, the condition leads towards chronic retention of pus in the mastoid with overflow. This is called **mastoid reservoir**.

The causative organism is usually a β-haemolytic streptococcus. There may be a steady progressive coalescence without the warning signs and symptoms of pain, fever, swelling and discharge. This is termed **masked mastoiditis** and is due to modification of inflammatory reactions by inadequate antibiotic therapy. In these types of cases, the patient will not feel up to the mark, the mastoid may be tender and X-ray mastoids will show haziness or a cavity.

It occurs most often in "slum" areas, where the poorer, overcrowded social conditions encourage a higher frequency of upper respiratory infections in children with low resistance.

The factors concerned in the development of acute mastoiditis may be summarized as follows:

1. Anatomical—highly pneumatised mastoids.
2. Existing otitis media—mastoiditis is an extension of otitis media to bone.
3. Inadequate drainage of pus.
4. Virulence and type of organism.
5. Resistance of patient—age, illness, environment.
6. Mishandled antibiotics.

Symptoms

1. Pain—generally throbbing in nature and may radiate down the neck or along the lower jaw.
2. Deafness.
3. Discharge—will be mucopurulent and increased in volume.
4. Gastrointestinal disturbance may be present in infants and children.

Signs

1. Pyrexia—high.
2. Tenderness—always present somewhere between root of zygoma and mastoid tip.
3. Swelling—retroauricular oedema or subperiosteal abscess.
4. Pinna will be pushed downward and forward.
5. Sagging of the posterosuperior bony meatal wall.
6. Tympanic membrane is always abnormal, and a combination of this sign with sagging of posterior meatal wall is sufficient for a diagnosis of acute mastoiditis.
7. Conductive deafness.
8. General condition—the patient looks ill, and feels ill. With the rise in temperature the patient has an anxious look. A common tendency in children to fall asleep for short periods at odd times. The tongue is furred and heavily coated despite regular bowels.

Investigation

1. Digital X-rays: Air cells are hazy or opaque with coalescence. Radiography can be of practical use in the diagnosis of infection of mastoids only in the cases of patients who crossed one year of age. This is because it is usually not until about the age of one year that the pneumatisation has proceeded to the point of radiological diagnosis.
2. Blood examination: Usually reveals polymorphonuclear leucocytes and an increase in the sedimentation rate.

Differential Diagnosis

1. Acute external auditory canal furunculosis.
2. Swelling or suppuration of retroauricular lymph glands. If a fluctuant abscess is present, incision and drainage will afford a certain means of differentiation. In adenitis the pus is never deep to the periosteum.
3. Other swellings over the mastoid, e.g. sebaceous cyst and lipoma.
4. Fibrositis in the sternomastoid muscle attachment, sub-occipital fibrositis, osteoarthritis of cervical joints may cause pain over the mastoid. The teeth of the lower jaw, the temporomandibular joint, the pharynx and larynx should be examined to exclude causes for referred pain.

Masked Mastoiditis

Masked mastoiditis is the result of inadequate treatment with antibiotics. It is associated with unresolved or latent otitis media. Early recognition and vigorous treatment prevent intracranial complications like meningitis or lateral sinus thrombosis in such a case.

Persistence of deafness is an important symptom. Mastoid tenderness and headache may be present. Temperature is slight. Tympanic membrane is usually congested and thickened. X-rays of the mastoid show opacity or haziness with loss of cellular outlines in some cases.

Treatment

Vigorous treatment with suitable antibiotics. If does not improve early, a cortical mastoidectomy should be performed.

Varieties of Subperiosteal Abscess

Postauricular subperiosteal abscess (Fig 6.2) is the commonest variety of acute mastoid abscess.

Other varieties include:

1. *Zygomatic abscess:* If the zygoma is highly pneumatised, the infection may extend to these air cells. It will cause swelling and tenderness in front of and above the external auditory meatus. The zygomatic abscess usually lies deep to the temporal muscle, may lie superficial to it at times.

2. *Luc's abscess:* Pus from zygomatic region may track outwards under the perio-steum of the roof of the bony canal and can reach the infratemporal region. This is called Luc's abscess.

3. *Bezold's abscess:* Perforation of inner surface of the tip of mastoid may give rise to an abscess deep to the sternomastoid muscle. Bezold's abscess

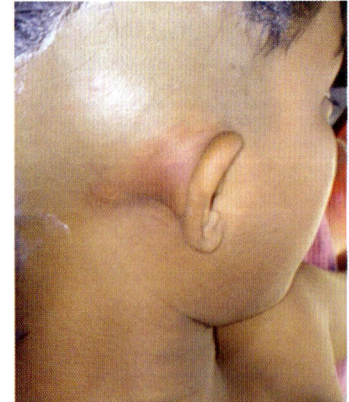

Fig. 6.2: Acute subperiosteal abscess (right)

is also known as "sinking abscess" of the neck. This causes a swelling in the neck below the mastoid tip.

4. *Citelli's abscess:* Perforation of the tip cells causing extension of abscess in the digastric triangle is called Citelli's abscess.

5. *Apisitis or petrositis:* This is due to the extension of infection into the body and apex of the petrous bone. This may be acute or chronic depending on the acute or chronic otitis media.

It causes

a. Unilateral headache—which is frequently retro-orbital. Neuralgic pain in the face, jaws and teeth due to the involvement of trigeminal ganglion, which lies immediately above the apex of the petrous bone.

b. Sixth nerve paralysis—resulting in internal squint and diplopia. When these symptoms are present in addition to usual signs and symptoms of acute mastoiditis, then it is called **Gradenigo's syndrome**.

The operation used for treating acute mastoiditis is cortical mastoidectomy or Schwartze operation. Suitable antibiotics and chemotherapy should be given in adequate doses.

Cortical Mastoidectomy

(Synonym: Schwartze operation, simple or conservative mastoidectomy)

Indications

1. Subperiosteal abscess formation, Bezold's abscess, or sagging of the roof of the external auditory canal.
2. Recurrence of pain and constitutional disturbances following apparent recovery after myringotomy or perforation.
3. Increase of discharge when associated with rising pulse rate and increasing oedema over the mastoid area.
4. Persistent or increasing deafness associated with plenty of discharge lasting for a period of several weeks.
5. Persistent headache and throbbing pain on the affected side when associated with thick creamy discharge.
6. Associated with threatened intracranial complication.

Cortical mastoidectomy is performed to remove the infected air cells of the mastoid process. The middle ear and its contents are not interfered with.

Anaesthesia

This operation is usually performed under general anaesthesia, if it is not contraindicated.

Steps of Operation

After aseptic dressing and draping, the incision is given. The postaural incision of Wilde is commonly used parallel to the postauricular groove given either in or 1/2 cm behind it. The incision begins at the tip of the mastoid process upward to the level of the upper attachment of the auricle and carried through the skin, subcutaneous tissue, and periosteum (Fig. 6.3).

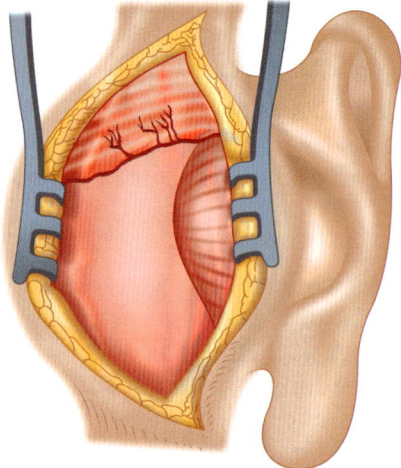

Fig. 6.3: Postaural mastoidectomy

In infants and younger children until the age of 2 years, a high posterior incision is given to avoid injury to the facial nerve. The facial nerve in infants lies very superficial at its exit from the stylomastoid foramen.

The periosteum is elevated forward and backward from the incision line. The suprameatal spine of Henle, the suprameatal triangle of McEwen and the posterior bony margin of the external auditory canal are exposed and defined. The self retaining retractor is then applied.

This keeps the soft tissue away from the field of operation and produces haemostasis.

The mastoid cortex is removed over the suprameatal triangle which is the landmark of the mastoid antrum with a drill until the antrum is entered (Fig. 6.4). The infected mastoid air cells are systematically removed until a cavity is left behind,

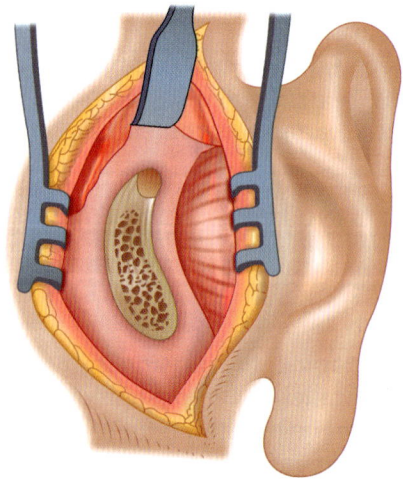

Fig. 6.4: Exposure of the area of operation after application of the retractor

bounded above by the bony plate covering the dura of the middle cranial fossa, behind by the bony plate covering the sigmoid sinus and in front by the posterior bony meatal wall and aditus ad antrum (Fig. 6.5).

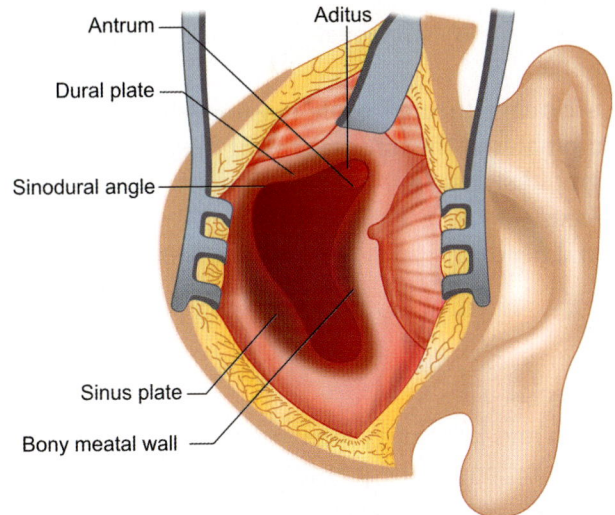

Fig. 6.5: Mastoid cavity of cortical mastoidectomy

The incision is closed by interrupted silk thread sutures. A drain of medicated ribbon gauze or corrugated rubber may be inserted at the lower end of the incision. The external auditory canal should be firmly packed with medicated ribbon gauze. The dressing is applied and bandaged firmly.

The dressing, the drain and sutures are removed between the fifth and seventh postoperative days.

Suitable antibiotics in adequate dosage and analgesics should be given during the postoperative period for about 7 to 10 days.

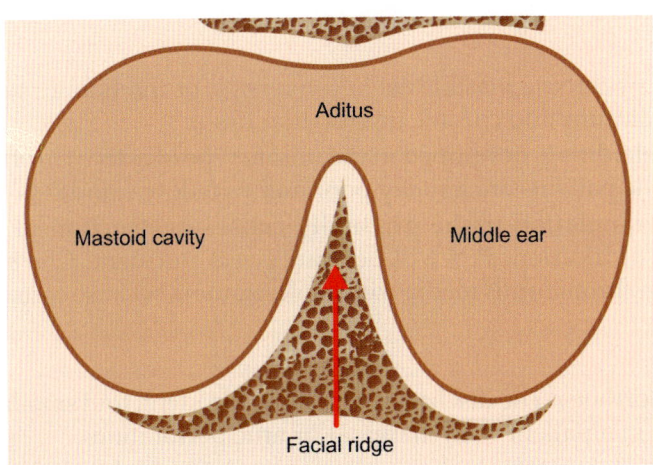

Fig. 6.6: Schematic diagram representation of cortical mastoid cavity

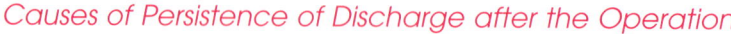
Causes of Persistence of Discharge after the Operation

1. Operation if performed before localization of the infection.
2. Inadequate removal of mastoid cells.
3. In petrositis or apisitis.
4. A simple mastoidectomy if erroneously performed for an allergic otitis media or for a cholesteatoma.

The following accidents during simple mastoidectomy can happen:
1. Injury to the duramater of the middle cranial fossa.
2. Injury to the sigmoid sinus.
3. Dislocation of incus.
4. Injury to the facial nerve.

Summary of Treatment

a. Acute mastoiditis
   1. Immediate antibiotics.
   2. Immediate swab and laboratory assay of discharge from ear.
   3. Immediate preparation for the possible surgery.
   4. If no response by conservative treatment in 48 hours do simple mastoidectomy.
b. Acute mastoiditis with subperiosteal abscess.
   1. Immediate antibiotic.
   2. Immediate simple mastoidectomy.
   3. Pus to laboratory for culture and sensitivity test.
c. Mastoid reservoir with overflow (subacute mastoiditis).
   1. Simple mastoidectomy.

Prognosis

Prognosis both regarding life and hearing is good.

Chronic Mastoiditis

Aetiology

The precursor of chronic mastoiditis is conversion of the lining membrane of the middle ear or antrum into chronic granulation tissue.

Chronic mastoiditis is developed in the unsafe type of active chronic suppurative otitis media. The patients are usually poor and with low standards of hygiene.

Persistent granulation tissue gradually causes destruction of bony wall by hyperemic decalcification. Pus will be scanty and purulent. Chronic mastoiditis also develops in chronic otitis media with cholesteatoma because of its erosive nature.

Clinical Features

1. Persistent otorrhoea. The discharge is creamy, purulent, foul smelling and scanty. These occur in a patient with marginal or attic perforations.
2. Severe conductive deafness due to destruction of ossicular chain.
3. Granuloma formation.

Treatment

Operation is the only choice of treatment. Radical or modified radical mastoidectomy will be required to cure these types of patients.

Conservative treatment in such cases is bound to fail. Cholesteatoma must be thoroughly removed. Following excision of diseased tissue, one should try to restore the function by plastic reconstruction of the conducting apparatus (tympanoplasty).

Radical Mastoidectomy

Radical mastoidectomy is performed to expose and remove the bone invading disease of the mastoid and middle ear, and to create a perfectly accessible and exteriorized cavity.

The radical mastoidectomy of the nineteenth century is rarely justified today. In the early years of twentieth century, modified radical mastoidectomy sought to exteriorise disease by performing an open procedure on the mastoid portion of the ear, but leaving behind the ossicles and tympanic membrane or their remnants if they were not involved with disease.

Today the term modified radical is used to describe a further modification of the open cavity procedure. The possibility to graft the tympanic membrane and reconstruction of the ossicular chain has broadened the scope of this type of surgery and today's procedure should better be described as "an open mastoidectomy with tympanoplasty" with adequate and wide meatoplasty.

There are two approaches to the procedure:

i. From within outwards or starting from the mastoid antrum (outside-in)

ii. Working forwards towards the attic and middle ear, i.e. the outside-in approach.

The inside-out procedure has the advantage of limiting the operation straightly to the diseased tissues and sparing healthy tissues.

The outside-in approach ensures total disease removal with a wider approach and a gentler exposure of the important middle ear structures.

Indications

1. Secondary acquired cholesteatoma.
2. Chronic otorrhoea due to osteitis or osteomyelitis without cholesteatoma formation.
3. For labyrinthectomy.
4. For certain cases of petrositis.
5. For removal of glomus jugulare tumour of the middle ear.
6. For carcinoma of the ear.
7. For facial nerve decompression and repair.
8. For many tympanoplasty operations.

Anaesthesia

The common practice to perform this operation is under general anaesthesia. In adults who are not apprehensive may perform the surgery under local anaesthesia.

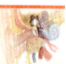

Steps of Operation

Incision: Usual postaural incision (see cortical mastoidectomy) may also be performed through end-aural incision. In sclerotic mastoid this is preferable as it gives better exposure of the middle ear cavity.

Elevation of periosteum and exposure of surgical field: The periosteum is elevated with the help of periosteal elevator. The self-retaining retractor is then applied. The cortex of the mastoid including the spine of Henle and suprameatal triangle is exposed.

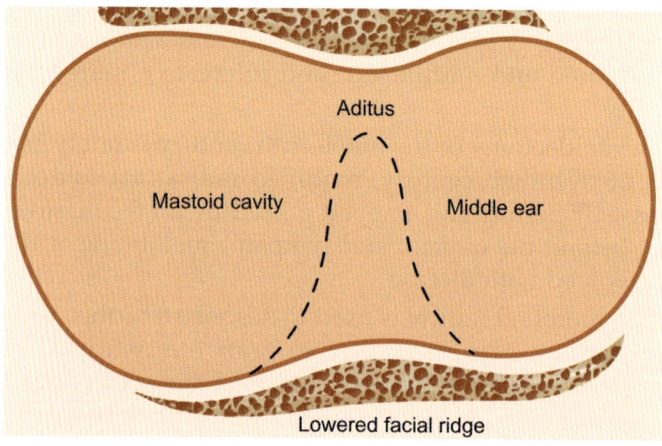

Fig. 6.7: Schematic diagram of radical mastoid cavity

Exploring the mastoid antrum and identifying the tegmen plate and lateral semicircular canal: The mastoid cortex is removed over the region of mastoid antrum with the help of electric burr to remove the bone. The tegmen anti and lateral semicircular canal are identified. The aditus ad antrum is explored with a blunt probe or by the cell seeker or by the Stacke's guide.

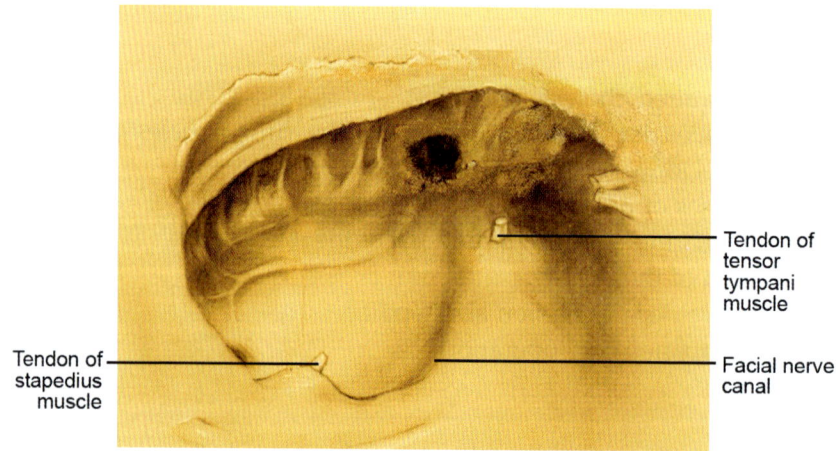

Fig. 6.8: The tympanomastoid cavity after completion of canal wall down mastoidectomy

Enlarging the aditus ad antrum and removal of middle ear pathology: The posterior meatal wall is gradually lowered until a thin bone remains over the aditus. This thin bone is called bridge of bone. The bridge is removed exposing the aditus. The short process of incus lies on the floor of it. The facial nerve and lateral semicircular canal are in relation with its medial wall. The cell seeker is placed on the medial wall of the aditus while removing the bridge. This prevents injury to the facial nerve and lateral semicircular canal.

Then the aditus is sufficiently enlarged by removing the anterior and posterior buttresses of the bridge. The posterosuperior meatal skin is utilised to make a lining of the mastoid bowl thus allowing easy entry into the mastoid cavity from the external and the middle ears.

The remnant of the tympanic membrane, the malleus, the incus and all diseased structures of the middle ear have been removed. The stapes is retained.

The mastoid cavity, antrum, the middle ear and the external ear have now become one cavity, which is fully accessible and exteriorized.

Preparation of the Meatoplasty

The skin and periosteum of the posterosuperior meatal wall may be used to cover the lowered meatal wall or facial ridge. The deepest bony ridge of the posterior meatal wall is called facial ridge as the vertical portion of the facial nerve lies just under this bone. The pedicle of this flap of skin is preferably at the floor of the meatus. The upper part is freed by a vertical incision at the tympano squamous suture. Korner's flap and Siebenmann's flap are the different ways of dealing with the posterosuperior meatal skin. A wide concho meatoplasty is created which should be proportionate to the size of the mastoid cavity (Fig. 6.9).

The cavity is packed with medicated ribbon gauze. The incision is closed with interrupted silk sutures and bandaged.

Aftercare

The patient can move about after 24 hours. The suitable antibiotic is given for about 7 to 10 days. The bandage, packing and stitches are removed on the 6th or 7th postoperative day. The packing is replaced at weekly interval till the epithelial covering of the operative cavity is complete. It usually takes 3 weeks to complete the epithelialization. In cases of a wide concho meatoplasty, no pack is required to place after the first dressing.

The patient is advised to come for review and cleaning of the waxy debris from the mastoid cavity as frequently as it is required.

Complication and Sequelae of Radical Mastoidectomy

1. Facial palsy.
2. Suppurative labyrinthitis.

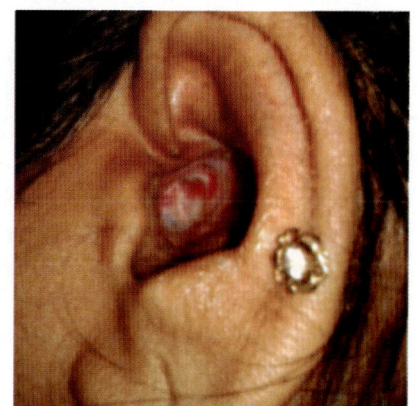

Fig. 6.9: Wide meatoplasty after modified radical mastoidectomy

3. Severe conductive deafness.
4. Unhealed cavity.

Disadvantages of Radical Mastoidectomy

The disadvantages of radical mastoidectomy are as follows: Remember 4 Ds.
1. Deafness—will persist.
2. Discharge—may persist.
3. Dizziness—may sometimes occur.
4. Dependence on doctor.

The mastoid bowl (cavity) after modified radical mastoidectomy requires regular toileting and cleaning. In cases with wide meatoplasty and tympanoplasty, the mastoid cavity heals rapidly and becomes dry by 3 weeks to 3 months in majority of patients.

Tympanoplasty

Plastic reconstruction of the damaged conductive apparatus resulting from chronic suppurative otitis media is called *tympanoplasty*.

To achieve this objective certain basic requirements must be fulfilled. These are:
1. Control of infection.
2. Good cochlear reserve.
3. Patency of the eustachian tube.
4. Mobility of the oval and round window membranes.

The objective of tympanoplasty is the preservation or recreation of the disproportionate conductivity of the two fenestra (oval and round window).

Types of Tympanoplasty

Long time ago Wullstein in 1952 published his article on tympanoplasty and described five types of operation for reconstruction of the middle ear (Fig. 6.10).

- *Type I:* Ossicular chain intact and mobile. Tympanic membrane perforation is central in type. Inspection of the attic and antrum is done through "control holes" before placing the graft. It is identical with myringoplasty. In myringoplasty "control holes" are not made.
- *Type II:* Ossicular chain is mobile and intact except for a small defect of the handle of the malleus that can be bridged by placing the graft to close the perforation against the incus and head of the malleus.
- *Type III:* Stapes is intact and mobile; malleus and incus are not usable. The graft is placed over the head of stapes (myringostapediopexy, columella type).
- *Type IV:* The stapedial crurae are necrosed; the footplate is mobile. A small closed middle ear cavity is constructed by placing the graft, including the eustachian orifice, hypotympanum and round window niche. The stapes footplate is left exposed, covered only by a thin tissue graft (total tympanoplasty).
- *Type V:* The stapedial crurae are damaged and the footplate is fixed. A closed middle ear cavity is constructed as in type IV tympanoplasty and a fenestra is made on the horizontal semicircular canal. The fenestra is covered by the free tissue graft either by fat or fasciae.

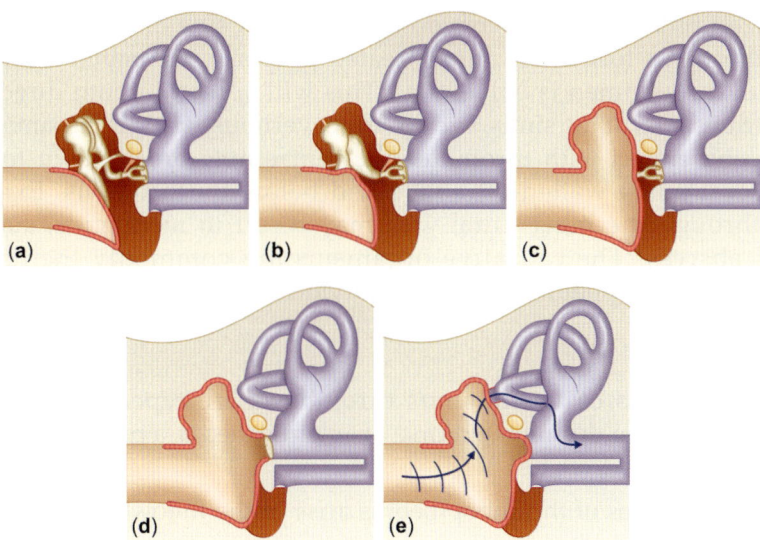

Fig. 6.10: The five types of tympanoplasty (Wullstein). (a) Type I, (b) Type II, (c) Type III, (d) Type IV, (e) Type V

In the absence of reinfection, useful hearing can be restored and maintained by this procedure in the majority of cases.

Types IV and V tympanoplasties are not practiced nowadays. In type IV artificial columella is used and in type V interposition cartilage or synthetic prosthesis is used after removing the footplate as done in stapedectomy operation for otosclerosis. In place of type V the interposition surgery is done in the second stage and not during the primary surgery (Fig. 6.11).

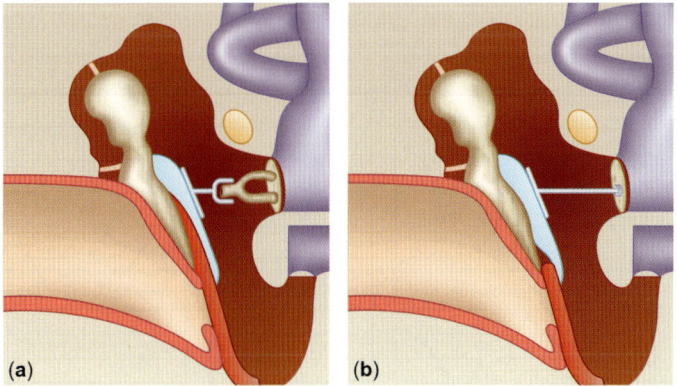

Fig. 6.11: Reconstruction of the middle ear sound conducting mechanism. (a) Partial ossicular reconstruction prosthesis (PORP); (b) Total ossicular reconstruction prosthesis (TORP)

Lateral Sinus Thrombosis

Infection from the middle ear cleft reaches the interior of the sinus in two ways:

1. Direct extension.
2. Retrograde venous thrombosis.

A localized phlebitis is developed on the venous side of the dura. This helps in mural thrombus formation. If not treated properly, thrombus formation will continue until the lumen is obliterated. This will spread in both directions and along the tributaries of the sinus, even to the cavernous sinus. If the sinus becomes filled and obliterated with thrombus, the centre may break down forming an abscess precariously walled-off above and below by thrombus. Extension of infection through the inner dural wall may result in meningitis, subdural or cerebellar abscess. The causative organisms are commonly the haemolytic streptococci, type III pneumococci or staphylococci.

Clinical Features

The clinical features of lateral sinus thrombosis are repeated hectic type of temperature occurring during the course of an otitis media, a positive blood culture and a positive Tobey-Ayer test.

The clinical features of thrombophlebitis arise in the following sequences:

1. Perisinus abscess—results in headache and malaise.
2. Infection of bloodstream—causes fever or rigors. Blood culture will be positive.
3. Occlusion of lumen—causes obstruction of venous return. These results in headache and retinal changes due to raised CSF pressure and a positive Tobey-Ayer test on lumbar puncture.
4. Extending thrombosis—causes thrombosis of the mastoid emissary vein resulting in oedematous swelling on the mastoid bone at the site of emergence of vein **(Griesingers' sign)**. Cavernous sinus thrombosis may occur resulting chemosis, proptosis, orbital swelling, ophthalmoplagia, papilloedema and pain.

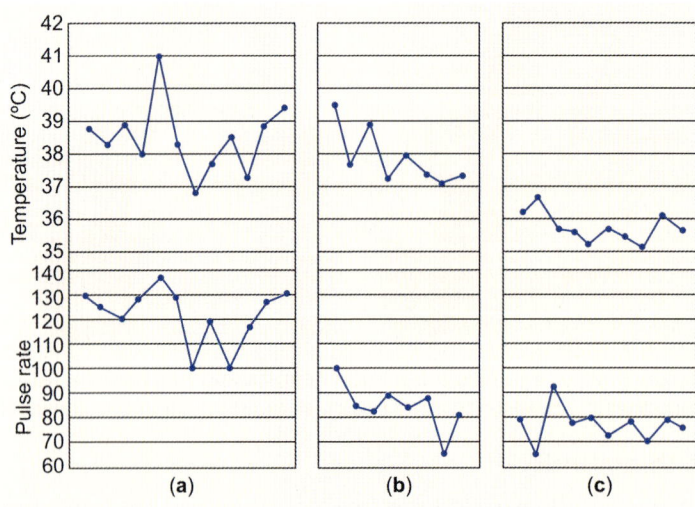

Fig. 6.12: Charts showing characteristic temperature in intracranial complications. (a) Lateral sinus thrombosis; (b) Otogenic meningitis; (c) Brain abscess

Diagnosis

In the presence of mastoiditis the diagnosis of lateral sinus thrombosis is not difficult. However, the following conditions should be considered and excluded:

1. *Meningitis:* Temperature is high and continued. Not hectic in nature. Neck rigidity and Kernig's signs are present and help to differentiate it from other intracranial complications. Lumbar puncture will be confirmative.
2. *Brain abscess:* Temperature is usually subnormal; pulse rate will be low (bradycardia). There may be presence of localizing signs. The patient will be drowsy.
3. *Fever:* Malaria and Typhoid fever may cause confusion if they occur in the presence of acute otitis media. History and blood examination will help to differentiate.

Treatment

Surgical exploration of lateral sinus and removal of the source of infection from the mastoid is a must. The nature of mastoid operation will depend on the type of otitis media. In the acute type with cellular mastoid, cortical mastoidectomy and in the chronic type, a radical mastoidectomy should be performed.

Suitable antibiotics in adequate dosage should be given parenterally.

Intrasinus abscess is required to be drained and infected clots from the sinus should be removed.

If the infection extends to the other sinuses, especially the cavernous sinus, the use of anticoagulants like heparin and phenindion should be considered if laboratory control to the dosage is available. Anticoagulant therapy is usually continued for 3 or 4 weeks or until the patient is fully ambulant.

Contraindications to the use of anticoagulants are as follows:

1. Hypoprothrombinaemia
2. Renal insufficiency
3. Active peptic ulcer
4. Active pulmonary tuberculosis

Ligation of internal jugular vein, once a routine procedure, has become unpopular since the introduction of antibiotics.

Prognosis

Prognosis is excellent if the disease can be diagnosed early and treated adequately.

Otitic Hydrocephalus

Hydrocephalus means enlargement of the ventricular system of the brain. But no enlargement of the ventricle occurs in otitic hydrocephalus, hence it is a misnomer. It is due to thrombosis of the lateral sinus extending into the torcular and superior sagittal sinus secondary to ear infection. The chocked arachnoid villi fail to absorb the cerebrospinal fluid resulting in raised intracranial pressure.

Clinical Features

1. Severe intermittent headache
2. Vomiting

3. Sixth cranial nerve paralysis
4. Papilloedema with blurring of vision.

The space-occupying lesion should be excluded. The only positive finding is markedly raised CSF pressure on lumbar puncture. The cell count and biochemical contents remain unaltered.

Treatment

The high intracranial pressure is reduced by administration of steroids and diuretics. Repeated LP with draining out of CSF helps in reduction of pressure. Subtemporal decompression or ventricular shunts are helpful.

Course: The condition may subside within one month or so. Prolonged treatment may be required sometime.

Labyrinthitis

It is the inflammation of the inner ear. It can occur in three forms as follows:
1. **Paralabyrinthitis** (also known as perilabyrinthitis, circumscribed labyrinthitis, and fistula of the labyrinth).

   In this variety the pathological fistula formation into the labyrinth threatens the spread of infection into the inner ear. It is a localized inflammatory process limited outside the endosteal lining.
2. **Serous labyrinthitis:** It is a diffuse intra-labyrinthine inflammation without pus formation. Only a few round cells are found in the perilymphatic space. In these two types, no organisms are present in the perilymph. This stage is not followed by permanent loss of vestibular and cochlear function. This condition, however, may lead to the next form of labyrinthitis.
3. **Suppurative labyrinthitis** (also known as purulent labyrinthitis). This is a diffuse infection of the peri and endolymphatic spaces in which organisms are present with pus formation. This is always associated with permanent loss of vestibular and cochlear function.

Treatment

In acute labyrinthitis
1. Antibiotics in adequate dosage.
2. Sedatives.

   In chronic infection: In addition to above, mastoid surgery is also necessary.

Labyrinthectomy

Opening the Semicircular Canals

Complete removal of the semicircular canals and all the soft tissues of the vestibule are required to eradicate labyrinthine vertigo. A complete simple mastoidectomy is performed. Posterior canal wall is left intact. The sinodural angle must be completely drilled out to provide adequate exposure of the area of the vestibule. The middle fossa plate must be thinned completely to provide access to the superior semicircular canal. A large cutting burr is used to open the sinodural angle posterior to the labyrinth. By cutting into the labyrinth fenestrate the horizontal semicircular canal. By enlarging this dissection unroof the posterior canal and the anterior portion of the superior canal.

Anterior to the horizontal canal, the external genu and horizontal part of the facial nerve can be skeletonised. Anterior wall of the horizontal canal is preserved for protection of these portions of the facial nerve. The largest burr should be used to enable bone removal with decreased frictional heat and prevent burr clogging. Profuse irrigation is necessary to remove vast quantities of bone dust and also to prevent frictional burning of the nearby bone.

The semicircular canals must be followed as they are the highways into the vestibule. Transection without following will leave "snake eyes" and create confusion about which direction to continue the dissection.

The superior semicircular canal arches in a posteromedial direction underneath the middle fossa plate. This canal is traced posteriorly and medially until it becomes the common crus in its junction with the posterior semicircular canal. The subarcuate artery usually penetrates the hard labyrinthine bone in the centre of the circle of the superior semicircular canal. The posterior canal is then followed inferiorly and anteriorly under the descending portion of the facial nerve. The endolymphatic duct courses from its opening in the medial wall of the vestibule next to common crus. It travels posteriorly in the medial wall of the common crus and then curves inferiorly and laterally as it passes under the posterior canal to enter the endolymphatic sac in the posterior fossa dura. The endolymphatic duct appears as a pearly white thread like discolouration in the hard labyrinthine bone. Follow the common crus into the vestibule and open it widely. The bone over the facial nerve is then thinned well to provide good visual access to the vestibule. Soft tissue is removed from the vestibule and the semicircular canals. Note the spherical recess of the Saccule in the anterior portion of the vestibule and the elliptical recess for the utricle posteriorly. Palpate the stapes footplate from its medial side.

Opening the Internal Auditory Canal

After removal of the bone as described above, the exposed dura of the internal auditory canal is slit along the long axis of the canal at its inferior border.

Within the internal auditory canal, the vestibular nerves are both posterior, whereas the facial nerve is antero superior and the auditory nerve antero inferior. The facial nerve is the principal landmark. The facial nerve is located anterior to the superior vestibular nerve on opening the medial wall of the superior ampulla with a diamond burr; the superior vestibular nerve is exposed as it enters the labyrinth at that point. If the bone has been removed from the superior border of the internal auditory canal for enough anteriorly, the facial canal may be seen descending through its labyrinthine portion from the geniculate ganglion into the internal auditory canal.

Directly inferior to the superior vestibular and facial nerves, a bony prominence (transverse crest) divides the canal into superior and inferior portions. The inferior vestibular nerve is identified lying laterally and the auditory nerve medially. The singular nerve to the posterior semicircular canal is a branch of the inferior vestibular nerve and lies within the internal auditory canal.

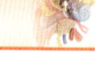
This method of exposure of the internal auditory canal is used for removal of the acoustic neuroma and for translabyrinthine section of the vestibular nerve.

If bone is removed from the fallopian canal starting at the Bill's bar, the facial nerve may be decompressed to the geniculate ganglion and internal genu (first genu) a few millimeters anteriorly.

Otogenic Brain Abscess

Brain abscess can be of cerebral or cerebellar type. The pyogenic organisms are derived from an infection of the middle ear cleft.

The infection from the middle ear may spread in the following ways:
1. Direct extension.
2. Venous thrombophlebitis.
3. Bloodstream infection.
   A brain abscess may progress through four clinical stages. They are as follows:
   i. Initial encephalitis (stage of invasion)
   ii. Latent or quiescent abscess (stage of localization)
   iii. Manifest abscess (stage of enlargement)
   iv. Terminal stage (stage of ruptured abscess).

Cerebral Abscess

Symptoms

Prior to the onset of symptoms of abscess, the discharge from the ear is either diminished or ceased.

The symptoms are to be considered under the following headings:
1. Suppuration and abscess formation. During this stage chills and rigor may occur. Pulse rate rises with temperature, vomiting and headache. After the establishment of the suppuration the condition steps into the latent stage. In this period the patient looks normal. The temperature becomes subnormal with a slow pulse rate. There may be occasional fits or convulsions.
   Careful lumbar puncture will confirm the diagnosis.
   CSF will be clear, protein is raised and lymphocyte count will be increased. If associated with meningitis, sugar and chlorides will be reduced.
2. Symptoms due to raised intracranial pressure: Headache will be severe. There will be occasional projectile vomiting. Ocular signs of raised tension, e.g. papilloedema, blurring of disc margins and dilatation of retinal veins will be present.
3. Focal symptoms and signs.
   a. Aphasia is present in cases of left temporal abscess if the patient is right-handed (Nominal aphasia). The patient cannot name common objects like a key or a coin, although he can describe them and explain their use.
   b. Paralysis—it is contralateral and a common symptom. Paralysis of the sixth cranial nerve with internal squint and diplopia is common in raised intra-cranial tension.
   c. Visual field changes—the abscess may cause homonymous hemianopia if the optic radiation is involved.

Cerebellar Abscess

The symptoms due to raised intracranial pressure mentioned above may occur in this type of abscess as well. Papilloedema occurs early.

Localizing Signs

Homolateral nystagmus of an irregular nature is found. Past pointing is present to the side of the lesion. Ataxia, atonia, asynergia, incoordination, indistinct speech, skew position of the head may be found. There may be homolatetal increase of the deep reflexes.

Special Investigations

1. CT scan will confirm the nature of the lesion and demonstrate its site.
2. Radiography: X-ray of the skull may reveal displacement of calcified pineal gland from the midline.
3. Angiography: By injection of thorotrast into the carotid artery the intracranial arterial tree can be visualized. This will be abnormal in temporal lobe abscess.
4. Ventriculography (air encephalography).
5. Electroencephalography: An abnormal EEG is present in a majority of cases of brain abscess.
6. Brain puncture.

Treatment

Adequate doses of antibiotic and chemotherapy should be administered to get maximum localization and encapsulation of the abscess. Aspiration of pus should then be effected either via a burrhole or through the mastoid. After aspiration of pus antibiotic and thorotrast are injected into the abscess cavity. This helps subsequent radiological checkup of the abscess.

If this fails to cure, the abscess must be excised. When the patient is fully fit, a radical mastoidectomy is indicated in chronic infection.

Facial Nerve

Structure of Nerve

A group of nerve fibres is enclosed in a sheath named perineurium and form a fascicle. The fascicles are bound together by a sheath called epineurium.

Classification of Nerve Injuries

Nerve injuries can be classified in five degrees:
1. *Neuropraxia:* Partial block to flow of axoplasm. It is fully recovered.
2. *Axonotmesis:* Loss of axons but the endoneural tubes remain intact. Recovery is good.
3. *Neurotmesis:* Injury to endoneurium. During recovery, axons can grow into another tube resulting in synkinesis.

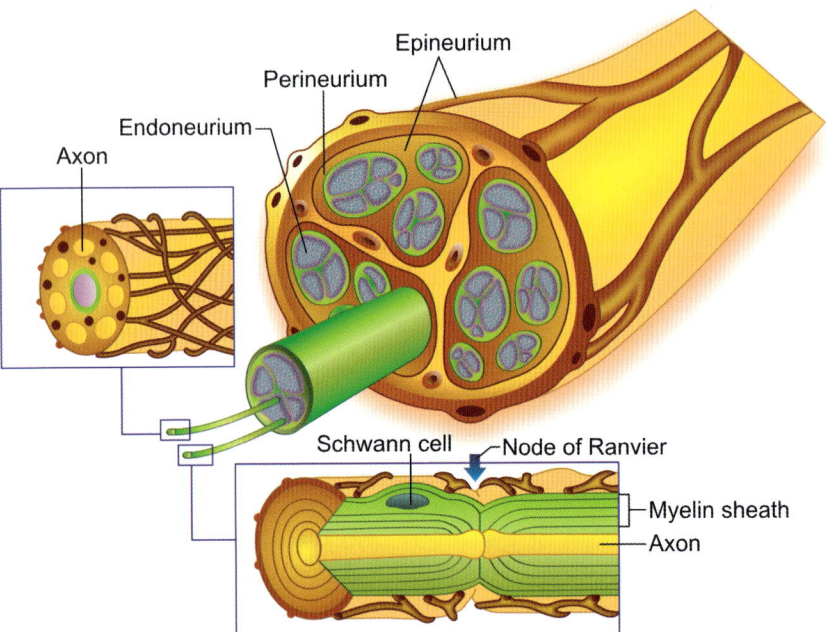

Fig. 6.13: Representation of a nerve fibre

4. Synkinesis means injury to perineurium along with above injury. Regeneration of nerve fibres is impaired due to fibrosis (partial transaction).
5. In addition to above the epineurium is damaged (complete transaction).

Etiology

1. Traumatic—skull fracture, after mastoid surgery.
2. Infective—in CSOM with cholesteatoma by erosion of bony wall to the Fallopian canal, in ASOM due to a congenital dehiscence of bony facial canal wall, tuberculous infection of the middle ear and herpes zoster oticus (Ramsay Hunt syndrome).
3. Neoplastic—glomus jugulare tumour, malignant tumours of the middle ear or parotid gland.
4. Idiopathic—Bells palsy.

Clinical Features

It may be an upper and a lower motor neuron lesion. In upper motor type, the voluntary movement of the lower half of the face is affected. The lower motor type affects both upper and lower parts of the face.

Clinical Grades of Facial Paralysis

House and Brackman from House Ear Institute, Los Angeles, California has classified the grading of facial paralysis as follows:

Grade	Dysfunction	Gross appearance	At rest	Forehead	Eyes	Mouth
I	Normal					
II	Mild	Slight weakness	Looks normal	Moderate to good function	Complete closure	Slight asymmetry
III	Moderate	Difference between two sides of face is obvious (Synkinesis)	Normal looking	Slight to moderate movement	Complete closure with no effort	Slight weakness with maximum effort
IV	Moderately severe	Disfiguring asymmetry of face	Normal symmetry or tone	Slight to moderate movement	Closure complete with effort	Asymmetry with effort
V	Severe	No perceptible movement of face	Asymmetry	No movement	Closure incomplete	Slight movement of mouth
VI	Total paralysis	Total paralysis	No movement of any part of face			

Tests of Facial Nerve Functions

1. *Nerve conductivity test:* This test is valuable after 3 to 4 days of onset of paralysis. In complete degeneration conductivity is lost and the progress of degeneration is indicated by increased threshold on the affected ear.
2. *Strength-duration curve:* In this case, the intensity of stimulation and the duration of stimulus required to elicit facial movement are measured.
3. *Electroneuronography:* The facial nerve is stimulated just outside the stylomastoid foramen by a bipolar electrode and the impulses generated are recovered by another bipolar electrode placed in the nasolabial fold. The test is effective 24 hours after the onset of the palsy. The nerve is stimulated by a square wave of 0.2 milliseconds with a 50 to 150 volt amplitude and a frequency of 1 per second. Summation of the responses is obtained by an averaging computer. A marked difference in the summated potentials in between the two sides indicates severe nerve damage.
4. *Electromyography:* It is useful after 12 to 14 days of the paralysis. It gives useful informations regarding denervation and reinnervation of muscle fibres.

Site of Lesion

The tests used to determine the site of the lesion in facial paralysis are:
1. *Schirmer's test:* It helps to know the function of the greater superficial petrosal nerve. Abnormal lacrimation indicates that the lesion is in or above the geniculate ganglion of the facial nerve.
2. *Stapedial reflex:* The absence of stapedial reflex in the presence of normal hearing suggests a lesion proximal to the origin of the nerve to stapedius muscle. It is done by impedance audiometry.
3. *Taste:* Loss of taste sensation in anterior two-thirds of the tongue suggests a lesion proximal to the origin of the chorda tympani nerve.

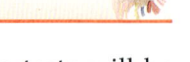

If the lesion is distal to the chorda-tympani nerve, all the above tests will be normal. The nerve conductivity test is abnormal.

These tests are necessary to decide upon the approach to the lesion during surgery. If the lesion is proximal to the geniculate ganglion, the approach is through the middle cranial fossa and if the lesion is distal to the geniculate ganglion it can be dealt with through the mastoid.

Site of Lesion of Facial Nerve in Bell's Palsy

The lesion involves the vertical part of facial nerve in the stylomastoid foramen.

Treatment

1. *In Bell's palsy*

Medical
1. Reassurance about the benign nature of the condition.
2. Physiotherapy.
3. *Eye care:* For prevention of exposure keratitis. Artificial tear is helpful. Use of dark sunglasses over an eye pad on the affected side is essential for outdoor work.
4. Vasodilators in the form of Nootropil 800 mg t.i.d. a for few weeks.
5. *Antiviral:* Acyclovir (Zovirax) 800 mg t.i.d. for 5 days in adults.
6. *Steroid:* To reduce or prevent the risk of degeneration or synkinesis. Steroid in the form of Deflazacort may be used safely even in diabetic patients (corresponding dose with Prednisolone 1 mg/kg of body weight).

Surgical
Nerve decompression after four days of the onset of paralysis. Electro-neuronography is performed and repeated every 3rd day until the 14th day. If degeneration is less than 90%, no surgery is necessary. If within a period of 2 weeks the degeneration is more than 90%, decompression is required.

Melkersson Rosenthal syndrome
Recurrent facial nerve paralysis along with angioedema of lips and face and fissured tongue. This paralysis is like a Bell's palsy clinically. A systemic steroid is the line of treatment.

Ramsay Hunt syndrome (viral)
Treatment: Free use of appropriate analgesics along with antivirals and corticosteroids as described in Bell's palsy.

Bell's phenomenon
Rolling of eyeball upwards and laterally on attempting eye closure in Bell's palsy is called Bell's phenomenon.
The absence of Bell's phenomenon, anaesthesia of cornea and dryness of eye are called BAD syndrome which needs lateral tarsorrhaphy to prevent exposure keratitis and its complications.

2. *In herpes:* Treatment is mainly symptomatic. Steroids and surgery have no value.

3. *In complicating otitis media:* In ASOM in addition to adequate antibiotics myringotomy and cortical mastoidectomy usually result in a return of function. In CSOM-radical mastoidectomy is indicated.

Paralysis due to operative trauma should be dealt with early by re-exploration of the mastoid. If electrical tests suggest no degeneration of the muscles, the facial nerve surgery may be delayed for a month or more.

Surgery for facial nerve paralysis are as follows:
   i. Decompression or apposition of the cut ends of the facial nerve.
   ii. Nerve grafting—autogenous greater auricular nerve or lateral cutaneous nerve of the thigh may be used. Recovery of function, if at all, usually occurs in 6 to 8 weeks. Full recovery may take 6 to 9 months or more.
   iii. In the presence of severe muscle atrophy—plastic surgery may be done in the form of muscle or a fascia lata graft.
   iv. Rerouting of the facial nerve may be done with an end-to-end anastomosis.
4. In tumours—surgical removal of the tumour.

The Facial Nerve: How to Find it?

Twelve different surgical techniques for the safe exposure and identification of the facial nerve throughout its course through the temporal bone were described.

The most common method to identify the facial nerve involves:
1. The direct exposure of the lower-half of the mastoid portion. Under operating microscope, suction irrigation and a large cutting drill bone can be removed directly from the lateral part of the mastoid segment inferior to the posterior semicircular canal and superior to the stylomastoid foramen.

The other methods are:
2. Bone removed along the sigmoid sinus inferiorly to the digastric groove and muscle and then anteriorly until the stylomastoid foramen and facial nerve are exposed. This method is more time consuming.
3. Facial recess approach. The facial nerve is identified in the mastoid as in method (1) and is then followed superiorly to the cochleariform process with a small drill and suction-irrigation.

NEOPLASMS OF THE MIDDLE EAR CLEFT

Classification

a. Benign glomus jugulare tumour
b. Malignant
   1. Squamous cell carcinoma.
   2. Adenocarcinoma.
   3. Sarcoma.
c. Secondary
   From nasopharynx, external auditory meatus and parotid.

Glomus Jugulare Tumour (Non-chromaffin paraganglioma)

It is a benign but locally malignant tumour of a slowly growing nature. It arises from the glomus tissue in the adventitia of the dome of the jugular bulb. This belongs to the chemoreceptor system. This tumour does not metastasize. It commonly occurs in females after the age of 40. Diagnosis can be confirmed by biopsy.

Treatment

1. Radiosurgery is the treatment of choice.
2. Surgery causes severe haemorrhage. The patient should be removed from the tumour mass instead of the tumour being removed from the patient.

Carcinoma

Squamous cell carcinoma is usually common. The ear discharge is bloodstained and facial nerve paralysis occurs early. Deafness of the conductive type with granulations and polypi, which bleeds to touch, are present. Pain appears in the later stage of the disease. Diagnosis is confirmed by biopsy.

Treatment

1. Radical excision of the growth as far as possible. This differs from radical mastoidectomy. In radical mastoidectomy bone-work starts from the diseased to the healthy area. But in case of malignant growth bone-work starts from the healthy to the diseased area.
2. Deep X-ray therapy: Cobalt (Co60) is suitable in this type of growth, which may be given before or after the surgery.

Acoustic Neurinoma

It is also described as 'acoustic neuroma', neurilemmoma, and schwanoma. It is a benign tumour. It arises from the schwann cells enveloping distal portion of the eighth cranial nerve from the point at which the neurological elements cease. This can arise from any point of the eighth cranial nerve between glial-neurolemmal junction and the cribrose area of the internal auditory meatus. A small percentage of these tumours arise medially in the cerebellopontine angle itself rather than the internal auditory canal.

Stages

1. Otological stage—stage I
2. Trigeminal nerve involvement—stage II
3. Brainstem and cerebellar compression—stage III
4. Increasing intracranial pressure—stage IV
5. Terminal stage—stage V

It causes pressure on the cochlear division of the VIIIth cranial nerve, the vestibular nerve, the facial nerve and the branches of the internal auditory artery. When grows bigger, it comes out of the meatus into the cerebellopontine angle.

Clinical Features

Otological
1. Deafness
2. Tinnitus
3. Vertigo.

Neurological
1. Facial pain and numbness
2. Diminution of lacrimal secretion on the affected side
3. Other cranial nerves may be involved if the tumour is large
4. VIth cranial nerve may be paralysed, with diplopia and internal squint
5. Pressure on the cerebellum and brainstem will cause ataxia with a tendency to fall towards the side of the lesion and ipsilateral spontaneous nystagmus. Headache, loss of vision and papilloedema occur late.

The earliest sign is the diminished corneal reflex due to Vth cranial nerve involvement.

Terminal phase: Raised intracranial tension with bulbar palsy result in death. Aspiration pneumonia due to loss of laryngeal reflex may be a cause of early death.

Diagnosis

Diagnosis should be made in the otological phase and in all patients of unilateral nerve deafness. The following investigations should be done in addition to usual clinical examination:
   i. Audiometry:
      1. Pure tone, SISI and TDT
      2. Speech audiometry SRT and SDS.
  ii. Corneal reflex
 iii. VIIth cranial nerve function
  iv. Spontaneous nystagmus
   v. Positional nystagmus
  vi. Caloric test, ENG.
 vii. Digital X-rays-of the internal auditory meati and contrast myelography
viii. Computerized axial tomography scan (CAT-scan) and MRI
  ix. Blood WR and VDRL test.
   x. Lumber puncture—CSF protein is raised in great majority of the patients with even smallest tumour.

Acoustic neurinoma has to be differentiated from basal meningitis, arachnoiditis, posterior fossa meningioma, tuberculoma, fifth cranial nerve neurinoma, cerebellar tumour and aneurysms, which may occur in the cerebellopontine angle.

Treatment

Surgical excision as early as possible, i.e. in otological phase through either of the following approaches:
1. Middle-fossa approach
2. Translabyrinthine approach
3. Combined suboccipital—translabyrinthine approach.

Histiocytosis

It is a rare condition, which involves mostly the head and neck region. Eosinophilic granuloma, Hand-Schuller-Christian disease and Letterer-Siwe disease were initially thought to be distinct clinical conditions. Major difference in the severity and prognosis of the disorders only served to be reinforced the belief that they were separate entities. They are, however, now regarded as different parts of the same disease spectrum. Underlined pathological lesions were similar, and constituted of an inflammatory reticuloendotheliosis. All the three are of histiocyte origin, and termed 'histiocytosis X. The aetiology is unknown. The mildest form of histiocytosis X is eosinophilic granuloma. It occurs in the children and younger adults with a male predominance. It usually appears as a solitary osteolytic lesion. Histopathology demonstrates sheets of benign histiocytes and small eosinophils. There may be areas of haemorrhage and necrosis with giant cells.

Treatment is by local curettage, steroids and radiotherapy and is invariably curative.

Hand-Schuller Christian disease is more severe than eosinophilic granuloma. The onset is typically in children and young adults. This form is fatal although spontaneous regression may occur. Aural suppuration with granulation tissue; fever, lymphadenopathy, hepatosplenomegaly and general malaise are the usual clinical features. Chemotherapy is the treatment of choice.

Letterer-Siwe disease is a rare acute illness of infancy and early childhood. The condition is fatal. It does not produce any otological manifestations.

7

Otosclerosis

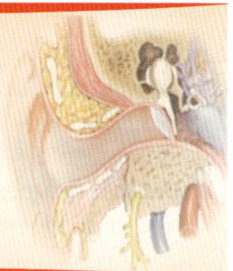

Otosclerosis is a primary progressive focal disease of the labyrinthine capsule. It causes ankylosis of the footplate of the stapes by the formation of new spongy bones (otospongiosis).

It is hereditary localised disease derived from the otic capsule characterized by alternating phases of bone resorption and formation. Mature lamellar bone is replaced by woven bone of greater thickness, cellularity and vascularity. Known sites of predilection are the oval and round windows, in areas where cartilaginous rests are normally found. It gives rise to conductive deafness.

Production of enzymes by the focus may result in sensorineural deafness and vestibular abnormalities.

"Otospongiosis" is considered as active vascular focus and "Otosclerosis" is the final inactive stage of the lesion. Neither of these terms is strictly accurate.

Aetiology

It is only seen in the human species. The exact aetiology of otosclerosis is not clearly understood.

This is found in the younger age group. Incidence in males and females is almost the same. The disease is quite prevalent in our country. In about 50 per cent of cases there is a family history of deafness which goes in favour of hereditary factor. Affected members of the family belong to the same blood group.

The condition aggravates during periods of endocrine activity, such as puberty, pregnancy and menopause but it never acts as an etiological factor.

It is a disorder affecting the growth of collagen.

Metabolic, and immune disorders, vascular disease, infection, trauma, anatomical and histological anomalies of the temporal bone are also considered as the aetiological factors.

A possible relationship is suggested recently between prior infection with the measles virus and later development of clinical otosclerosis. Antigen study, however failed to detect any viral antibodies in otosclerotic stapes.

Incidence

It is seen in 0.5 to 2% of the people.

In recent years it has become quite clear that the number of patients seen in clinics and operated on by stapedectomy has fallen dramatically and this is unlikely to be the result of patients failing to attend for treatment as the results of surgery are good and widely known to be highly successful.

The most likely explanation is that the original pool of patients has been reduced by energetic otologists, keen to operate on those patients who come to them with a conductive deafness caused by otosclerosis.

Greater stringency in the selection of patients suitable for operation is also likely to have been contributory.

If the measles virus is confirmed as an aetiological agent, the effect of vaccination on the incidence of otosclerosis may already be in progress.

Sex Incidence

The incidence is the same in both sexes. Hormonal influences may cause the disease to advance more rapidly in women.

Asymmetric deafness is more common in men and those working in a noisy environment.

Genetic Factors

It is a simple autosomal dominant inheritance with incomplete 'penetrance' or manifestation.

Otosclerosis belonged to a group of hereditary disorders of collagen, with a similar mode of inheritance, incomplete manifestation, varying degrees of expressivity, and possibly an abnormal enzyme system (Fig. 7.1).

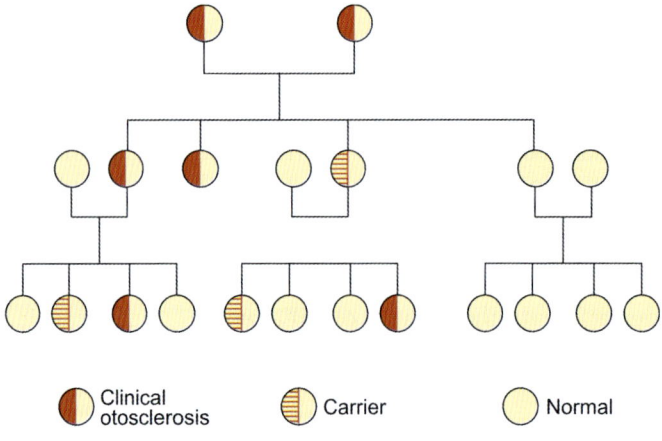

Clinical otosclerosis   Carrier   Normal

Fig. 7.1: A typical family tree

Familial Incidence

Dominant inheritance with manifestation of clinical otosclerosis is half of the expected ratio. "Carriers" may transmit the disease.

Effect of Noise in Otosclerosis

It is unimaginable that a marked conductive deafness does not protect the individual from the damaging effects of a high level of industrial noise, although it is also possible that otosclerosis may make the cochlea of the affected person more sensitive to the damaging effects of noise in the early stages of the disease with minimal hearing loss.

It is common in Caucasians and Aryans. In India it is predominant in people of eastern coastal region. It is uncommon in Mongolians and in African countries.

Pathology

The disease is caused by spongy bone formation replacing the normal bone around the oval window and the promontory. This type of bone formation occurs in the middle layer (endochondral layer) of the bony labyrinth. The commonest site is the fissula antefenestrum which lies just in front of the oval window. It causes fixation of the stapes. The condition may also involve the cochlea.

Clinical Features

1. Deafness—usually slowly progressive and bilateral. It is conductive in type.
2. Tinnitus—is frequently present and sometimes to a severe degree.
3. Paracusis Willisii is usually present—the patient hears better in noisy surroundings.
4. Giddiness is rare and not disabling.
5. Voice is soft.
6. The tympanic membrane is usually normal. In some cases of rapid progress, a "Flamingo pink" tinge may be seen through the membrane, which is called Schwartz's sign. "Honey-combing" appearance of the tympanic membrane is present in about one-third of the cases.
7. Tuning Fork test—Rinne's test is negative, i.e. BC>AC in both ears and Weber's test is not lateralised in majority of the cases (80%).
8. Gelle test is negative.
9. Audiometry
   a. Pure-tone audiogram shows a considerable degree of air-bone gap, bone conduction curve being at the normal level. Air conduction curve shows a slope to the left indicating low frequency loss in early stage.
   b. Speech audiometry—shows above 90% speech discrimination score.
   c. Impedance audiometry—shows normal middle ear pressure with low compliance due to increased acoustic impedance.
   Stapedius reflex is absent.

Radiography

CT scan may show thickening of the stapes footplate and/or evidence of bony cochlear involvement.

Differential Diagnosis

1. Chronic non-suppurative otitis media
2. Healed suppurative otitis media

3. Ossicular disconnection or fixation, congenital, traumatic or inflammatory.
4. Sensorineural deafness in young adults.

Treatment

The treatment can be (a) medical and (b) surgical.

If otosclerosis is associated with eustachian tube dysfunction due to adenoids, sinuses, nasal septum defect or tonsils, the treatment of these should be undertaken first.

Medical

"Hearing aid" in otosclerosis is considered as medical treatment. The function of hearing aid is to amplify the sound waves and thus overcome the resistance of transmission. It improves the hearing. Disease is not cured.

Sodium fluoride reduces osteoclastic bone resorption and increases osteoblastic bone formation. It has an antienzymatic action on proteolytic enzymes, which are cytotoxic to the cochlea and produce SN deafness. With fluoride very few experience improvement of the SN element of deafness, but it has become stabilized in over 80% of patients.

Indications of Sodium Fluoride

1. Otosclerosis with progressive SN deafness.
2. SN deafness with family history, age of onset, audiometric pattern and good auditory discrimination indicate the possibility of chronic otosclerosis.
3. Polytomographic evidence of spongiotic changes in the cochlear capsule.
4. Patients with a positive Schwartze sign.

Contraindication to Fluoride Therapy

1. Chronic nephritis
2. Chronic rheumatoid arthritis
3. Pregnant or lactating mother
4. In children
5. Hypersensitivity
6. Patients with skeletal fluorosis

Surgical

Rapid advances have taken place in recent years. The surgery has three main directions:

1. Mobilisation of stapes (Rosen, 1953)
2. Replacement of stapes by artificial prosthesis (Shea, 1958)
3. Bypassing the stapes (Lempert, 1938)

The general choice of treatment nowadays is stapedectomy by:

- Shea method or its modifications.
- The mobilization of stapes is no longer performed. In this technique the gain in hearing is partial and temporary owing to re-ankylosis of the stapes.

Fenestration (bypass operation) of the lateral semicircular canal has become unpopular for the following reasons:
1. Postoperative mastoid cavity which requires permanent care
2. Severe postoperative vertigo
3. Long convalescent period.

Stapedectomy (Shea technique)

One should have the facilities of operative microscope in performing stapedectomy (Fig. 7.2).

A vein graft from the back of the hand is first prepared.

The middle ear is exposed through endomeatal incision of Rosen.

Incision is taken from 12 o' clock to 6 o' clock position posteriorly maintaining about 6–8 mm distance from the annulus tympanicus. This may be required to be extended up to 1 o' clock position in the right ear and 11 o' clock position in the left ear. The skin of the meatus is elevated from the bone until the attachment of the tympanic membrane is reached. The fibrous annulus is lifted out of its bony sulcus and the middle ear is thus exposed (anterior tympanotomy).

The stapedius tendon is cut followed by dislocation of the incudostapedial joint. The superstructure of stapes, i.e. head, neck and crurae of stapes are removed. A suitable opening is made on the footplate-preferably at its centre or posterior part and prosthesis is applied between the oval window and the lower end of the long process of incus. The length of the prosthesis should be measured appropriately by the help of a gauze so that it does not dip into the vestibule for more than 0.5 mm. Prosthesis can be introduced to a depth of 0.5 mm into the vestibule over the entire surface of the stapedial foot plate without risk.

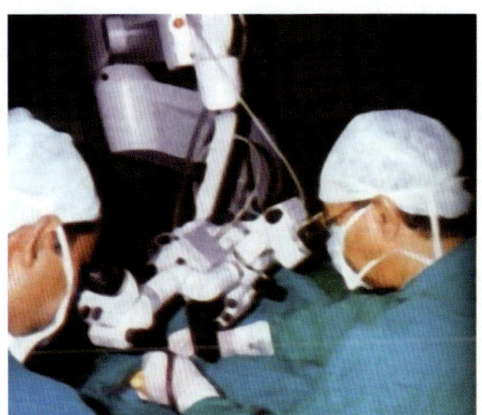

Fig. 7.2: Stapes surgery being performed under operating microscope

The middle ear is then closed by replacing the flap. The external auditory canal is packed by medicated cotton wool. The pack is removed after 5 days.

Problems Found at Operation

1. Facial nerve abnormality
2. Persistent stapedial artery
3. Perilymph flooding
4. Floating and submerged footplate
5. Presence of blood in the vestibule
6. Tympanic membrane tear
7. Obliterative otosclerosis
8. Narrowed oval window niche
9. Damage to the chorda tympani nerve

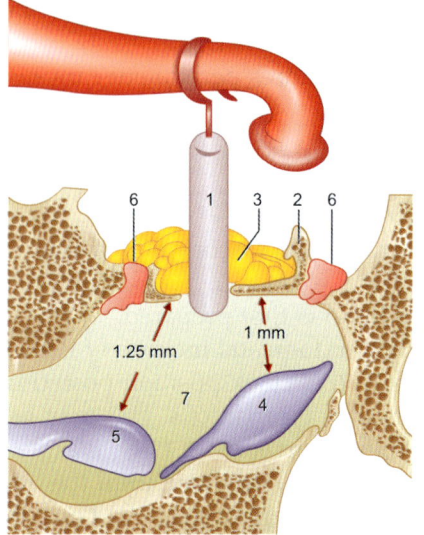

1. Piston
2. Anterior crus
3. Fat or gelfoam
4. Saccule
5. Utricle
6. Otosclerotic focus
7. Scala vestibuli

Fig. 7.3: Depth of perilymphatic space from the undersurface of footplate of stapes to the utricle and saccule, which is 1.25 mm and 1 mm respectively

If the chorda is cut in addition to the loss of taste, there is loss of the secretomotor supply to the submandibular and sublingual salivary gland; producing an uncomfortable dry mouth.

The modifications of this operation are as follows:

1. Platinectomy (Portmann, 1959). In this the posterior crus of stapes is not removed and the incudostapedial joint is not disturbed. The anterior crus and footplate are removed and the posterior crus of stapes is placed on the vein graft over the oval window.
2. Interposition with stainless steel wire. Fatty tissue is placed over the footplate fenestration instead of vein graft (Schuknecht, 1960).
3. Interposition with wire and gelfoam (House, 1960).
   Shea (1963) developed a new technique. In this a Teflon piston of 3 to 5 mm in length and 0.5 to 0.8 mm. in diameter is passed through a hole made on the footplate of the stapes. The other end is made to hook on the long process of the incus. This causes less trauma to the inner ear and is easy to perform. The rate of successful hearing gain is also much high.
4. Stapedotomy—it means small fenestra stapedectomy where less than 25% of footplate is removed.
5. Stapedotomy with preservation of stapedius tendon and incudostapedial joint followed by anterior and posterior crurotomy (neostapedotomy).

Postoperative Care

The patient should not blow the nose hard, should sneeze with the mouth open, should avoid any kind of strenuous work, carrying heavy load and should avoid getting water in the ear—for 3 weeks.

Broad-spectrum antibiotics are given for about a week.

Diligan, avomine or stemetil should be given to control the giddiness.

8

Miscellaneous Diseases of the Inner Ear

MENIERE'S DISEASE

Meniere (1861) drew attention to a syndrome characterized by paroxysmal attacks of vertigo, deafness, tinnitus and vomiting. The seat of the disease is the inner ear. Meniere's disease is nothing but recurrent attacks of endolymphatic hydrops. This may lead to permanent distension of the cochlear duct and sometimes of saccule and utricle.

Meniere's disease is characterized by a fluctuating sensorineural hearing loss, with the hearing deterioration during each attack and partly recovering between attacks. In a variant of Meniere's disease—**Lermoyez's syndrome** the hearing drops before an attack, recovering as the vertigo begins.

Movement tends to make vertigo of peripheral origin worse. The best known example of this is the sudden onset of rotatory dizziness associated with certain head movements in patients with benign paroxysmal positional vertigo. Vertigo associated with coughing and sneezing suggests a presence of a perilymph fistula. Tullio's phenomenon is the vertigo caused by loud sounds and may be due to endolymphatic hydrops, a third labyrinthine window, as in a labyrinthine fistula.

Central lesions tend to produce less intense vertigo. Positional changes have less effect but the patient tends to have more disturbance of gait.

Aetiology

1. Genetic
2. Anatomical
3. Traumatic
4. Viral infection
5. Allergy to either food or inhalants
6. Psychosomatic and personality features
7. Autoimmunity

Aetiology of secondary endolymphatic hydrops

1. Developmental insult
2. Abnormal metabolic and endocrine states
3. Syphilis
4. Chronic otitis media
5. Viral infection

6. Autoimmunity
7. Otosclerosis
8. Abnormal fluid balance
9. Leukaemia.

The most acceptable theory is psychosomatic disturbance. In the majority of cases no aetiological factor can be found and only one ear is usually affected. It is common in males than in females between 35 and 55 years of age and prevalent in countries of high socioeconomic status.

Pathology

Endolymphatic hydrops in the inner ear is the most significant change. The histological change is gross dilatation of scala media and saccule. Sulcus endo-lymphaticus is not dilated. It shows fibrosis. Reissner's membrane bulges into the scala vestibuli and may eventually rupture.

Clinical Features

1. Vertigo is sudden and severe.
2. Deafness is perceptive in type.
3. Tinnitus—a constant hissing noise.
4. Vomiting and nausea.
5. Nystagmus spontaneous and to the healthy side.

Investigation

1. Otoscopy—reveals normal tympanic membrane.
2. Tuning fork test:
   - Rinne test—positive.
   - ABC—reduced in the affected ear.
   - Weber's test—lateralised to the healthy ear.
3. Ocular sign—nystagmus-quick component is directed towards the healthy ear.
4. Pure tone audiometry—reveals perceptive deafness.
5. Recruitment is usually present.
6. Caloric test—the response is reduced on the affected side. Differential diagnosis:
   a. Eustachian tube blockage.
   b. Cerebral anaemia.
   c. Central vestibular lesion, e.g. disseminated sclerosis or a tumour of the brain-stem or cerebellum.
   d. Serous or suppurative labyrinthitis.
   e. Postural vertigo.
   f. Cerebellopontine angle tumour, e.g. acoustic neurinoma.
   g. Sudden labyrinthine deafness.
   h. Cogan's disease, a rare collagen disorder affecting the eyes as well as the labyrinth.
   i. Vestibular neuronitis.

Treatment

The septic foci should get attention and the patient is reassured regarding the benign nature of the disease. Smoking is prohibited. Any psychological illness is investigated and treated.

Medical

1. Electrolyte and water balance.

   Fluid and salt restricted diet. Diuretics can be helpful.

2. Sedatives—many cases can be controlled by anti-histamine. Relaxation and freedom from stress are essential. In an acute attack promethazine theoclate, cinnarizine, dimenhydrinate, perphenazine, proclorperazine, or promethazine hydrochloride may be given. Phenergan 25 mg twice a day gives very good result.

   During quiescent period phenobarbitone and diazepam are helpful.

3. Strial permeability

   a. Histamine sensitive group is treated by desensitization.

   b. Histamine insensitive group is treated by nicotinic acid and vasodilator drugs.

   Nicotinic acid in doses of 50–250 mg three times a day. Betahistine (8 mg), cyclospasmol (100 mg) three times a day is a good average.

Surgical

If medical treatment fails

1. Conservative surgical treatment

   a. Control of endolymph formation—stellate ganglion block or cervical sympathectomy.

   b. Control of endolymph absorption–decompression of the labyrinth by opening the sulcus endolymphaticus, Ficks operation and endolymphatic shunt operation.

   Endolymphatic Sac Ballooning Surgery (ESBS): A 0.005-inch thick ribbon of silastic sheet is inserted into the sac lumen and then fanfolded within the lumen to dilate the sac. The ribbon tail is left outside the sac. Intraductal capillary tube implantation (ICTI) and ESBS produce the best clinical results.

   c. Control of sensory nerve impulses—by electrocoagulation of the lateral semicircular canal or destruction of the vestibular endorgans by ultrasonic beam of Aslant and cryosurgery.

   d. Grommet insertion (Tumarkins, 1966).

   e. Microvascular decompression (Janetta, 1986)

2. Radical surgical treatment

   a. Intratympanic Inj. of streptomycin (Schuknecht, 1957), gentamycin (Beck, 1978).

   b. Membranous labyrinthectomy—mainly indicated in unilateral severe Menniere's disease with deafness.

   c. Division of vestibular nerve by way of middle fossa approach, by a retrolabyrinthine approach, or by a posterior fossa approach.

BENIGN PAROXYSMAL POSITIONAL VERTIGO

Benign paroxysmal positional vertigo (BPPV) is defined as recurring paroxysmal attacks of vertigo in certain critical positions of the head in space.

Aetiology

1. After minor head injury.
2. Associated with surgery to remove a parietal lobe tumour.
3. Associated with viral labyrinthitis, Meniere's disease, vertebrobasilar insufficiency.
4. Idiopathic.

Pathology

Defect in posterior semicircular canal, cupulolithiasis, degeneration of the utriculo-otolithic membrane (traumatic), ischaemia, infection

- Release of otoconia
- Deposition over cupula of PSC
- Altering specific gravity of cupula
- Converting to a gravity receptor
- Provoke rotatory nystagmus on rapid changes of head position.

Canalolithiasis: Otoconial debris forms a floating clot in PSC. Air bubbles in the endolymph.

Causes of Short-lived Episodic Vertigo

1. Benign paroxysmal positional vertigo
2. Labyrinthine fistula
3. Caloric effect
4. Alternobaric vertigo
5. Post-concussional syndromes
6. Vertebrobasilar insufficiency
7. Cervical vertigo
8. Coriolis phenomenon

BPPV and other CNS lesions		
	BPPV	*CNS lesions*
Latent period	A few seconds	Nil
Distress	Present—may be severe	Nil
Direction of nystagmus	Usually rotatory Anticlockwise—right ear down Clockwise—left ear down	Variable
Duration of nystagmus	Less than 30 secs	Persists while position maintained
On sitting up again	Similar events with nystagmus in opposite direction	Nystagmus stops
Fatigability	Nystagmus and dizziness stop on repeated testing	Nystagmus persists on repeated testing

Investigations

1. Audiometry—PTA otoadmittance testing, acoustic reflex thresholds (auditory brainstem responses, click-evoked otoacoustic emissions, speech audiometry if indicated).
2. Vestibular tests—bithermal caloric tests, ENG; rotational tests (sono ocular test, galvanic test, posturography if indicated).
3. Imaging—gadolinium enhanced MRI scan.
4. Blood—Hb/TC/DLC/ESR, serology including FTA-HbsAg/Abs, TSH–other specific tests as clinically indicated.

Positional Test

Patient sitting—test explained to the patient.

- Instructed to keep eyes open—to look at the centre of the observer's forehead
- Patient's head held gently with both hands
- Turned slowly to one side—45° from sagittal plane as he/she is slowly laid down
- Wait for a latent period of 20 secs
- Rotatory nystagmus seen in the cases and held just 30° below the horizontal plane—directed towards undermost ear
- Lasts for several seconds—gradually fades—associated with vertigo of the same quality as experienced
- Nystagmus fatigues on repetition of test. Nystagmus in reverse direction may occur on sitting.

Treatment

Basic principles:

1. Treat or eliminate the cause.
2. Suppress the vestibular system.

Labyrinthine sedatives: Cinnarazine, cyclizine, dimenhydrinate and prochlorperazine. Diazepam is a potent labyrinthine sedative as well as anxiolytic.

Notes of Caution

1. These drugs may not only delay central compensation but can make it incomplete; therefore, they should be used for only a few days (no longer than a week when there is a destructive lesion).
2. In the elderly these drugs will simply increase the unsteadiness.
3. Suppress the patient's emotional reaction. These patients need strong reassurance both about the nature of their dizziness and prognosis.
4. Wait for compensation
5. Eliminate the offending labyrinth
6. Acceptance of the problem

Surgery for Vertigo

Being a self-limiting disease and is only rarely sufficiently severe, surgery is required rarely.

1. Section of the posterior ampullary nerve (singular nerve)
   Risks
     i. SN hearing loss in 10% of patients
     ii. Opening into the labyrinth–persistent unsteadiness
     iii. CSF leak from the singular canal.
2. Occlusion of the posterior semicircular canal (Parnes and McClure, 1990)—probably the best procedure with reduced risk to hearing and the facial nerve.
   Prognosis: Spontaneous cure may be delayed for several months. Recurrences are common.

PRESBYACUSIS

'Senile' deafness after 55 years of age is called presbyacusis. It is always bilateral and symmetrical with equal sex ratio. Individual susceptibility and hereditary predisposition play important role as the causal factors besides age. Vascular insufficiency due to sclerosis or thrombosis results in degeneration of the epithelial tissue in the basal turn of cochlea, neural tissue in the spiral ganglion cells, stria vascularis and loss of elasticity of the basilar membrane. These changes cause sensori-neural deafness with high tone loss, recruitment and loss of speech discrimination.

Treatment

Does not help much. Modern hearing aids with automatic volume control (AVC) or pick clipping arrangements may be useful. One should talk with these persons in a clear, relatively slow and soft voice. Lip reading and auditory training may be helpful. Programmable digital type of hearing aids have been recently proved to be very satisfactory in improvement of hearing in these type of deafness.

OTOTOXICITY

Drug induced damage of the cochlea and/or vestibule of the inner ear is called ototoxicity.

The offending drugs produce degeneration of the stria vascularis, sensory epithelia of the organ of Corti and vestibule, and spiral ganglion cells. Outer hair cells are affected more than inner hair cells and the degenerative changes diminish from base to apex of cochlea. The ganglion cells are degenerated secondary to degeneration of the sensory epithelia. Ototoxic drugs are:

1. Aminoglycoside antibiotics, e.g. streptomycin and gentamycin (mainly vestibulotoxic); neomycin, kanamycin, vancomycin, framycetin and tobramycin (mainly cochleotoxic)
2. Diuretics, e.g. ethacrynic acid, frusemide (Lasix)
3. Antiprotozoal agents, e.g. quinine, chloroquine
4. Salicylates
5. Cisplatin
6. Phenytoin may cause disequilibrium.

Aminoglycoside antibiotics are responsible for the damage of sensory epithelia of the cochlea and vestibule. Degeneration of the stria vascularis occurs by all the ototoxic drugs.

No treatment is useful in these cases. Preventive treatment in the form of avoidance or discontinuation of ototoxic drugs, monitoring hearing with regular audiometric check up and monitoring treatment with regular estimation of drugs and/or creatinine in serum are essential. It is generally considered that topical aminoglycoside antibiotics, as used in eardrops in discharging ears, do not cause hearing loss. However, in CSOM with large or subtotal perforations ototoxic drugs do cause sensory neural deafness if used as ear drops.

COCHLEAR IMPLANTS

Cochlear implant is made of electrodes, which are implanted into the scala tympani of the cochlea. The electrodes stimulate the spiral ganglion cells and axons in the modiolus of the cochlea. Cochlear implants are one of the very useful developments for use in persons who are severe to profoundly deaf bilaterally and who are not benefited with the best possible hearing aids available. It is useful both in prelingual and postlingual bilateral deafness. Prelinguals are those who are either born deaf or developed deafness before learning speech and language. Postlingual patients are those who had normal hearing and speech and language development but due to any reason they have lost their hearing bilaterally.

Cochlear implants used nowadays are with multichannel electrodes with 22 to 24 electrodes. This type helps in excellent improvement in hearing and also excellent development of speech and languages. Regular rehabilitation procedures by a team of well-versed audiologists and speech and language pathologists are needed. The prelingual cases if implanted before the age of six years get maximum benefits. They become, though late, just like one of the normally developed children who had normal hearing and speech and language.

In the beginning the ENT surgeons used to use single channel implants (in sixties) which was obviously of a very limited benefit, in the sense that those patients used to hear the sounds only but speech and language development was very poor.

CROS HEARING AIDS

Contralateral routing of signals (CROS) aid is a type of hearing aid where the microphone is placed near the deaf ear. The microphone picks up the signals from the deaf ear side and routes them to an ear phone mounted behind the normal hearing ear. Therefore, the patient gets the sound from the deaf ear side and never feels any difficulty to appreciate the sound coming from that side.

BONE ANCHORED HEARING AID (BAHA)

It is an implantable hearing aid. It is a temporal bone stimulator. Cochlear stimulation by this aid is similar to that of a conventional bone conducting hearing aid. It is indicated in patients of CSOM with a conductive or mild sensorineural deafness and in patients with bilateral ear canal atresia in whom reconstruction is contraindicated.

Patient whose SDS (speech discrimination scores) are above 60% and bone conduction loss is less than 40 dB are better candidates for BAHA implantation.

Rhinology

(Nose and Paranasal Sinuses)

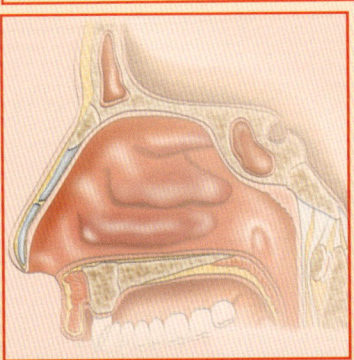

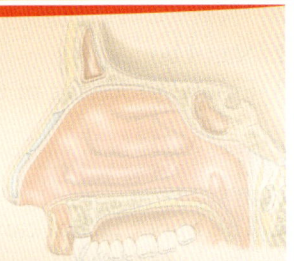

9

Anatomy of the Nose

Development

Primitive nasal cavity and anterior nares are developed from the dorsal extension of the lateral and medial nasal processes. These processes are formed around olfactory pits by division of the frontonasal process. Primitive nasal septum is formed from the frontonasal process and Rathke's pouch. The lateral process by the union of the maxillary process forms the palatine process. From the deep part of the frontonasal process primitive palate is developed. The palate fuses with maxillary palatine processes of both sides from before backward.

Due to defective union of different processes the cleft palate, harelip, unilateral or bilateral choanal atresia, deviated nasal septum, bifid nose, probosis, bifid uvula, submucous cleft palate, etc. may develop (Fig. 9.1).

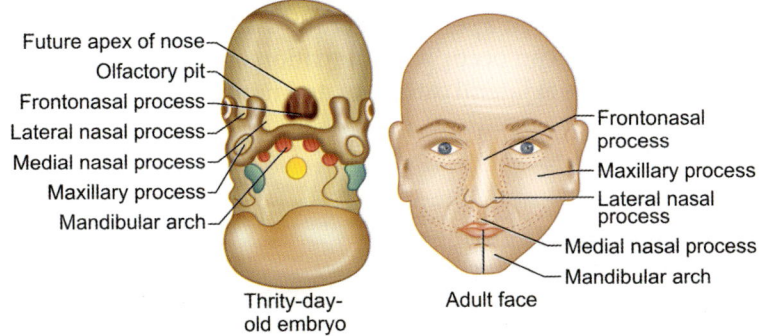

Fig. 9.1: Development of nose showing 30-day-old embryo and adult face

The external nose is pyramidal in shape composed of bone, cartilage and soft tissue. The base of the pyramid is perforated by two orifices, called anterior nares or nostrils. They are separated by a median partition called columella. The root of the nose is the junction of it with the forehead. The tip of the nose is called the apex. The dorsum of the nose is the anterior border joining the root and the apex. The upper bony part of the dorsum is called the bridge of the nose. The rounded eminences at the lower end of the sides are named ala nasi. The free edge of the ala forms the lateral boundary of each nostril.

Bony Parts

1. Nasal process of the frontal bones.

2. Nasal bones.
3. Frontal processes of the maxillae.

Cartilaginous Parts

Paired

1. The upper lateral cartilages.
2. The lower lateral cartilages.
3. Lesser alar cartilages.

Unpaired

Cartilage of the septum, is quadrangular in shape. This is attached to nasal bones and maxillae by firbrous tissue. The cartilage of the septum is interposed between the lateral cartilages.

The lower lateral cartilages lie surrounding the nostrils. They maintain the patency of nostrils. Each cartilage has a medial and a lateral part. The two medial parts together form the lowest part of the nasal septum. The lateral parts are attached to the upper lateral cartilages and to the maxillae by fibrous tissue. In this fibrous tissue the lesser alar cartilages are buried. The lower part of the ala has no cartilage and it is composed of subcutaneous fibrofatty tissue (Fig. 9.2).

Nasal Valve

Nasal valve complex is the narrowest part in the nasal cavity and is an angle between the upper lateral cartilage and nasal septum above, the anterior end of the inferior turbinate behind, the pyriform aperture laterally and the floor of the nose below. Obstruction of nasal valve can occur with deviation of the anterior septal cartilage, distortion of upper and lower lateral cartilages and hypertrophied inferior turbinates.

Muscles of the Nose

They are:

1. Dilators and compressors of the nostrils.
2. Depressors and elevators of the alae nasi.

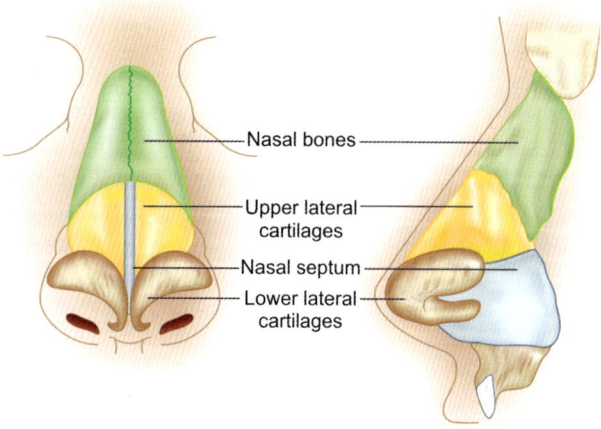

Nasal bones

Upper lateral cartilages

Nasal septum

Lower lateral cartilages

Fig. 9.2: Skeleton of external nose

The dilators and elevators tend to disuse atrophy in mouth breathers resulting in pinched-up nose of adenoid facies.

Blood supply of the external nose is from the facial and ophthalmic arteries.

Veins drain in the anterior facial and ophthalmic veins. Ophthalmic vein is one of the tributaries of the cavernous sinus.

Lymphatics drain into the submandibular and preauricular lymph glands.

The nasal cavities lie below the cranial cavity, above the oral cavity, and in between the orbits. The nasal cavity is divided into two parts by nasal septum. Each nasal cavity communicates with the nasopharynx posteriorly through the posterior nares or choana and with the paranasal sinuses. In adult the anteroposterior length is 7.5 cm and height is 5 cm. Each nasal cavity is bounded by:

1. Lateral wall.
2. Medial wall.
3. Roof.
4. Floor.

Lateral wall is mainly formed by medial wall of maxilla and the lateral mass of ethmoid and lacrimal bone. Other smaller parts are:

1. Ascending process of maxilla.
2. Perpendicular plate of palatine bone.
3. Medial pterygoid process of sphenoid bone.

Three ridges known as the conchae or turbinates spring from the lateral wall. The space in between the turbinates is known as the meatus. The turbinates are named inferior, middle and superior. The inferior one is a separate bone but the middle and the superior turbinates are parts of the ethmoid bone.

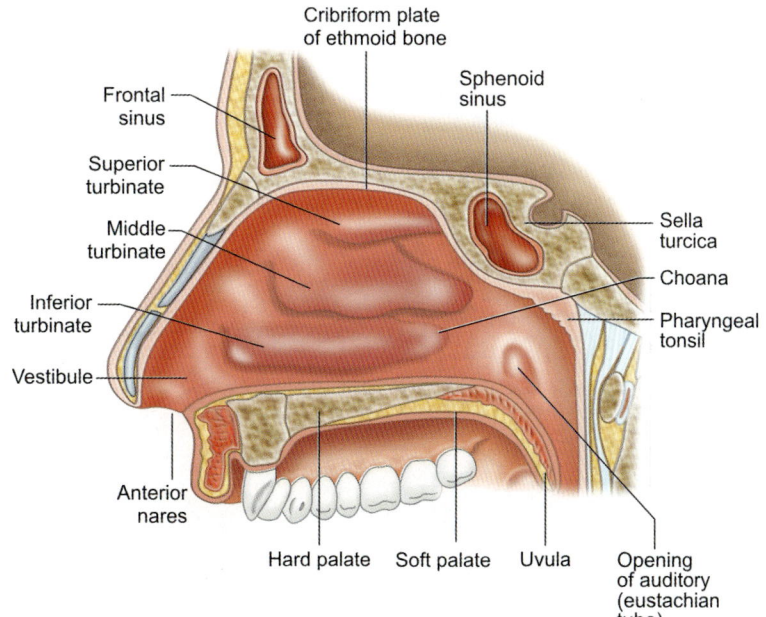

Fig. 9.3: The nasal cavity showing different parts

Each meatus lies below and lateral to the corresponding turbinate. The space above the superior turbinate is named sphenoethmoidal recess and receives the ostium of the sphenoidal sinus.

Superior meatus receives the posterior ethmoidal cells.

The most complex and important of the meati is the middle one. The anterior group of paranasal sinuses, e.g. maxillary, frontal and anterior ethmoidal drain in the middle meatus. The middle meatus is continuous with a depressed area immediately above the nasal vestibule. This area is called atrium nasi. There is a curved ridge above the atrium named agger nasi. This may contain some small cells (agger cells). Anterior ethmoidal cells form a bulge, called "Bulla ethmoidalis". These cells sometimes open on the surface of the bulla. Anteroinferior to the bulla lies the uncinate process of the ethmoid bone. Between these two structures is hiatus semilunaris (semilunar gap which leads forwards into the infundibulum). Maxillary sinus communicates with the most inferior part of the infundibulum.

The inferior meatus receives at its anterior end close to the attachment of the inferior turbinate, the opening of the nasolacrimal duct.

The medial wall is formed by the nasal septum. The septum is partly bony and partly cartilaginous. The main constituents of the septum are three. They are:

1. Perpendicular plate of ethmoid, above and behind.

2. Vomer, below and behind.

3. Quadrilateral cartilage-in between 1 and 2.

Other minor constituents of the septum are:

   i. Anterior nasal spine of maxilla.

  ii. Nasal crest of maxillary and palatine bones.

 iii. Rostrum of sphenoid bone.

 iv. Nasal spine of frontal bone.

  v. Crest of nasal bones.

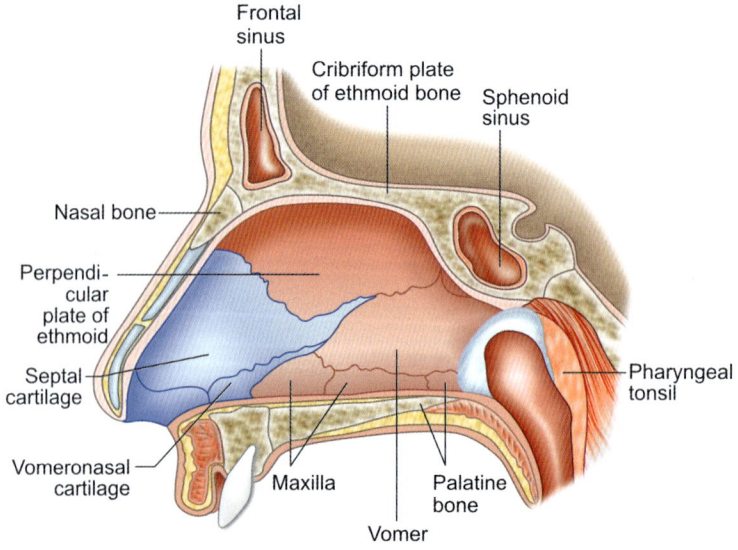

Fig. 9.4: Medial wall of nasal cavity

vi. Medial crus of lower lateral cartilages.

vii. Vomeronasal cartilages.

The vomeronasal cartilages lie on either side of the posteroinferior edge of the septal cartilage as narrow bands. They remain attached to the vomer.

The septum is covered with perichondrium and periosteum according to the situation of cartilage and bone respectively. The septal branch of the sphenopalatine artery (the artery of epistaxis) courses along the surface of the vomer. This artery anastomoses at the anteroinferior part of the septum with the following arteries:

1. Greater palatine artery.

2. Septal branch of the superior labial artery.

3. Septal branch of the anterior ethmoidal artery.

This anastomosis forms the Kiesselbach's plexus, 'bleeding area' or Little's area of the nose (Fig. 9.5). It is situated about 6 to 8 mm within the vestibule and 6 mm above the floor of the nose. Owing to increased vascularity, the slightest trauma causes bleeding from this site.

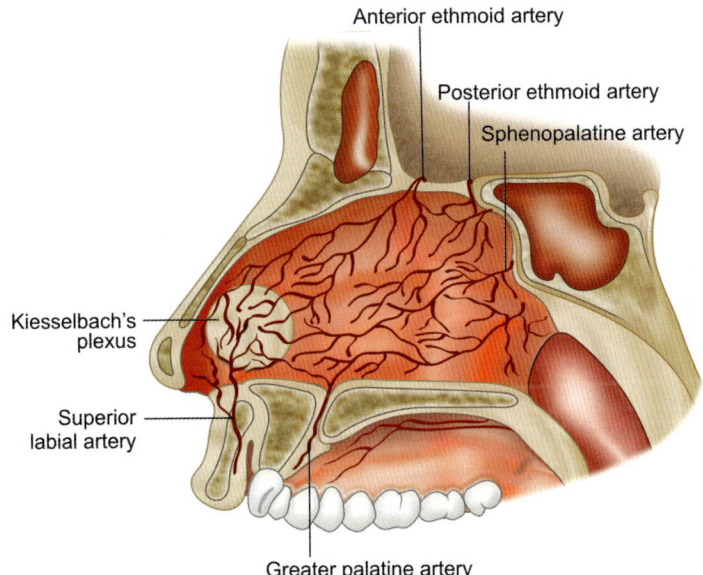

Fig. 9.5: The nasal septum showing "Little's area" (Kiesselbach's plexus) and its anastomosing blood vessels

The roof of the nasal cavity is formed by the nasal process of frontal bone anteriorly, cribriform plate of the ethmoid bone at the middle, and body of the sphenoid bone posteriorly.

DANGEROUS AREA OF NOSE

This is the upper one-third of the nasal cavity bounded above by the cribriform plate of the ethmoid bone, laterally by the lateral wall of the nose up to the superior concha and medially by the corresponding part of the nasal septum. The other name of this region is the **olfactory area** of the nasal cavity and a potential danger zone.

The olfactory filaments (about twenty in number) from olfactory bulb enter the nasal cavity through the foramina of cribriform plate. They get pia and arachnoid sheaths (perineural sheaths) having a subarachnoid space, which is continuous with the same of the cranial cavity. This communication is responsible for spreading infection from a septic focus within the nose to the intracranial leptomeninges following injury to the olfactory filaments. This fact should be kept in mind during intranasal operations.

DANGEROUS AREA OF THE FACE

Confusion may be there with the dangerous area of nose. Dangerous area of the face is a triangular area formed by the upper lip and the vestibule of the nose. Infection from this area may spread to the cavernous sinus resulting fatal cavernous sinus thrombosis through its tributaries like the anterior facial vein and angular veins.

The floor of the nasal cavity is formed by:
1. The palatine process of maxilla, major portion (anterior 3/4) of hard palate.
2. The horizontal part of the palatine bone.

MUCOUS MEMBRANE

The mucous membrane is of two types:
1. *Respiratory:* Pseudostratified ciliated columnar epithelium, pinkish in colour, lines the lower two-thirds of the nasal septum, the lateral wall of the nose below the superior turbinate and the floor of the nasal fossa. This epithelium consists of tall ciliated cells with some mucus secreting goblet cells in between. Irregular basal cells lie on the basement membrane and fill up the gaps between the ciliated cells. The cilia move from before backwards, towards the choanae. This epithelium is separated from the subepithelial tissue by a fibro elastic membrane. Subepithelial tissue is loose and highly vascular. It contains many mucous and serous glands. A localized thickening of the respiratory mucous membrane of the septum opposite the anterior end of the middle turbinate is specially named tubercle of the septum.
2. *Olfactory:* A specific sensory epithelium containing a network of nerve endings of bipolar olfactory cells, supporting and basal cells. It lines the upper one-third of the nasal septum, the roof of the nose and the upper part of the lateral wall including superior turbinate. This epithelium is of non-ciliated columnar cells and is yellowish in colour. It contains Bowman's glands whose secretion is serous.

Nerve Supply

The nerve supply of the whole nasal cavity may be described in three headings. They are:

1. Nerves of Common Sensation

　　a. Maxillary division of the trigeminal through the branches arising from the sphenopalatine ganglion. The sphenopalatine foramen lies posterior to and immediately above the posterior end of the middle turbinate.

　　b. Ophthalmic nerve through its lateral and medial internal nasal branches. These supply the anterior portion of the lateral wall and of the nasal septum.

2. *Nerves of Special Sensation*

The olfactory nerves of about twenty filaments arise from bipolar cells of the olfactory mucosa. They pass through the foramina of the cribriform plate and enter the under-surface of the olfactory bulb. They carry the sense of smell. These filaments receive arachnoid and pia mater of the cranial cavity. The perineural subarachnoid spaces communicate directly with the cranial subarachnoid space.

3. *The Autonomic Nerve Supply*

It controls the vascular reaction of the nasal mucous membrane.

a. Sympathetic causes vasoconstriction and diminished secretions. This is deep petrosal nerve that derives from the plexus around the internal carotid artery. The fibres pass from the superior cervical sympathetic ganglion.

b. Parasympathetic produces vasodilatation and increased secretion. They are carried via the greater superficial petrosal nerve, a branch of facial nerve.

The vidian nerve or the nerve of the pterygoid canal is formed by the union of deep petrosal and greater superficial petrosal nerve and carries postganglionic sympathetic fibres and preganglionic parasympathetic fibres. Stimulation of vidian nerve causes vasodilatation.

Blood Supply

Blood supply of the nose derives both from the external and internal carotid arteries.

Venous Drainage

The veins from the nasal cavity mostly terminate in the pterygoid venous plexus through the sphenopalatine foramen. Some join the superior ophthalmic vein and inter-communicate with the anterior facial vein.

Arrangement of Blood Vessels of Nasal Mucous Membrane

The vascular arrangements of nasal mucous membrane are peculiar and needs a special note.

The dilated blood spaces in the subepithelial connective tissue called sinusoids receive blood from the subepithelial and periglandular capillary network. From the sinusoids blood is drained into the venules through the venous plexuses.

This arrangement forms the erectile tissue. It is more marked in the inferior turbinate, adjacent part of the septum and the posterior part of the middle turbinate. The autonomic nerves control the vascular reactions of the mucous membrane of the nose.

Lymphatic Drainage

From the most anterior part of the nasal mucosa lymphatics drain in the submandibular glands. The efferent of these glands drains into the upper deep cervical glands.

The lymphatics from the rest of the nasal mucosa pass backwards and drain into the upper cervical gland either directly or through the retropharyngeal glands.

10

Anatomy of the Paranasal Sinuses

PARANASAL SINUSES

On the lateral surface of the primitive nasal cavity three ectodermal projections appear. With the migration of mesenchymal tissue into these projections, the three turbinates are formed: the superior, middle and inferior turbinate.

The sinuses are developed by the extensions of mucosal pouches into the surrounding bone. The maxillary sinus develops as a mucosal depression below the middle turbinate and grow into the maxilla. The frontal sinus develops as an extension of the mucosal pouch that forms the anterior ethmoid cells.

Paranasal sinuses are the spaces filled up with air in certain skull bones in relation to nose. These develop as outpouchings of the mucous membrane of the nasal fossae. They start developing at about the third or fourth month of foetal life. The development is completed by 20 to 25 years of age. They may be divided into two groups as follows:

Anterior Group

1. Maxillary sinuses (antrum of Highmore) (Fig. 10.1).

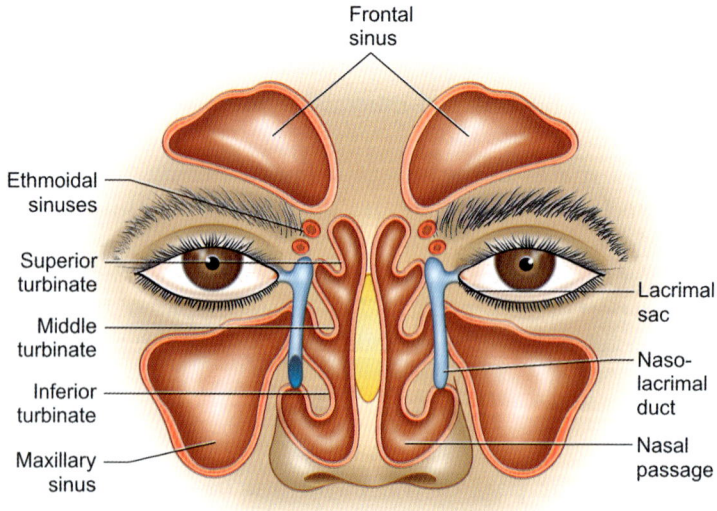

Fig. 10.1: Coronal section showing anterior group of paranasal sinuses and nasal cavity

2. Frontal sinuses.
3. Anterior group of ethmoidal sinuses.

Posterior Group

1. Posterior group of ethmoidal sinuses.
2. Sphenoidal sinuses.

The anterior group of sinuses drains in the middle meatus and the posterior group drains in the superior meatus of which the sphenoidal sinuses drain via sphenoethmoidal recess.

All the sinuses are lined with respiratory epithelium, i.e. pseudostratified ciliated columnar epithelium. The movement of the cilia in the paranasal sinuses is directed towards the nasal cavity.

THE MAXILLARY SINUS (ANTRUM OF HIGHMORE)

It is pyramidal in shape and occupies the body of the maxilla. The base of the pyramid lies medially. The apex lies in the zygomatic portion of the maxilla. It is the largest of all the paranasal sinuses. The average capacity of this in adult is 15 ml. It has five walls.

Medial wall: It is the base of the pyramid and is the part of the lateral wall of the nose. The bone is the thinnest immediately below the attachment of the inferior concha. The opening of the sinus lies immediately beneath the roof of the antrum. This is unfavourably placed for the drainage of the cavity. Sometimes there may be presence of an accessory opening lying posteroinferior to the normal opening.

Apex: It may extend to the zygomatic process of the maxilla.

Anterolateral wall: It separates the sinus from the skin of the cheek. The space between the canine root and the zygomatic process is the canine fossa.

Posterior wall: It is a thin plate of bone separating the sinus from pterygopalatine and infratemporal fossae.

Roof: It is a thin plate of bone forming the floor of the orbit. This wall is grooved by infraorbital nerve.

Floor: It is formed by the alveolar process of maxilla. In adults it lies half an inch below the floor of the nasal cavity. In children it lies at, or above the level of the floor of the nasal fossa. The bicuspid and tricuspid teeth are related to the floor of the maxilla.

Development: The sinus exists as a definite small cavity at birth. It reaches its maximum dimensions around the twenty-fifth year of age. These sinuses are liable to attain surgical importance as early as the third and fourth years of life.

Relations: The roof is related to the orbit. The floor is related to the premolar and molar teeth. The second premolar and first molar teeth are commonly related. The upper part of the antrum is related to the middle meatus of nose. This helps in operations in the ethmoidal labyrinth through the antrum (Horgan's transantral ethmoidectomy). The posterior wall is related to the maxillary artery and maxillary division of the fifth cranial nerve lying in the pterygopalatine fossa. The maxillary artery may be approached through this wall of antrum if it is required to be ligated.

Medial wall is related to the nasolacrimal duct, which opens into the inferior meatus of the nose. The lumen of the duct may be obstructed by the new growth of the nasal cavity and the maxillary antrum.

THE FRONTAL SINUS

The frontal sinuses, right and left, are nothing but the upward extensions of the anterior ethmoidal sinuses. They occupy the frontal bone. The capacity of the sinus is about 7 cc in adults. It has three walls, and a partition in between the two sinuses.

Anterior wall is formed by the outer table of the frontal bone which contains the marrow spaces.

Posterior wall is formed by a thin compact bone separating the frontal lobe of brain from the sinuses. It is partly vertical and partly horizontal.

Floor is the thinnest of the three walls. It lies in the horizontal plane and forms part of the orbital roof.

The opening of the sinus is situated in the floor of it and favourably placed for the better drainage of the inflammatory products.

Development: The frontal sinus is absent at the time of birth. The development of the cavity in the early years of life is subject to considerable variation but a well-formed sinus has been recognised and opened for the relief of suppuration between the third and fourth years. It is usually well developed between the seventh and eighth years.

THE ETHMOIDAL SINUS (LABYRINTHS)

There are two groups of cells:
There are about 7 to 15 thin walled ethmoid cells in each ethmoidal labyrinth.
1. *Anterior* open into the upper part of the hiatus semilunaris. Sometimes open on to, or above the bulla ethmoidalis. These are usually small and numerous.
2. *Posterior* open into the superior meatus. The cells are large and a few.

Relations: Anterior cranial fossa lies above the roof of the upper ethmoidal cells.

The orbit is separated from the labyrinth by the lamina papyracea (thin orbital plate of the ethmoid). Lacrimal sac is related laterally to the anterior cells. The optic nerve lies very close to the posterior group of cells.

Development: The anterior group of cells are present at the time of birth.

THE SPHENOIDAL SINUS

They occupy the body of the sphenoid bone. The capacity of each sinus is about 7 cc. in adults. The two sinuses are separated by a thin plate of bony partition. The opening of the sinuses is situated in the upper part of the anterior wall. It drains in the superior meatus through the sphenoethmoidal recess.

Relations: The lateral wall is related to the cavernous sinus with the internal carotid artery and the optic nerve. The cavernous sinus contains the third, fourth, sixth cranial nerves and ophthalmic and maxillary division of fifth cranial nerve.

The roof is related from before backwards to the frontal lobe and the olfactory tract, the optic chiasma, the pituitary body, and sometimes the pons.

The lower part of the anterior wall is related to the vessels and nerves from the sphenopalatine foramen.

The floor is related to the vidian nerve:

The posterior wall or basisphenoid is related to the basilar artery and brainstem.

Development: The sinus attains the size of a bean as early as the sixth year and is fully developed by 12 to 14 years of age.

Anatomy of the Nose and Paranasal Sinuses Related to Endoscopic Sinus Surgery (ESS)

The anatomy of the paranasal sinuses was among the most poorly described areas in the human body.

The technological advancements in the form of microscope and endoscope have helped to see and operate more precisely inside the nose and paranasal sinuses.

The knowledge about the nose and paranasal sinuses was rediscovered following the advancements in imaging modalities such as CT, MRI, operative instrument technology and the work of the sinus surgeons like Wigand in 1978, Messerklinger in 1985 and Stamberger in 1985.

Middle Turbinate

The middle turbinate has three parts:
1. The anterior third
2. The basal lamella or middle third
3. The posterior third

The anterior third lies in the **sagittal plane** and attaches vertically to the lateral lamella of the cribriform plate above.

The basal lamella lies in the **coronal plane** inserted into the lamina papyracea and separates the anterior from the posterior ethmoidal sinuses.

The posterior third of the middle turbinate lies in the **horizontal plane** and attaches with the lamina papyracea. Its superior surface is separated from the posterior ethmoid sinuses by a narrow slit.

Ethmoid Sinuses

The ethmoid bone is considered the "Keystone in the paranasal sinus system". In adults the ethmoid sinus forms a pyramid with the apex lying anteriorly and the wider base posteriorly measuring 4 to 5 cm anteroposterior, 2.5 cm inferosuperior, 0.5 cm wide and 1.5 cm posteriorly.

The roof of the ethmoid articulates with the lateral lamella of the cribriform plate. Lateral lamella is the thinnest bone in the entire skull base and determines the depth of olfactory fossa. Keros (1965) has described three forms of olfactory fossa.
- Type I—shallow fossa (1 to 3 mm deep).
- Type II—due to long lateral lamella the fossa is 4 to 7 mm deep.
- Type III—the fossa is 8 to 16 mm deep.

The ethmoidal air cells are of two types: intramural (cells within the ethmoid) and extramural (cells outside the ethmoid).

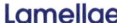
Lamellae

There are 5 lamellae which are as follows:
1. Lateral extension of the uncinate process is the anterior most lamella
2. The plate of the bulla ethmoidalis
3. The attachment of the middle turbinate
4. The attachment of the superior turbinate
5. The supreme turbinate when it is present

Fovea

Fovea or Fovea ethmoidalis are the pits overlying the superior clefts or spaces in the roof of the ethmoid bone. Fovea is not considered for the entire roof of the ethmoid sinus. The cribriform plate articulates with the frontal bone, i.e. lateral lamella of the cribiform plate which is the thinnest bone in the skull base. The anterior most part of the middle turbinate is attached superiorly to the lateral lamella.

Ostiomeatal Complex

Ostiomeatal complex is a region with a functional entity comprising anterior ethmoidal complex representing the final common pathway for drainage and ventilation of the frontal, maxillary and anterior ethmoidal cells.

Uncinate Process

Uncinate process is one of the most important surgical landmarks in the lateral nasal wall for endonasal surgery and in addition it forms the anterior boundary of ostiomeatal complex.

The maxillary sinus ostium usually opens into the inferolateral aspect of the ethmoid infundibulum in the middle or posterior third. The natural ostium of the maxillary sinus remains hidden lateral to the uncinate process in the ethmoid infundibulum.

Hiatus Semilunaris

Hiatus semilunaris introduced by "Zuckerkandl" is a two-dimensional space between the posterior edge of the uncinate process and the anterior aspect of the ethmoid bulla, which lead into the ethmoid infundibulum superiorly.

Hiatus semilunaris superior: Hiatus semilunaris superior is a cleft between the bulla ethmoidalis and the middle turbinate. The suprabullar and retrobullar recesses can be entered through this.

Hiatus semilunaris inferior: Hiatus semilunaris inferior is a two-dimensional slit between the free posterior margin of the uncinate process and the anterior surface of the bulla ethmoidalis. To reach the ethmoid infundibulum one must pass through this.

Ethmoidal Infundibulum

It is a three-dimensional pouch or trough-like space that ends superiorly in the frontal recess. It lies anterior to the bulla ethmoidalis and is bounded medially by the middle turbinate and the lamina papyracea laterally. It is the site of drainage for frontal sinus and anterior ethmoidal cells.

Infundibular cells range from 1 to 7 cells and are the second most anterior cells. The most constant of these cells is the extramural pneumatisation of the lacrimal bone which gives rise to a prominence on the lateral nasal wall anterior to the attachment of the middle turbinate named agger nasi.

Retrobullar Recess

The retrobullar recess or lateral sinus lies posterior to the bulla ethmoidalis and anterior to the basal lamella. The roof of the ethmoid forms the superior boundary.

Suprabullar Recess

The suprabullar recess is a space bounded inferiorly by the bulla ethmoidalis, laterally by the lamina papyracea and above by the roof of the ethmoid.

Lateral Sinus

It is also known as the sinus lateralis of Grunwald and the Subbullar cell of Mouret. When the posterior wall of the bulla lamella is not in contact with the basal lamella of the middle turbinate, the suprabullar and retrobullar (synonym: infrabullar recess) recess form one space known as the lateral sinus.

Haller Cell

Sometimes a bony process develops from the attachment of the middle turbinate and projects laterally towards the orbit. Pneumatisation of this process is termed a Haller cell.

Conchal Cell

These are ethmoid air cells that invade the middle concha termed a concha bullosa.

Onodi Cell

Migration of the posterior ethmoid cells to the medial aspect of the optic nerve within the sphenoid bone is called postreme cells. When these cells are located superiorly and inferiorly to the optic nerve they are known as Onodi cells. These are the extramural extension of ethmoidal cells.

11

Physiology of the Nose and Paranasal Sinuses

Functions of the Nose

1. *Olfaction:* Odoriferous materials on reaching the olfactory area by diffusion stimulates the receptor cells for olfaction. Only about 10% of inspired air reaches the olfactory area in normal respiration which increases to about 25% on sniffing. The poor ventilation of the olfactory cleft does not hamper the sensation of smell as the odoriferous materials reach this area by diffusion.

2. *Respiration: Inspiration:* Inspiratory air passes from before backward forming a parabolic curve.
   Expiration: Expiratory air passes from behind forward forming an eddy current.

3. *Protective function:* The lower respiratory tract is being protected by the nose by purification, warming and moistening and reflex sneezing. Purification of the inspired air is done by:
   i. Vibrissae of nasal vestibule—removes the coarse particles.
   ii. Cilia—expels the fine objects.
   iii. Lysozymes—has bacteriostatic action.
   iv. Reflex sneezing.
   Warming of cold air is done by radiation. Moistening of dry air is done by transudation of fluid through the epithelium and secretion from mucus glands and goblet cells.

4. Vocal resonance.

5. The nose acts as the drainage cavity for the paranasal sinuses and lacrimal apparatus.

6. The nose acts as the ventilating shaft for the eustachian tube.

7. *Reflex functions:* like sneezing, salivation and gastric secretion, and reflex inhibition of respiration during exposure to irritating fumes.

Mucociliary Action

The cilia have an effective and recovery stroke and beat before backwards about 10 times per second. The viscous sheet of mucus on to the cilia is moved from before backwards as a "conveyor belt" into the nasopharynx and then swallowed. The complete sheet of mucus is cleared into the pharynx about twice an hour. Ciliary movement stops rapidly with drying. The bacteria, finer dusts and other objects in the inspired air get stuck on the mucus blanket and are ultimately thrown out into the nasopharynx.

Functions of the Paranasal Sinuses

There are several theories regarding the functions of the paranasal sinuses. They are:

1. The sinuses develop owing to the rapid growth of the facial bones. The process can be compared with mastoid pneumatization.
2. Warming and moistening of the inspired air to some extent.
3. Lightening of the skull.
4. Resonance of voice.

However, the functions of the paranasal sinuses are still uncertain. The daily volume of nasal transudate and secretions is about 1 litre.

Rhinolalia

Rhinolalia is the nasal intonation of voice. Rhinolalia is of two types:

1. Rhinolalia aparta—hyperventilation of the nose due to incomplete closure of the nasopharyngeal sphincter, e.g. cleft palate, short palate; paralysis of the soft palate due to bulbar poliomyelitis, post diphtheritic paralysis, mechanical impedance causing limitation of the palatal movement.
2. Rhinolalia clausa—obstruction of the nose and nasopharynx resulting hypoventilation, e.g. common cold, adenoids, nasal polyp, DNS.

Smell Sensation

- Anosmia is defined as the absence of smell sensation.
- Cacosmia is defined as foetid smell.

Common causes of cacosmia are:

1. Maxillary sinusitis of dental origin.
2. Old forgotten foreign bodies in the nose.
3. In unsafe type of CSOM.

- Parosmia is defined as perverted sensation of smell. It usually occurs in hysteric patients. It is a subjective sensation of nonexistent smell.
- Hyposmia is defined as lowering of the acuity of smell.

Causes of hyposmia are:

1. Nasal obstruction
2. Vasomotor rhinitis
3. Peripheral neuritis—particularly from influenza
4. Atrophic rhinitis
5. Trauma to the base of the skull
6. Intracranial lesions, e.g. abscess, tumour and meningitis
7. Exposure to noxious gases, e.g. bromine.

OLFACTION

Olfaction is a sensation of smell of the odorous substance. The odour of a substance is related to the shape of its molecules and to some extent to its molecular vibrations.

THEORIES OF SMELL

There are different types of primary receptors in the olfactory mucosa responsible for the sensation of limited number of primary odours. They are etherial, camphoraceous, musty, floral, pungent and putrid. All smells can be accounted for by permutations of these primary receptors, stimulated to varying degrees. Theories of smell can be grouped into two main divisions:

1. The Corpuscular Theory

This explains that the olfactory region of the nose is stimulated by odorants which are carried in the air in particulate form. On coming in contact of these odorants with the sensory surface a sort of chemical reaction takes place.

2. The Wave Theory

Like the light and sound waves the odorant substances emit waves which stimulate the olfactory organ.

The smell is a complex process. Stimulation of the olfactory epithelium by air borne odoriferous molecule, sets up a transmitted electrophysiological impulse along the olfactory pathways.

Smell can be tested by asking the subject to sniff from bottles of coal tar, concentrated essences of coffee or lemon and to name them if he can.

Quantitative sense of smell is termed olfactory spectrometry. It has a diagnostic potential no doubt but the practical clinical work for this assessment is rarely done. The olfactory mucous membrane is of nonciliated columnar cells and is yellowish in colour. It contains the serous glands of bowman.

There are three types of cells:
1. Olfactory cells
2. Supporting cells
3. Basal cells.

Olfactory Pathway

Olfactory cells are bipolar cells. The superficial process ends at the surface of the mucous membrane in a bulbus process, which bears the olfactory hairs. The central processes of the bipolar cells are the non-myelinated filaments pass to the olfactory bulb through the cribriform plate of the ethmoid bone. From olfactory bulb a new set of filaments arises to form the olfactory tract, which passes backward in the neighbourhood of the anterior perforated substance at the base of the brain where it divides into two diverging striae, forming the olfactory trigone. From the lateral striae it reaches to the uncus, which is a part of the hippocampal gyrus. It is situated on the medial aspect of the temporal lobe, close to the optic chiasma and pituitary fossa.

12

Method of Examination of Nose and Paranasal Sinuses

EXAMINATION OF NOSE

Examination of the nose includes:
1. Examination of the external nose.
2. Examination of the nasal cavity.

Nasal Airway Assessment

Indirect rhinometry: Indirect test for patency of nasal airways. Rhinometry may be indirect or direct.

Direct rhinometry: Helps to assess the airway resistance, and pressure difference in addition to measurement of the rate of nasal airflow.

The nasal airways or the patency of the nasal cavity can be checked by directing the patient to take a deep breath and expirate through the nose on a cold metallic or glass spatula. The accumulation of moisture over the spatula indicates the patency of both nasal cavities simultaneously.

Subjective assessment of the nasal airway is the commonly relied on system. For quantification of the nasal airway, the following methods have been used:
1. Peak nasal inspiratory flow.
2. Rhinomanometry. It is an important objective assessment of the nasal airway.
3. Acoustic rhinometry. It gives an accurate measurement of the cross-sectional area of the airway from the nasal vestibule to the nasopharynx. Examination of the vestibule of nose is one of the preliminary steps towards the examination of the external nose. The vestibule of nose is examined by lifting the tip of the nose upwards.

Anterior Rhinoscopy

Examination of the anterior part of the nasal cavity is called anterior rhinoscopy.

It is done by means of a nasal speculum under good illumination. The speculum either Thudicum or Duplay's variety should preferably be held by the left hand and inserted into the nostril with the blades closed. Then the blades are opened gently to dilate the nostril. After examination the speculum is removed with the opened blades to prevent pulling out of the hairs from the vestibule of nose.

The following structures are visible by anterior rhinoscopy:

1. Part of the nasal vestibule, which is not covered by the blades of the nasal speculum.
2. The lower and the anterior part of the nasal septum.
3. The anterior portions of the inferior and middle turbinates with their corresponding meati.
4. The anterior portion of the floor of the nose.

Most often the view of the nasal cavity is obstructed by the swollen turbinates. To get a proper view the vasoconstrictive drugs like 1% ephedrine saline or any decongestive nose drop should be applied. Anterior rhinoscopy is not complete unless the middle meatus is properly seen. The superior turbinate and meatus are not seen by this method.

The method of examination of the posterior part of the nose and nasopharynx is called posterior rhinoscopy.

Posterior Rhinoscopy

In this method the dorsum of the anterior two-thirds of the tongue is gently depressed with a tongue depressor. A posterior rhinoscopic mirror after being slightly warmed is slipped over the tongue as shown in Fig. 12.1 and placed in between the soft palate and posterior pharyngeal wall. Light is focussed on to the mirror. The reflected image of the posterior part of the nasal cavity and nasopharynx will be seen. The mirror should not touch the soft palate, the palatal arches, the posterior one-third of the tongue, and the posterior wall of the pharynx, as it will cause reflex gagging. During this procedure the patient is asked to breathe through the nose or to sniff.

The following structures are seen by posterior rhinoscopy:

1. The posterior free margin of nasal septum.
2. Choana on either side of the septum.
3. Posterior ends of the inferior, middle and superior turbinates.
4. Posterior portion of the superior and middle meati. The inferior meatus will not

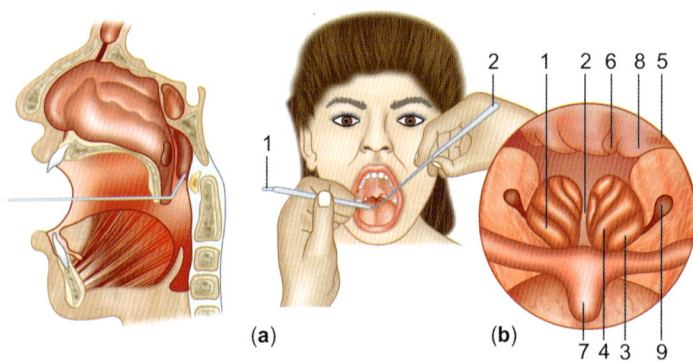

Fig. 12.1: Posterior rhinoscopy. (a) Method of holding the tongue depressor (1) and the mirror (2); (b) Composite picture of the nasopharynx composed of individual view: 1. choana, 2. posterior edge of the septum, 3. inferior turbinate, 4. middle turbinate, 5. superior turbinate, 6. adenoid, 7. uvula, 9. tubal ostium

be seen owing to the soft palate, which will obstruct its view unless retracted forward.

5. The nasopharyngeal vault—with pharyngeal tonsil or adenoids in children.
6. The pharyngeal openings of the pharyngotympanic tubes on the lateral wall of the nasopharynx with tubal tonsils.

In some hypersensitive patients the pharynx may have to be anesthetized by spraying or painting 4% xylocaine or other local surface anaesthetics.

Posterior rhinoscopy may also be done by electric nasopharyngoscope, fibre-optic rigid nasopharyngoscope—all the walls (normal or with pathology) may be visualized with the help of 0°, 30° and 70° scope, flexible nasopharyngoscope and also by Yankauer speculum which is not used nowadays. It is very big in size.

Palpation

1. Digital: The external nose, the postnasal space and the nasopharynx should be palpated with the right forefinger. During palpation of the postnasal space and nasopharynx the left cheek of the patient is pressed by left index finger in between the jaws so as to prevent biting. The examiner stands on the right-hand side of the patient (Fig. 12.2). The tenderness over the sinuses should be elicited by finger palpation.

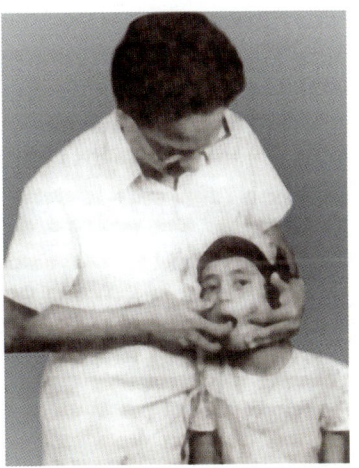 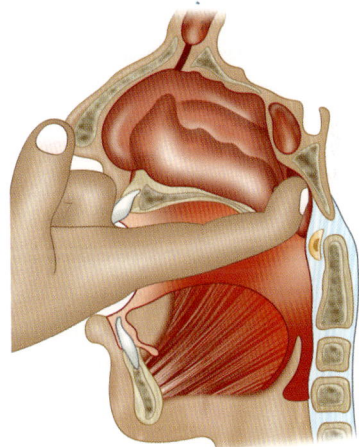

Fig. 12.2: Digital examination of the nasopharynx

2. Probing: The results of the examination of the nose should be verified by probe test with a nasal probe.

EXAMINATION OF THE PARANASAL SINUSES

Maxillary and frontal sinus tenderness requires to be ascertained. In acute sinusitis the frontal and maxillary sinuses are found tender depending on the sinus involved.

Transillumination Test

This method is possible only for the maxillary and frontal sinuses. The test may help in some cases in spite of its various fallacies. The fallacies are: the cavities of the sinuses may be asymmetrical or the walls may be unusually thick giving rise to lack of illumination. Antral polypi and dental cyst may produce a brighter illumination on the diseased side. This test has therefore been largely discarded in favour of X-rays and CT scans.

The examination room should be darkened. For the maxillary sinus, a small lamp of low voltage attached to narrow handle, is placed inside the oral cavity with the lips firmly closed. The test for the frontal sinuses is performed by placing the lamp against the floor of the sinus in the inner corner of the orbit.

The transmission of light rays through the walls of the sinuses produces a crescentic tache in the region of the lower eyelids and a cherry red glow through both the cheeks and pupils. The presence of pus or inflammatory changes in the lining mucosa interferes with the transmission of light rays (objective sign) and loss of patient's perception of light sensation (subjective symptom).

Posture Test

This method is helpful for the diagnosis of maxillary and frontal sinusitis. Decongestive drug is applied in the middle meatus after cleaning it by means of cotton tipped probe. Then the middle meatus is examined with the patient in erect position. If pus appears in the middle meatus after cleaning, it is presumably coming from the frontal sinus.

The reappearance of pus in the middle meatus after the head is bent forward with the vertex dependent, and the cheek of the suspected side is uppermost, is strongly presumptive of its escape from the maxillary sinus. This position is to be maintained for about five minutes. Occasionally the patient gets a disagreeable odour (subjective sensation), which is a valuable diagnostic aid.

Nasal Endoscopy and Fibreoptic Sinoscopy

The scope of different degrees may be introduced into the maxillary sinus through the special type of trochar and cannula. The cannula may be passed either through

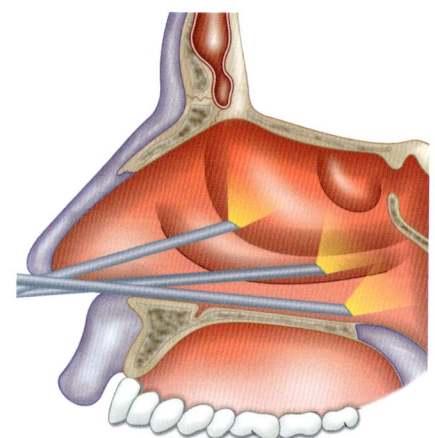

Fig. 12.3: Rhinoscopy using an endoscope

inferior meatus or through the canine fossa. Endoscopic examination of nose and paranasal sinuses nasal endoscopy is now the standard method of examination with the help of either rigid endoscope or flexible fibre optic endoscope (Fig. 12.3).

Wigand (1978), Messerklinger (1985), Stammberger (1985), are the pioneers of using endoscope in the diagnosis and surgery of nose and paranasal sinuses.

Rigid endoscope is preferred because of the superior image quality and angular viewing ability. Rigid endoscopes of 4 mm or 2.7 mm diameter and of 0° or 30° angulation tip are commonly used.

Fibreoptic Nasal Endoscopy

1. Rigid 4 mm or 2.7 mm diameter endoscope is used for diagnostic endoscopy and sinoscopy for endoscopic sinonasal surgery. The endoscopes may be of wide-angle 0°, 30°, 45° or 70°.
2. Flexible endoscope is used for examination of nose nasopharynx and for sinoscopy.

Indications for Endoscopy of Nose

To examine the parts of the nose which are not visualized by anterior rhinoscopy with nasal speculum. It helps to diagnose the diseases, which cause nasal obstruction.

For diagnostic nasal endoscopy a solution of 4% xylocaine with any decongestant nasal drop like oxymetazoline or xylometazoline solution are used for local anaesthesia and decongestion of nasal cavity mucosa. A wide angled 0° or 30° rigid endoscope or a flexible nasopharyngoscope is used for endoscopy. An antifog solution like savlon is used to keep the lens of the endoscope fog free. The nose is examined by following the three standard passes:

The first pass: The endoscope is passed along the floor of the nose and the following structures are visualized: Inferior turbinate and meatus, the nasal septum, the eustachian tube orifice, the cartilaginous cushion of the eustachian tube at the posterosuperior part of the orifice and the fossa of Rossenmuller behind the eustachian cushions and in front of the posterior nasopharyngeal wall.

The second pass: In this pass the endoscope is passed along the middle meatus to visualize:

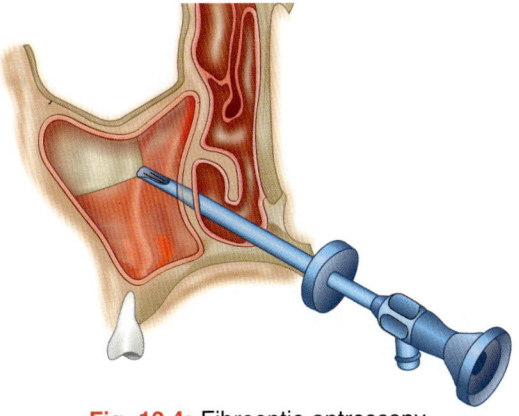

Fig. 12.4: Fibreoptic antroscopy

i. Middle turbinate and meatus

ii. Uncinate process

iii. Bulla ethmoidalis

iv. Frontal recess

v. Accessory ostium of maxillary sinus

The third pass: In this the endoscope is passed along the superior meatus to visualize the spenoethmoidal recess and the superior turbinate and meatus.

Endoscopic Documentation

Endoscopic photographs for documentation has been a major advancement in the world of medicine. With the help of light source and the endoscope mounted on a telezoom adapter and a centre weighted or spot metering camera is probably the easiest method of taking photographs.

Radiological Examination of Paranasal Sinuses

The standard views are the following:

i. Occipitomental or Water's view.

ii. Frontooccipital or Caldwell view.

iii. Lateral.

iv. Submentovertical.

v. Right oblique.

vi. Left oblique.

vii. *Orthopantomography (OPG):* OPG is done by a panoramic X-ray machine. The X-ray tube and the film cassette of the machine move synchronously and reciprocally around the lower part of the head of the patient. It gives a complete picture of all the bony structures in both lower and upper jaws as well as of all teeth: erupted and unerupted on one film.

In an OPG the maxillary antra, the temporomandibular joints, styloid processes and parotid regions are also visualised.

Computerised Tomography (CT)

The computed tomography scanning was developed in the late 1970s and 1980s. The unit of measurement in CT is a Hounsefield unit (HU) with a range of -1000 to $+3000$. After a single exposure to X-rays the raw data obtained can be manipulated by the computer within different "window" settings. Outside the window settings higher densities such as bone will appear white and lower densities such as air will appear black. A wide window setting should be used for imaging the paranasal sinuses in a patient with benign inflammatory diseases usually between 2000 and 3000 HU. If imaging of the soft tissue is required, a narrow window setting of 300 HU should be selected.

The images can be produced in axial or coronal planes. The plane and the thickness of slice in which the image is acquired is demonstrated on a lateral topogram which is named a "scout image". For paranasal sinuses the thickness of the slice is usually between 4 and 5 mm. Imaging for preoperative radiological assessment for benign inflammatory diseases of the paranasal air sinuses should be in the coronal plane. To assess the posterior ethmoid or sphenoid sinus, anatomy and pathology imaging in the axial plane is indicated. The axial images can be reconstructed to provide coronal and sagittal plane images. Intravenous contrast is required in lesions that have increased blood flow and intracranial abscesses.

The superiority of CT over other measures of imaging sinuses can be summarised as follows:

1. The bony walls of the sinuses are demonstrated as well by CT in the high resolution mode.
2. An excellent anatomical display of soft tissue density including fluid levels and polypoid masses within the normally airfilled cavities of the sinuses, nasal cavity and postnasal space is provided.
3. Most important of all is that the diseases extending beyond the bony perimeters of the sinuses into the adjacent soft tissue of the orbit, brain and infratemporal fossa can be imaged.

Magnetic Resonance Imaging (MRI)

MRI is a very important imaging tool since the late 1980s. The major advantage of MRI is that it does not cause any ionising radiation. MRI involves magnets, radiofrequency coils and a computer processing system. It is dependant on the presence of water and fat. Two sequences are commonly used in the head and neck MRI: T1-weighted and T2-weighted.

The T1-weighted images demonstrate static fluids, oedema and tumour as black. Fat, blood proteinaceous cysts and gadolinium contrast agents give a bright signal, whereas T2-weigted images of tendons, muscles and cartilages show dark or black images. Fluid, oedema and tumours are revealed as white or bright.

The bony margins of the sinuses appear as a plain of the absent signal on MR scans and these limits the usefuless of the technique for examination of the sinus. Moreover, the immense signal from the high fat content of bone marrow as in the basisphenoid and petrosquamous and around the frontal sinus can be very confusing for the radiologist interpreting the scans. This is particularly so as retained fluid within the sinus gives a similar intense signal from the high water content. It is difficult or impossible on a CT scan to differentiate tumour tissue from the retained fluid in sinuses where the drainage of a sinus is blocked by obstruction from the tumour. Differentiation on a MR scan is simple and clear. Extension of sinus tumour into the cranial cavity is shown very well by MR and the ability to image in any plain is a considerable advantage.

Summary

Plain X-rays continue to have a role in the initial investigation of the diseases of paranasal sinuses. Good radiographic method and positioning of the patient are important as is the ability of the observer to detect early signs of disease such as erosion of the sinus walls. High resolution CT gives an excellent demonstration of both fine bone and soft tissue anatomy on the same sectional picture and is now the investigation of choice. The CT can demonstrate a neoplasm early in the course of

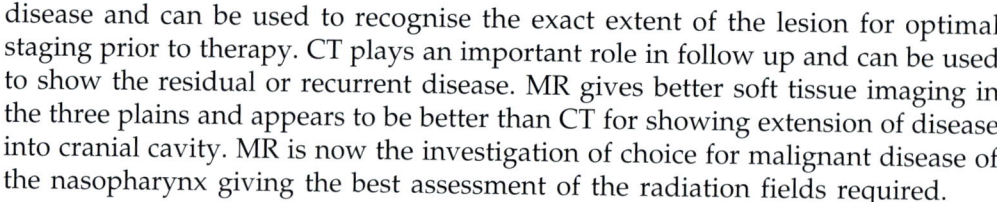

disease and can be used to recognise the exact extent of the lesion for optimal staging prior to therapy. CT plays an important role in follow up and can be used to show the residual or recurrent disease. MR gives better soft tissue imaging in the three plains and appears to be better than CT for showing extension of disease into cranial cavity. MR is now the investigation of choice for malignant disease of the nasopharynx giving the best assessment of the radiation fields required.

Sinogram

This means taking the X-ray of sinuses after introducing the radiopaque dye. The introduction of the radiopaque material may be done either by:
1. Injection through a cannula into the maxillary antrum.
2. Proetz's replacement method.

Proof Puncture

This is also called diagnostic antral lavage. It is commonly carried out for the confirmation of the clinical and radiological diagnosis of chronic maxillary sinusitis.

Test of Smell

The acuity of smell is determined by using various odours-like those of camphor, oil of cloves, ashafoetida, etc. One nostril should be tested at a time. No pungent material should be used to avoid stimulation of the nerves of general sensation.

13

Diseases of the External Nose and Nasal Apertures

TRAUMATIC

Fracture of the Nasal Bones

Aetiology

The nasal bone fracture is caused by direct trauma on the nose or face. This may also be involved in injury of the base of skull.

Clinical Features

1. Deformity in the form of lateral displacement, depressed bridge of nose and external swelling is often accompany injury.
2. Subconjunctival haemorrhage and "black eye" are common.
3. Bleeding from within the nose (epistaxis) is often profuse.
4. Nasal obstruction may be present in case of dislocation or haematoma of the septum.
5. Pain and tenderness are sometimes severe.

Diagnosis

The fracture of nasal bones is often compound and the extent of injury may not be ascertained owing to external swelling but X-ray examination will reveal the bony injury.

Treatment

1. *Early:* If the patient is seen at once or within a week of the accident, the displaced bones should be immediately reduced under general anaesthesia. If the swelling is marked, nothing should be done till the swelling has subsided.
2. *Late:* If the patient is seen between 7 and 14 days when the swelling subsides, reduction of nasal bones should be undertaken by Walsham's forceps under general anaesthesia. The septal fracture and dislocations are corrected at the same time by means of Asch's septum forceps.
   As a rule no packing or splint is required.

Fracture of the Bones of the Middle Third of Face

The bones of the face from supraorbital ridge to the upper teeth are involved. The middle third fracture of the face may be of the following types:
1. The central middle third fracture
2. The lateral middle third fracture

The central middle third fracture: It involves the maxilla and is classified into the following types:
  i. Alveolar
 ii. Le Fort I (Guerin type): It runs above the floor of the nasal cavity through the nasal septum, the maxillary sinus and the medial and lateral pterygoid plates.
iii. Le Fort II (Fig. 13.1): It starts from the floor of the maxillary sinus and ascends up to the infraorbital margin. Then it passes upwards and medially, across the lacrimal bone to the nasion.
 iv. Le Fort III (Fig. 13.1): This fracture starts at the root of the nose and goes to the superior orbital fissure by crossing the medial wall of the orbit and then ends in the zygomaticofrontal suture by traversing the greater wing of the sphenoid bone.

The lateral middle third fracture: It involves the malar zygomatic complex. In depressed fracture at this complex due to direct trauma from the side, the fractures occur at three sites (tripod fracture) like at the frontozygomatic suture, the fronto-orbital rim and the zygomatic buttress.

Clinical Features

1. Collapse of the bridge of the nose.
2. Step deformity of the infraorbital margin.
3. Malocclusion—the middle 1/3 of the face may be mobile and may drop.
4. Swelling of the soft tissues and complete closure of the eyelids with subconjunctival haemorrhage.
5. Epistaxis.
6. Numbness of the cheek due to involvement of the infraorbital nerve.
7. Diplopia, which may be permanent due to gross misalignment of the bony orbital floor. It is usually transient if caused by extravasation of blood into the orbit.
8. Nasal obstruction.
9. "Dish-face" deformity.
10. Anosmia.
11. Concussion.
12. Epiphora if the nasolacrimal duct is involved.

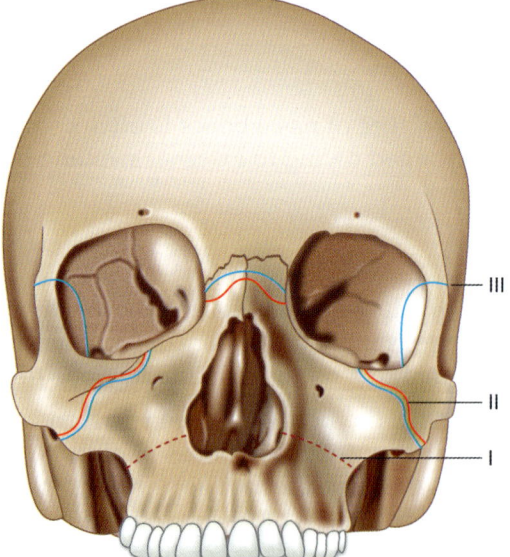

Fig. 13.1: Le Fort I, II and III classification in fractures of the middle third of face

Diagnosis

X-ray will show the fracture lines.

Treatment

Reduction–splinting

Lateral Type (Malarmaxillary Complex) Fracture

It develops by the blows from the side.

Clinical Features

1. Flattening of malar eminence
2. Swelling of soft tissues
3. Step deformity of the infraorbital margin
4. Diplopia in some cases
5. Trismus
5. Anaesthesia of cheek

Treatment

1. Elevation of the zygomatic arch through a small vertical incision above the zygoma.
2. In severe cases reduction should be done through the Caldwell-Luc approach. Elevation of zygoma and orbital floor are done. Gauze packing or inflatable balloon in the antrum keeps the reduced fragments in position. An intranasal antrostomy is essential.

Fractures Involving Paranasal Sinuses

Maxillary Sinus

Blunt trauma to the eyeball by a round object results in increased pressure inside the orbit. The floor of the orbit being the weakest of all the other walls, it fractures. This does not involve the rim of the orbit. The contains of the orbit may herniated into the maxillary sinus (antrum) resulting in enopthalmos with downward displacement of the eyeball, diplopia, periorbital echhymosis and loss of sensation at the area of distribution of the infraorbital nerve.

X-rays and/or CT scan confirm the diagnosis.

Treatment is to elevate the floor of the orbit. It may be done by a Caldwell-Luc approach.

Ethmoidal Labyrinth

Involves in the fracture of nasal bone and anterior cranial fossa. CSF rhinorrhoea follows if duramater is torn. May cause meningitis, surgical emphysema and aerocele.

Treatment consists of systemic antibiotics, avoidance of nose blowing and fascial graft if CSF rhinorrhoea persists by endonasal route.

Frontal Sinus

Caused by direct violence. Treated by systemic antibiotics and elevation of the depressed anterior wall through a small incision under the eyebrow. If the posterior wall is involved with formation of an intracranial aerocele, a fascial graft must be applied via craniotomy as soon as possible. It may be left alone if there is no aerocele. The sinus may require to be obliterated if both anterior and posterior walls are involved and an aerocele is present.

Haematoma and Abscess of the Septum

The trauma may be followed by extravasation of blood and it causes a smooth round swelling on both sides of the septum.

The haematoma may be transformed into abscess after infection. This causes bilateral nasal obstruction associated with pain and tenderness.

Treatment

Incision and drainage under local or general anaesthesia. Incision over the swelling is horizontally placed from behind forwards and as low as possible. The incision is given on one side. A small piece of ribbon gauze is loosely introduced through the incision. It is changed daily till the condition subsides.

INFLAMMATORY

Furuncle or Dermatitis of the Nasal Vestibule

This is due to infection of the hair follicles by *Staphylococcus aureus* and often occurs because of nasal discharge and picking the nose by infected fingers. It causes pain and nasal obstruction owing to crust formation and swelling. If it is squeezed, it may lead to cavernous sinus thrombosis by intracranial extension of infection via venous channels like the angular vein and superior ophthalmic veins.

Treatment

Local application of hot fomentation and antibiotic ointment. Systemic suitable antibiotics and analgesics are necessary.

In dermatitis the affected portion is cleaned after removing the crusts. Then painted with 5% silver nitrate solution followed by application of neomycin with steroid skin ointment.

14

Diseases of the Nasal Septum

Deviation and Spurs of the Septum

Straight septum of the nose is rare in the adults. Some persons with even gross deviation of the septum do not give any symptoms. Deviated nasal septum requires surgical interference.

Aetiology

Predisposing causes

1. Age: Rare in children before the second dentition.
2. Sex: Common in males than in females.
3. Racial: Fairly common in our country and in Europeans (Caucasian). It is rare in the more primitive races.
4. Heredity: The majority of cases are hereditary.

Exciting causes

a. Intranasal
   1. Defective development of the septum and hard palate, i.e. high-arched palate. The developing septum if grows faster than its surrounding skeletal framework it ought to bend. The position of the foetus in pregnancy may have an influence on these deformities (birth moulding theory).
   2. Excessive development of middle and inferior turbinates.
b. Extranasal
   Traumatic: It is the most common cause of the deviation of the septum. Compression of the nose during birth may cause septal deformity.

Abnormal intrauterine posture may result in compression forces acting on the nose and upper jaws. Moulding pressures vary with the type of delivery and are minimal in cases of elective caesarian section, moderate with normal vertex presentation and severe with a persistent occipitoposterior presentation.

Neurological changes: Pressure exerted by septal deviations of adjacent sensory nerves produce pain. Sluder first elaborated this concept and the resultant condition has been called *anterior ethmoidal nerve syndrome.* The very severely impacted nasal septum can exert pressure on the more sensitive structure of the lateral nasal wall and cause referred trigeminal pain and chronic headache.

The deformities of the septum are classified into deviations and spurs or a combination of the two.

Pathological Anatomy

Nasal deformity can be classified as follows:

1. Spurs: Sharp angulations, which may occur at the junction of the vomer below with the septal cartilage and/or ethmoid bone above. This type of deformity is usually the result of vertical compression forces. Fractures through the septal cartilage may also produce sharp angulations.
2. Deviations: This can be either "C" or "S" shaped either in the vertical or in horizontal plane. These usually involve both the cartilages and bone of the nasal septum.
3. Dislocations: The lower border of the septal cartilage is usually displaced from its medial position and projects into one of the nostrils.

Anterior septal deviations are often associated with the deviations in the external nasal pyramid (Fig. 14.1).

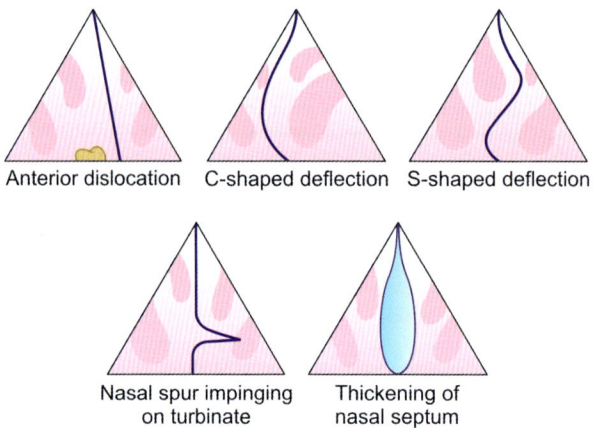

Anterior dislocation   C-shaped deflection   S-shaped deflection

Nasal spur impinging on turbinate   Thickening of nasal septum

Fig. 14.1: Deformities of the nasal septum

Secondary Changes

The turbinates on the deviated side are atrophied or ill-developed. The increased room in the concave side leads to compensatory hypertrophy of the inferior and middle turbinals. Sometimes atrophic changes in the roomy side are seen. The external nose may become crooked.

Infection of the sinus is common owing to their defective ventilation and drainage by deviated septum.

Symptoms

Nasal deformity may not be associated with any symptom. The common symptoms are:

a. Nasal obstruction—unilateral or bilateral.
b. Supraorbital neuralgia—in high deviation.
c. Vacuum headache.
d. Recurrent attacks of cold.
e. Epistaxis.

Diagnosis

Anterior rhinoscopy is sufficient to diagnose deviation or spurs of the septum.

Coronal NCCT scan of the nose and paranasal sinuses give details of septal deviation.

Indications of Treatment

1. External deformity, crooked nose.
2. Mouth breathing: Nasal obstruction.
3. Rhinitis: Recurrent attacks of cold.
4. Epistaxis.
5. To permit aeration of accessory sinuses.
6. To carry out treatment of the accessory sinuses.
7. Eustachian tube obstruction.
8. Atrophic rhinitis to the roomy nasal fossa.
9. Closure of septal perforation.
10. Source of grafting material in rhinoplasty and tympanoplasty operations.
11. To obtain surgical access in
    i. Hypophysectomy
    ii. Vidian neurectomy

Contraindications

1. Before the age of eighteen if SMR operation is planned.
2. Elderly persons.
3. Presence of acute infection.
4. Specific diseases like syphilis and tuberculosis.

Treatment

Septal correction may be done even without symptoms to prevent secondary effects of deviated nasal septum.

Treatment is correction of the septal deviation by submucous resection (SMR) of the septum or septoplasty. The septoplasty operation may be done after six years of age.

SUBMUCOUS RESECTION OF THE SEPTUM (SMR OPERATION)

This operation is preferably done in semi propped-up position under local or general anaesthesia. A good sedation is essential for this procedure, which is usually, achieved by Pethidine and Phenergan injection one hour before the operation.

An incision is given usually in the deviated side through the mucoperichondrium up to the cartilage. This is given just beyond and parallel to the mucocutaneous junction (Killian incision). The mucoperichondrium is then elevated from the deviated portion of the septum by a suitable elevator. Then the cartilage is incised along the first incision line. This is carefully done to avoid injury to the mucoperichondrium of the opposite side. The opposite mucoperichondrium is elevated by introducing a suitable elevator through the incision over the cartilage (Fig.14.2).

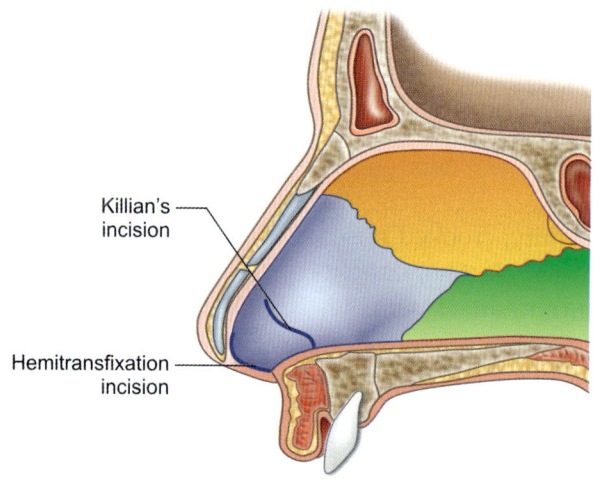

Killian's incision

Hemitransfixation incision

Fig. 14.2: Incisions for correction of the deviated nasal septum

After the elevation of both sides mucoperichondrium, a long-bladed nasal speculum is inserted and the two mucoperichondrium are kept apart by the outer surfaces of the blades, keeping the bare septum in between them. Then the cartilaginous deviation is resected either by Ballanger's swivel knife or septal punch forceps preserving a portion of cartilage in the anterior and superior parts to prevent collapse of the dorsum of the nose. The bony deviation and spurs are removed by means of a punch forceps and a bayonet-shaped gouge. The long-bladed speculum is now withdrawn and the flaps fall together. Stitching of the incision line is not required. The flaps are held in position by packing the cavities lightly by means of lubricated ribbon gauze or merocel of 8 cm length. The packs are removed after 20–48 hours (Fig. 14.3).

Decongestive nose drop, medicated steam inhalation and systemic antibiotics are preferably given after removal of the packs (Fig. 14.4).

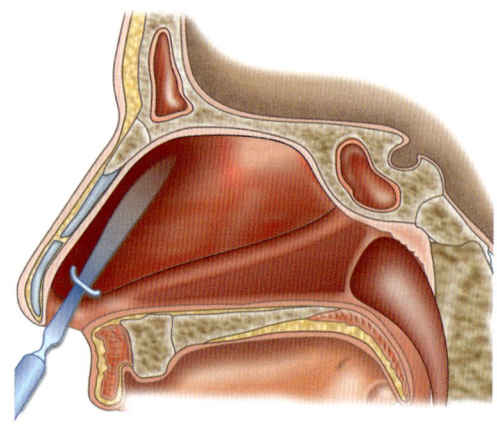

Fig. 14.3: Elevating the mucoperichondrium on the deviated side

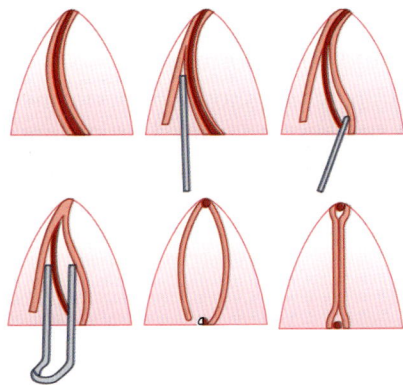

Fig. 14.4: Steps of submucous resection of the septum

Aftercare

The patient should be warned to avoid trauma for about 3 months. He should neither play football nor take part in boxing or any outdoor games for a few months.

Complications

1. Haemorrhage.
2. Septal haematoma.
3. Septal abscess.
4. Septal perforation.
5. Adhesion of the septum with the lateral wall of the nose.
6. Collapse of the dorsum of nose (Saddle nose).
7. Flappy septum.
8. Neuralgic pain.
9. Intracranial complications such as meningitis, cavernous sinus thrombosis, etc.

Cottle's Test

Septal deviations in the region of the nasal valve area cause the greatest obstruction, because this is the narrowest part of the nasal cavity. The Cottle's test confirms the obstruction in the valve area. In this useful and simple test, the patient pulls the cheek outwards and opens up the nares and thus reduces blockage.

Small septal deviations in the anterior part of the nose can cause significant obstruction, whereas large deviation can be present in the nasal cavity without affecting airflow resistance. Positive Cottle's test indicates nasal airflow obstruction due to deviation of the septum in the anterior part. The septoplasty operation is mostly suitable in these cases.

SEPTOPLASTY

It involves straightening of the nasal septum by conserving its cartilage and bones. The technique is more elaborate than SMR operation and especially suitable in children. The children with DNS between 6 and 18 years should preferably be dealt with septoplasty operation more. So if DNS is associated with deformity of the nose, septorhinoplasty should be performed.

Septoplasty is an operation, which should be performed under direct vision. This operation should not be a single standardised procedure, but should be tailored to the needs of the individual patient. For example, if the deviation is confined to the caudal border of the septum anteriorly, there is no need to touch the posterior part of the septum. However, the general principles of septoplasty include:

1. Incision
2. Exposure
3. Mobilization
4. Fixation.

Incision

The incision is best made at the lower border of the septal cartilage as was originally advocated by Freer. An unilateral hemitransfixation incision is adequate for a septoplasty. This is usually most conveniently made on the left side if the surgeon is right handed (Fig. 14.5).

Exposure

Exposure of the cartilaginous and bony septum is usually done by elevating the mucosal flap on the concave side. One **anterior tunnel** is produced by elevating mucoperichondrium over the septal cartilage above chondrovomerine junction. The two **inferior tunnels** are produced by elevating the mucoperiosteum over the anterior nasal spine on both sides over the premaxillary crest, and the vomer keeping below the chondrovomerine suture. The anterior and inferior tunnels are united under direct vision using a sharp dissector or knife. This is called "maxilla-premaxilla" approach of Cottle.

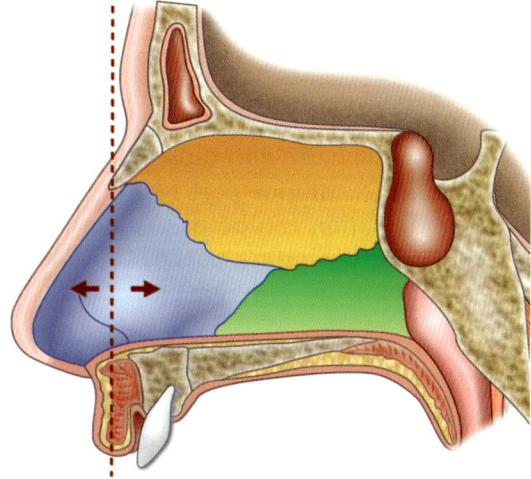

Fig. 14.5: Vertical line passing between the tip of nasal bone and maxillary bones

Mobilization and Straightening

Initially lower border of the septal cartilage is separated from its bony attachment. Then a strip of cartilage about 3–4 mm wide is removed from its lower border. The length of this cartilage may be up to 4 cm long. Then the vomerine crest is lowered and straightened. If the anterior nasal spine is deviated, it can be fractured and repositioned in the midline. In patients with deviation of external nasal pyramid, it is important to separate the skin and subcutaneous tissue from the underlying upper lateral cartilages through classical intercartilaginous incision. This allows the skin to be elevated easily over the straightened cartilaginous dorsum without the risk of cutaneous traction on the upper lateral cartilages producing the recurrence of the deviation.

Fixation

At the end of the operation the overriding of the segments is corrected by a Wright suture by applying through-and-through mattress suture with one arm passing between the segments of the cartilage and the other through all three layers of the septum. A figure of 8 suture immobilizing the lower border of the septum to the anterior nasal spine is then inserted. Finally the septocolumeller incision is closed with a few sutures. Intranasal splints and/or merocel packs are then used. This method is proved to be of no additional help in stabilizing septum postoperatively. Moreover, there is a definite risk of developing the **toxic shock syndrome**. This syndrome is multisystem disease characterised by fever, rash, hypotension, mucosal hyperemia, vomiting, diarrhoea, and multisystem organ dysfunction. It is caused by entrotoxine producing staphylococcus infections, which may be very serious and sometimes fatal.

PERFORATION OF THE NASAL SEPTUM

The perforation of septum may be either in the cartilaginous part or in the bony part. The commoner cause is trauma in the form of septal operation (SMR operation) though rare in expert hands, nose picking, and erosion by chromic acid fumes in chromium-platers.

Septal perforation may also develop secondary to lupus, tertiary stage of acquired and late form of congenital syphilis, haematoma or abscess of septum, malignant granuloma, rhinitis sicca and caseosa.

Except in syphilitic patients the perforation is found in the cartilaginous part of septum in all other cases.

Diagnosis is not difficult. It is diagnosed by anterior rhinoscopy.

Treatment: Keep the margin of perforation clean. Treatment of the causes is essential. Surgical closure may require in some percentages of patients.

15

Epistaxis, Snoring, Sleep Apnoea and Foreign Bodies in Nose

EPISTAXIS

Epistaxis is the bleeding from within the nose. It is a symptom as well as a sign. In majority of the cases it is due to a local condition. It may occur due to general causes also.

Causes of Epistaxis

Local

Congenital: Unilateral choanal atresia, meningocoele, encephalocoele, glioma

Acquired

Infective

    Acute: Viral, bacterial, fungal

    Chronic: Specific—tuberculosis, syphilis, leprosy, rhinoscleroma.

Non-specific—ozaena

Inflammatory: Rhinosinusitis (allergic/vasomotor disturbance), nasal polyposis

Traumatic

Iatrogenic (nose picking), facial trauma, foreign body, surgery

Idiopathic

Neoplastic

    Benign: Transitional cell papilloma, angiofibroma, others

    Malignant: Squamous cell carcinoma, adenocarcinoma, adenoid cystic carcinoma, olfactory neuroblastoma, melanoma, lymphoma

Drug-induced

Rhinitis medicamentosa (topical decongestants/cocaine)

Inhalants

Tobacco, cannabis, heroin, chrome, mercury, phosphorus, wood dust

General

1. Bleeding disorders
    a. Coagulopathies
        i. Inherited: Coagulation factor deficiencies, i.e. factor VIII (haemophilia A,B) and factor IX deficiency

   ii. Acquired: Anticoagulants, liver disease, vitamin K deficiency, disseminated intravascular coagulation (DIC)
 b. Platelet disorders
   i. Thrombocytopenia
      Congenital: Bone marrow failure, i.e. aplasia
      Acquired: Drugs, infiltration, increased consumption, i.e. immune modulated diseases (SLE), DIC, hypersplenism, massive blood loss
   ii. Platelet dysfunction
      Congenital: von Willebrand's disease, Bernard Soulier syndrome, Glanzmann's thrombasthenia
      Acquired: Myeloproliferative disease/leukaemia, uraemia, dysparaproteinaemias
      Drugs: Aspirin, NSAIDs, acquired storage pool disease, i.e. bypass
   iii. Blood vessel disorders
      Congenital: Osteogenesis imperfecta
      Acquired: Hereditary haemorrhagic telangiectasia, amyloid, vasculitis, vitamin C deficiency
   iv. Hyperfibrinolysis
      Congenital: X2 antiplasmin deficiency
      Acquired: Malignancy, DIC, fibrinolytic therapy, i.e. streptokinase
2. Drugs: Aspirin, anticoagulants, chloramphenicol, methotrexate, immunosuppression, alcohol, dipyridamole
3. Neoplasms
4. Idiopathic inflammatory disorders: Sarcoidosis, Wegener's Lethal midline granuloma
5. Others: Liver failure, hypothyroidism, HIV

Sources of Bleeding

1. In 90% of cases the source of bleeding is the Kiesslebach's plexus located on the anterior portion of the septum. The mucosa in this area is very fragile and adhered tightly to the underlying cartilage, thus offering a little resistance to mechanical or frictional stress.
2. Another source is capillary haemangioma occasionally found on the anterior third of the septum.
3. Bleeding from the posterior part of the nasal cavity or from the middle or superior meatus is difficult to locate. It may arise from anterior or posterior ethmoidal artery or sphenopalatine artery.

Pathology of Nasal Arteries

There is a progressive replacement of the muscle tissue in the tunica media by collagen. This change varies from interstitial fibrosis to almost complete replacement of the muscle by scar tissue. This accounts for the lengthy duration of arterial haemorrhages presumably because of a failure of the vessel to contract down in the absence of sufficient muscle in the tunica media. It seems that persons giving a history of epistaxis exhibit the more severe changes. It is also apparent that larger vessels of the calibre of the maxillary artery are prone to calcification (Monckeberg's Sclerosis). The resulting lack of elasticity could well contribute to the pathogenesis of small vessel rupture by the creation of a local systolic hypertension.

The precise mechanism of bleeding is thought to be a dissecting aneurysm of the nasopalatine artery or one of its branches, but the factors initiating this process have, so far, not been identified.

Diagnostic Steps for Epistaxis

1. History
2. Localisation of the source of bleeding by nasal endoscopy and determination of its cause
3. Blood pressure check up and assessment of the circulation.
4. Analysis of blood coagulation
5. CT scan of nose and PNS
6. Examination by general physician

Clinical Management of Spontaneous Epistaxis

Young Person with Recurrent Bleeding

Careful history taking to exclude bleeding secondary to systemic disease, the nose is carefully examined for the signs of recent bleeding and for local abnormalities. Examination should be as extensive as possible including flexible and rigid endoscopy. In the absence of any obvious local disease, attention is turned to the septum, which will often reveal an engorged vein at the anterior end of Little's area just behind the columella. If bleeding has been quite recent, a micro-aneurysm may be seen in the mucosa overlying the vein. Prominent vessels may also be seen within Little's area itself. After topical anaesthesia cauterization with a silver nitrate stick may be done. The important advice is to avoid "nose picking", to avoid blowing one nostril at a time and to use vaseline in the nasal vestibule and Little's area twice a day for a long time.

Some patients who bleed in spite of adequate attempts at cauterization, the best policy is to coagulate the offending vessel with diathermy under general anaesthesia.

Adult Person with Recurrent Bleeding

The history and examination is similar to that in the child. However, it is important in the history to ask about alcohol, current medication and blood pressure problems. Bleeding disorder should be screened, assessment of the cardiovascular system is important.

Treatment is initially with nasal cautery using silver nitrate under local anaesthesia followed by a week's course of antibiotic cream and to avoid nose picking. Resistant cases can be treated by electrocautery or diathermy under general anaesthesia. Alternative treatments include submucosal resection, transaction of varicose vessels and diathermy and excision of haemorrhagic nodules.

Management of Acute Epistaxis in the Young

The management of epistaxis at any age is well summarized by the age-old dictum: Resuscitate the patient, establish the site of bleeding, stop the bleeding, and treat the cause. Pinching the nostrils is the time-honoured method of stopping venous bleeding from the caudal end of the septum. Once bleeding has ceased, the offending vessel is cauterized under local anaesthesia. Advice them to follow as for the young person with recurrent bleeding. Occasionally, the bleeding persists despite simple measures and this often occurs in children with associated haematological problems. The nose should then be packed with vaseline gauze, a BIPP pack, nasal balloons of calcium sodium alginate. The latter is particularly useful in the very young since it can be inserted without local anaesthetic. It is relatively atraumatic and is absorbed locally. In sustained bleeding despite adequate packing, this should be treated with postnasal packs, diathermy under general anaesthesia and arterial ligation. Specialist's advice may also be required regarding haemotological replacement therapy (i.e. factor-VIII).

Management of Acute Epistaxis in Elderly

Resuscitation becomes a paramount consideration in the elderly patients with epistaxis. Observation of pulse, blood pressure and general condition are made in order to gauge the extent of any blood loss. Subsequent estimation of the packed cell volume in conjunction with the haemoglobin will guide the clinician as to the need for replacing any blood loss. If a blood dyscrasia is suspected, concurrent investigation of bleeding and clotting times along with a platelet count should be requested.

The nose is examined, preferably with the patient sitting upright in a chair. Proper precautions to avoid HIV contamination should be taken in high-risk individuals. After application of a vasoconstrictor drug (xylometozoline or oxymetozoline) try to locate the site of bleeding. In a case if the bleeding stopped already, the suspect areas can be gently rubbed with cotton tipped probe in an attempt to cause further bleeding. Formal examination should be completed with the use of flexible nasopharyngoscope, rigid endoscopes or the microscope. The accessible bleeding points are cauterized.

If the bleeding cannot be stopped or recurs, then the nose should be packed. When the bleeding is deemed to be posterior (or both anterior and posterior), then it is advisable to use a balloon catheter, such as a Foley, as an additional postnasal pack. The balloon is inflated with 15 ml of sterile water or air. Both the nasal cavities are then packed anteriorly. The old-fashioned method of controlling epistaxis by sitting the patient up with a cork between his teeth (Trotter's method) should allow him to bleed until he becomes hypotensive, is to be condemned.

Postnasal packing may be helpful in those cases where anterior packing alone has failed to control the bleeding. They may be sedated to lower their anxiety and lower their blood pressure. Sedatives should not, however, be used overzealously since heavy sedation not only increases the risks of confusion but may also allow blood to drip unnoticed into the pharynx, larynx and tracheobronchial tree with the possibility of subsequent bronchopneumonia and its inevitable consequences.

When elevated blood pressure is a significant problem, sublingual nifedipine may be helpful. If bleeding persists in spite of anterior and posterior nasal packing, then serious consideration may be given to the need for surgical intervention.

SURGICAL INTERVENTION

A patient who continues to bleed every time the pack is removed or when bleeding persists with the pack in situ will generally have to be transfused. If over a period of 4–5 days bleeding is not stopped or sooner in case of profuse haemorrhage, surgical intervention should be considered. In the absence of definite knowledge about the whereabouts of the bleeding point, it is reasonable to interrupt the external carotid system, since this supply as much as 90% of the nasal mucosa. Bleeding from the ethmoidal region is, in fact, very uncommon and is rarely severe to merit arterial ligation, in spite of the occasional report describing severe ethmoidal bleeding.

Submucous Resection

It may be helpful when bleeding originates behind a prominent septal spur, to improve access for inspection, cautery and packing and to interrupt the blood supply to Little's area haemorrhagic nodules and the septal turbinate.

Endoscopic Cautery and Ligation

The advent of endoscopic nasal surgery using rigid endoscopes has facilitated greater diagnostic accuracy regarding nasal bleeding sites and can facilitate both endoscopic cautery, unipolar diathermy or the laser as well as endoscopic ligation of the sphenopalatine artery. The carbon dioxide, argon, potassium titanyl phosphate (KTP), neodymium: yttrium-aluminium garnet (Nd: YAG) and KTP-YAG lasers have all been used.

Angiography and Embolization

The success rate in experienced hands is reported to be 90% or more. Embolization is contraindicated in the presence of angiographic evidence of significant anastomoses with the internal carotid system, severe atheromatous disease and allergy to contrast material.

Angiography may be performed directly via a percutaneous route or indirectly using digital substraction techniques. Materials, such as polyvinyl alcohol, gelfoam particles of different sizes and coiled springs can all be used for embolization

Summary of Management of Epistaxis

Local Procedures

1. Coagulation and chemical cauterization of Kisslebach's plexus
   a. Bipolar coagulation
   b. Chemical cauterization with $AgNO_3$ or chromic acid beads
2. Endoscopic ligation and coagulation of sphenopalatine artery, anterior and posterior ethmoidal artery by bipolar diathermy.

3. Selective embolisation during angiography or digital substraction angiography
4. LASER in recurrent epistaxis: Their method of action is determined according to their wavelength.
   a. Argon and Nd: YAG (Neodymium: Yttrium-aluminium garnet) LASERS are absorbed selectively by haemoglobin, resulting in a photothermolytic effect that makes them suitable for the so called "optical purse string sutures" and to treat recurrent haemorrhages in Rendu-Osler-Weber disease.
   b. CO_2 and diode lasers produce coagulation
5. Postnasal packing: The original posterior nasal packing described by Bellocq is quite stressful for the patient. The part of the nasopharynx can be closed off from the nose more easily by using a catheter with an inflatable cuff. This type of catheter should always be at hand in every hospital and ENT practice.
6. If the bleeding cannot be arrested by any other means, the following blood vessels may be ligated:
   a. Maxillary and sphenopalatine artery in the pterygopalatine fossa

Flow chart 15.1: Epistaxis management

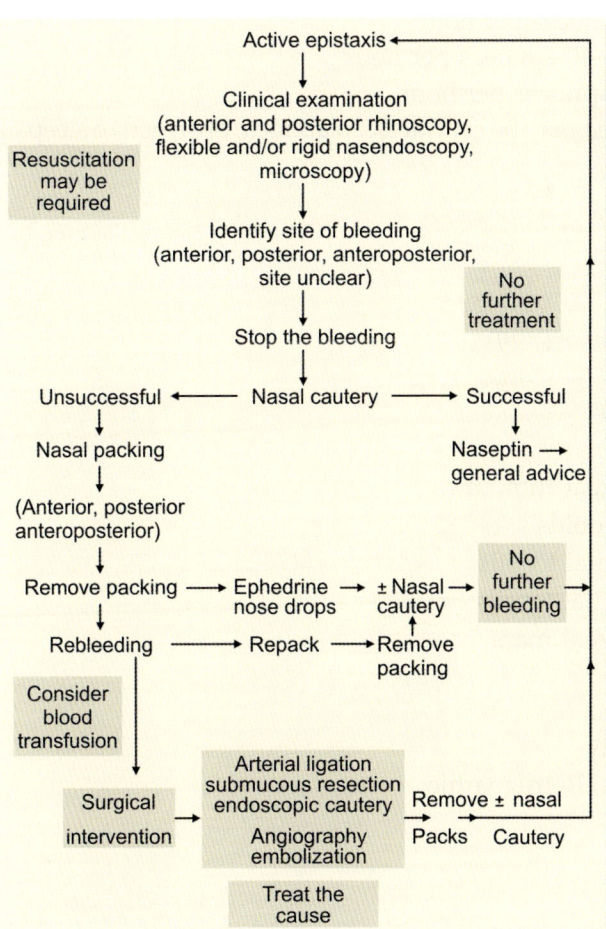

b. Anterior and posterior ethmoidal arteries
c. External carotid artery above the origin of the lingual artery.

SNORING AND SLEEP APNOEA

Definition

Snoring: A noise generated from the upper airway due to partial upper airway obstruction.
Apnoea: It is the cessation of airflow at the nostrils and mouth for at least 10 seconds.
Apnoea index (AI): It is defined as the number of apnoeas per hour of sleep.
Hypopnoea: It is a reduction in tidal volume.

The Sleep Apnoea Syndrome (SAS)

30 or more apnoeic episodes during a 7 hour period of sleep or with apnoea index equals to or greater than 5.

Grade of Sleep Apnoea

a. Mild: 5–20 apnoeas per hour
b. Moderate: 20–40 apnoeas per hour
c. Severe: > 40 apnoeas per hour

A sleep apnoea may be central sleep apnoea, obstructive sleep apnoea and mixed apnoea.

Causes of Obstructive Sleep Apnoea

Nose
• Nasal polyps
• Deviated nasal septum
• Rhinitis
• Nasal packing

Pharynx
• Nasopharyngeal tumour
• Enlarged adenoids
• Enlarged palatal tonsils
• Enlarged lingual tonsils
• Retropharyngeal mass
• Large tongue
  – Myxoedema
  – Acromegaly
• Micrognathia/Retrognathia
• Obesity

Larynx
• Tumours
• Edema

Clinical Features of Obstructive Sleep Apnoea Syndrome

Common
- Snoring
- Excessive daytime sleepiness
- Obstructive episodes

Less common
- Morning headaches
- Personality change
- Intellectual deterioration
- Poor memory
- Difficulty in concentrating
- Abnormal body movements
- Frequent waking
- Nocturnal choking
- Nocturnal enuresis
- Impotence
- Systemic hypertension
- Pulmonary hypertension
- Right heart failure
- Cardiovascular mortality

Examination

Important aspects of the examination are:
- General appearance
- Weight
- Height
- Blood pressure
- Craniofacial morphology
- Nasal airway
- Tongue size
- Soft palate/uvula/tonsils
- Nasopharynx—adenoids/polyps/cyst/tumour
- Hypopharynx—lingual tonsils, vallecula, epiglottic or supraglottic cysts/tumour
- Larynx—vocal cord mobility

Investigations

1. *To assess the patient's general condition*
    i. Full blood count: To look for polycythaemia/anaemia/mean corpuscular volume (MCV)
    ii. Thyroid function tests
    iii. Chest X-ray: To detect cardiomegaly or pulmonary disorders
    iv. ECG
    v. Blood gases: Arterial PO_2 and PCO_2

2. *To differentiate between simple snoring and sleep apnoea and determine the presence, type and severity of any apnoeic or hypopnoeic episodes.*

   Polysomnography: Parameters measured during polysomnography are:
   - Electroencephalogram (EEG)
   - Submental electromyogram (EMG)

   Electro-oculogram (EOG): These three measurements are needed for sleep staging and allow differentiation between sleep and wakefulness. The EEG allows the division of non-REM sleep into stages 1–4, the EOG detects REM stage sleep and the EMG allows the differentiation between REM sleep and arousal.

   Oxygen saturation (PO_2): Modern pulse oximeters are very reliable at measuring arterial oxygen saturation. Probes can be attached to ear lobe, finger or toe electrocardiogram (ECG).

   To monitor apnoea associated arrhythmias

   Nasal and oral air flow: Airflow is usually detected using heat sensitive thermistors. These are not able to quantify airflow but simply detect its presence or absence. Absence of airflow for greater than 10 seconds will be counted as an apnoea. It is also possible to have a CO_2 analyser that pulls expired air through a nasal or oral cannula.

   Chest and abdominal movements: Patients wear an elasticated belt around the chest and abdomen into which strain gauges are incorporated that measure changes in circumference. This information allows differentiation between central and obstructive apnoea.

   Tracheal microphony: Oesophageal balloon manometer. Allows measurement of respiratory effort as opposed to respiratory movement but obviously requires nasal intubation.

   Anterior tibialis EMG: Allows the diagnosis of periodic movements during sleep which can be a cause of excessive daytime sleepiness.

   Sleeping position detector

3. *To assess the site of obstruction.*

Tests performed on awake patients
   i. Muller manoeuvre: Patient performs a reverse valsalva during nasal endoscopy to check vellopharyngeal sphincter
   ii. Lateral cephalometry
   iii. CT scan

Tests performed in sleeping patients
   i. Fibreoptic nasendoscopy
   ii. Somnofluoroscopy
   iii. Cine CT
   iv. Pharyngeal manometry

Treatment

The choice of treatment depends on the following factors:
1. Simple snoring or obstructive sleep apnoea
2. What does the patient want?

3. The severity of the obstructive sleep apnoea and the presence of complications, i.e. apnoea index/degree of oxygen desaturation/apnoea associated cardiac arrhythmias/associated cardiopulmonary pathology.
4. The level of obstruction.

Medical Treatment

- Exclude hypothyroidism/acromegaly
- Alcohol avoidance
- Drug review
- Weight loss
- Nasal medication
- Nosovent
- Drug treatment (e.g. protriptyline)
- Positional advice
- Mandibular positioning device
- Tongue retaining device
- Nasal continuous positive airway pressure (CPAP)

Surgical Management

1. Anaesthetic considerations: Sedatives and narcotics should be avoided in the premedication. Paralysing agents should be avoided. The patient should be extubated when he is fully awake leaving a nasopharyngeal airway in place, constant PO_2 monitoring and the avoidance of narcotic analgesia.
2. Nasal surgery
3. Uvulopalatopharyngoplasty (UPPP)
4. Palatal procedures: It involves an attempt of stiffen the soft palate by removing a longitudinal strip of mucosa from its oral surface by using a Nd:YAG laser.
5. Maxillofacial techniques
6. Midline laser glossectomy: After a covering tracheostomy, carbon dioxide laser is used via an operating microscope and rectangular area of the tongue base excised down to the vallecula. Further the tongue base, hypertrophic lingual tonsils or abundant aryepiglottic folds are also excised using the laser.
7. Tracheostomy: Tracheostomy cures 100% of patients of obstructive sleep apnoea. Postoperatively patients will need extensive support and education about tracheostomy care. They can wear a speaking valve during day and leave the tube open at night. A tracheostomy will allow many patients to return to a near normal lifestyle.

FOREIGN BODIES IN NOSE

The foreign bodies in nose are commonly seen in children. They may enter by the following routes:
1. Anterior nares.
2. Posterior nares or choanae during an attack of vomiting and in paralysis of the soft palate.
3. Penetrating wounds.

Type of Foreign Bodies

These may be inanimate or animate. The common inanimate foreign bodies are-paper, beads, buttons and pebbles. Maggots and leeches are living foreign bodies in the nose.

Swabs or cotton-wool pledgets may be left inside the nose accidentally. In case of syphllis or malignancy bony sequestrum may be found. Rhinolith is another type of foreign body which forms inside the nasal cavity around a foreign body like, blood clot or mucus. This is formed of phosphates and carbonates of calcium and magnesium.

Clinical Features

In many patients the history of introducing foreign body is not obtained. In cases of forgotten foreign bodies the most important symptom is unilateral nasal obstruction with discharge, which may be foul smelling, and blood stained. The foreign body is commonly found on or near the floor of the nasal cavity. X-ray of the nasal cavity may confirm in some obscure cases if the foreign body is radiopaque.

Treatment

The treatment is removal of the foreign body under direct vision through the anterior nares by a nasal foreign body hook. If the patient is not cooperative, it should be removed under general anaesthesia. During this procedure the respective choana should be blocked by a suitable method to prevent the foreign body from slipping into the respiratory tract.

A rhinolith may require crushing and removal in piecemeal.

16

Nasal Allergy, Nasal Polyp and Cerebrospinal Rhinorrhoea

NASAL ALLERGY

An abnormal response of the tissues to certain substances is known as allergy. The causal substance which is often a protein (antigen) is called "allergen". They produce antibody. In the sensitive subjects the reticuloendothelial system reacts to foreign proteins by producing a specific antibody. The sensitive or susceptible people produce additional reaginic antibodies (IgA, reagin) associated with IgE immunoglobulins. These allergic subjects show a high IgE level in the blood. This immunoglobulin reaginic antibody combines with tissue mast cells to produce sensitization reaction.

The allergens may be classified as:
1. Exogenous—from outside the body.
2. Endogenous—from within the body.

Exogenous

i. Inhalants: These are dusts, feathers, fumes, and pollens.
ii. Ingestants: These are foods such as eggs, fish, lobster, milk, and other milk products, chocolate, etc.
iii. Contactants: Nasal drops used for relief of symptoms may produce an allergic reaction.
iv. Drugs: These include aspirin, iodine, penicillin and sulphonamides. Injections of liver extract and insulin also may cause allergic reactions.
v. Bacteria: *Streptococcus* and *Staphylococcus aureus* are said to be the most commonly responsible organisms. Fungi and parasites also may produce the same effect.

Endogenous

These include proteins from injured tissues, transudates and exudates. Heredity, endocrine disturbances, psychological upset, physical changes in the inspired air, and infection predispose to allergy.

Pathology

There will be local mucosal oedema due to increased permeability, eosinophils and plasma cells infiltration, thin watery discharge, dilatation of blood vessels with venous stasis resulting in purplish discolouration of the turbinates, and polyp formation. Secondary infection occurs with reddish discolouration of the mucosa. The discharge eventually becomes mucopurulent to frankly purulent in nature.

In the paranasal sinuses the lining mucosa becomes grossly thickened with effusion of straw-coloured fluid into the maxillary antrum. There may be formation of either ethmoidal or antrochoanal polypi.

Clinical Types

1. Seasonal.
2. Non-seasonal (perennial)

Symptoms

1. Nasal itching.
2. Sneezing, which occurs in paroxysms.
3. Nasal discharge, which is profuse, clear and watery.
4. Nasal obstruction is alternating in nature and occurs intemittently.
5. Anosmia is an occasional complaint even in the absence of obstruction.

Signs

The nasal mucosa is pale and oedematous. Excessive mucoid discharge is present. In chronic condition the mucosa becomes hypertrophied and there may be polyp formation. The mucosa shrinks considerably after application of decongestive drugs.

Diagnosis

1. History is the most important aid to a correct diagnosis.
2. Clinical findings.
3. Microscopical examination of nasal secretion, nasal mucosa or polypi will reveal plenty of eosinophils.
4. Prick and scratch tests of the skin with solutions of various allergens or blood allergy profile of specific IgE are confirmatory.
5. Elimination tests are helpful in food allergies.

Treatment

1. Removal of allergens, if possible.
2. Desensitization.
3. Antihistamine drugs—they are effectively given by mouth.
4. Local treatment:
    a. Cauterization of trigger points, e.g. the "tubercle" of the septum, and the antero-inferior border of each inferior turbinate.
    b. Submucous diathermy (SMD) of the inferior turbinate may be required if the nasal airway is obstructed by their enlargement.
5. Surgery: This should be avoided in case of nasal allergy as far as possible. If there is gross nasal obstruction, surgery may be required for the relief of it, for the drainage or removal of infected material:
    a. Removal of polypi.

b. Submucous resection of the septum may be indicated when a marked deviation of the septum is present.
c. Reduction of hypertrophied inferior turbinates (turbinoplasty).
d. Drainage of infected sinuses.
e. Removal of tonsils and adenoids. As a rule, this should be avoided unless infection is obvious.

NASAL POLYP

These are the protrusions of the hypertrophic and oedematous mucosa of the nose or paranasal sinuses. They are not regarded as neoplasms.

Types

There are two main types: simple type and neoplastic type.

Aetiology

1. Simple

   The simple type of polyps may be:
   a. Allergic: In this type the polyps are usually multiple. Eosinophils and plasma cells are found in large numbers.
   b. Infective: This is due to bacterial or viral infections. They may be
      i. Acute, i.e. of recent origin usually associated with influenza. The polypous is usually single, soft and slightly haemorrhagic.
      ii. Chronic simple, i.e. long-standing. These polypi are often multiple.
      iii. Chronic specific—rhinosporidiosis.
   c. Mixed (infective and allergic): This is probably due to secondary infection in the allergic type.
2. Neoplastic
   a. Benign: The bleeding polypous of the septum is a misnomer for "fibroangioma" or granuloma. Neurofibromata and fibromas may appear as polypoid tumours. Glioma in infants and meningioma in adults may also resemble a polyp.
   b. Malignant: These may be either carcinomatous or sarcomatous. They may simulate "mucous" polypi, but are usually more solid, friable and haemorrhagic.

There have been a number of different theories put forward for the pathogenesis of nasal polyps. There are five main theories of pathogenesis:

The Bernoulli's phenomenon, polysaccharide changes, vasomotor imbalance; infection and allergy. All may contribute polyp formation but none is obviously the commonest aetiology.

Antrochoanal polyps are an entity of unknown aetiology. They are not associated with allergy. Proetz suggested that they may contribute to a faulty development of a maxillary sinus ostium since it is always large. The ostium may be large because of expansion by the polyp but this is unlikely since there is no expansion of the posterior choana by a large polyp nor is there any erosion or displacement of the middle turbinate medially.

Pathology

Macroscopic

The nasal polypi consist of soft smooth bluish-white masses arising most commonly from the mucosa of the ethmoidal air cells and maxillary sinuses. Sometimes the mucosal covering of the turbinates and septum may undergo polypoidal degeneration.

Microscopic

They are oedematous hypetrophied masses of mucous membrane, covered by ciliated columnar epithelium. Sometimes the ciliated epithelium may undergo squamous metaplasia due to chronic irritation. The stroma is fibrillar and oedematous due to intercellular serous fluid. The glands are scanty but dilated. Lymphocytes, plasma cells and eosinophils are seen in varying numbers in the submucous layer.

Site of Origin

1. Ethmoidal: Polypi arising from the ethmoidal air cells or the middle turbinate are multiple and tend to grow forward towards the anterior nares. These may develop at any age but common in adults. They have a tendency to recur.
2. Antral or antrochoanal polyp arising from the lateral wall or floor of the maxillary antrum is usually single though multiple polypi may be present in the antrum. Antral polyp comes into the nasal cavity usually through the accessory ostium and then extends backward to the choana or posterior nares and as such is named antrochoanal polypous. These are commonly found in childhood or adolescence than in adult life. They do not recur if removed completely from the base.

Clinical Features

The symptoms usually start slowly but may be sudden and rapid after an acute infection.

1. The chief symptom is nasal obstruction. This may lead to anosmia, epiphora, postnasal drip, headache, snoring and nasal speech.
2. Sneezing and watery nasal discharge are common in allergic cases.
3. Mucopurulent discharge is common in infective cases.
4. Broadening of the nose due to expansion of the nasal bones is common in ethmoidal polypi.

Anterior Rhinoscopy

The ethomoidal polypi look like a bunch of grapes with a gelatinous appearance. The surface is smooth. The shape is oval, the colour is usually pale or bluish white but may become pink or dark red owing to transformation of the mucosa to the squamous epithelium due to constant exposure to atmosphere with its dust and irritation.

The antrochoanal polyp cannot be seen in most of the cases by anterior rhinoscopy.

Posterior Rhinoscopy

Antrochoanal polyp looks rounded, smooth, greyish-blue in colour. Sometimes it may be so enlarged that it is seen in the oropharynx hanging from above and posterior to the soft palate (Fig. 16.1).

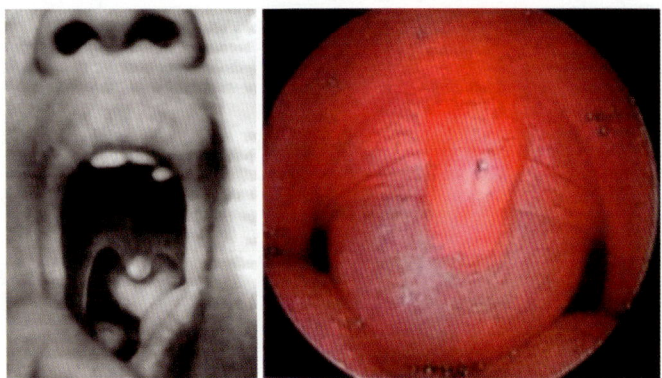

Fig. 16.1: Giant antrochoanal polyp hanging into the oropharynx from behind the soft palate

Probe Test

With the probe both ethmoidal and antrochoanal polypi are found to be mobile and soft. The antrochoanal polyp is free from attachments in the nasopharynx, which should be palpated by right index finger. They are insensitive to touch. The stalk or pedicle of the polyp may be identified in the middle meatal region.

Diagnosis

Squamous or transitional cell papilloma sometimes look like polypi. They may be smooth, pinkish and fleshy.

Unilateral and haemorrhagic polypi should be submitted for histopathology. Radiography in the form of X-ray and CT scan of the sinuses helps in diagnosis by widespread changes due to infection or allergy. Bony erosion by antral neoplasms may also be visualized. A meningocele may be mistaken for a polypous.

Prognosis

In simple type the prognosis is good regarding life and not favourable regarding recurrence. In malignant neoplastic type the prognosis is bad.

Treatment

When diagnosed the treatment involves removal of the polypi which should be followed by thorough investigation and treatment of causal factors. In allergic type antihistaminic preparations are applied locally or given by mouth and other antiallergic regimen should be followed. Nasal spray in the form of fluticasone, mometasone, etc. for a prolonged period reduce the polyps and prevent recurrences.

In the infective type local decongestants are used as drops or sprays. Proetz displacement therapy with 1% ephedrine saline solution has been found beneficial.

Differential diagnosis of nasoantral or nasal polyps

	Antrochoanal polyp	Adenoids	Hypertrophied inferior turbinate	Nasopharyngeal fibroma	Malignant growth	Rhinosporidiosis
Age	Children	Children	Adult	Young adult	Common in elderly	Any age
Colour	Greyish white	Pink	Pale in allergy	Red	Reddish with slough	Reddish with white spots on the surface
Surface	Smooth	Irregular with ridges and furrows	Smooth or irregular mulberry appearance in long-standing cases of allergy	Smooth and lobulated	Irregular	Finely granular
Site of origin	Maxillary antrum	Junction of roof and posterior wall of nasopharynx	Lateral wall of nose at its lower part	Near spheno-palatine foramen	Any wall of nasopharynx	Usually from septum also from other parts of nasal cavity
Mobility	Mobile	Fixed	Fixed	Fixed	Fixed	Mobile
Consistency	Soft	Soft rubbery	Firm	Firm to hard	Hard indurated	Soft
Bleeding on touch	Nil	Nil	Nil	Present	Present	Present
Lymph node involvement	Nil	Nil	Nil	Nil	Present	Nil
X-ray sinuses	Opacity maxillary antrum	No abnormality	No abnormality	No abnormality Bony erosion in long-standing cases	Bony erosion present	No abnormality
CT scan	Confirmative	Confirmative	Confirmative	Confirmative	Helpful	Helpful

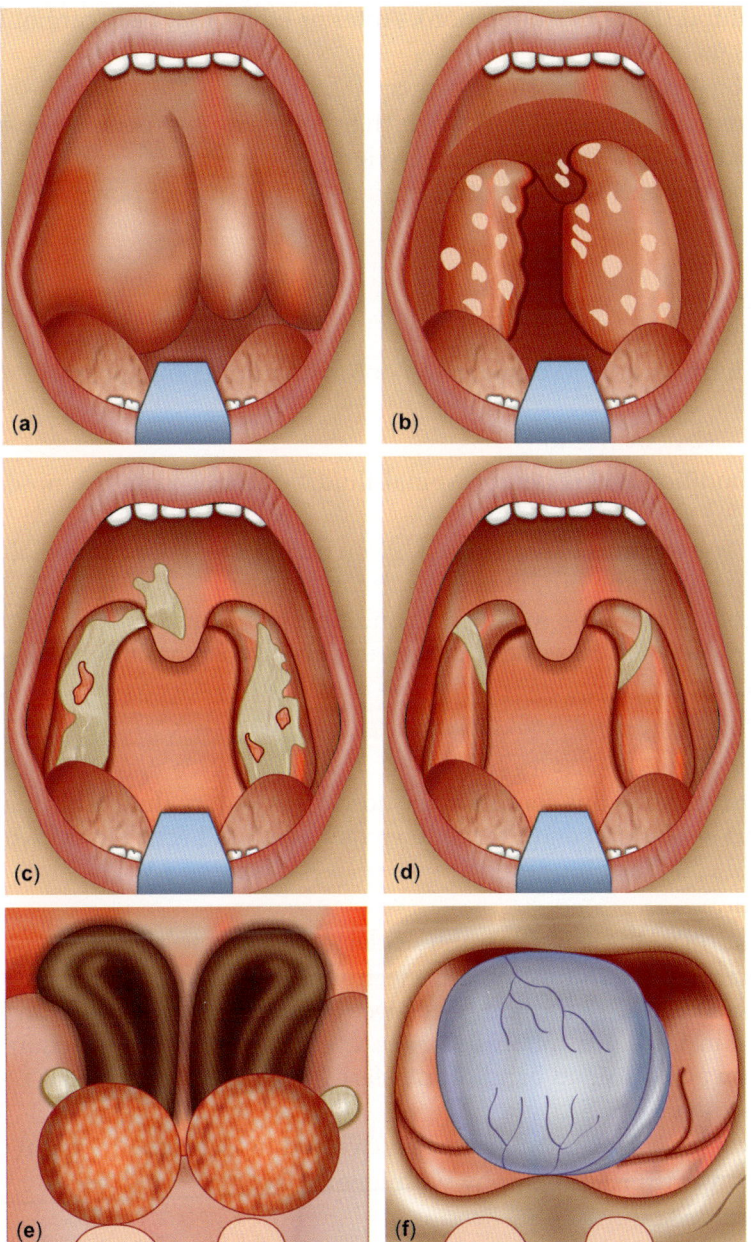

Fig. 16.2: (a) Acute peritonsillar abscess; (b) Acute follicular tonsillitis; (c) Faucial diptheria; (d) Vincent's angina; (e) Papillary hypertrophy of the posterior ends of the inferior turbinates; (f) Antrochoanal polyp (right) as seen by posterior rhinoscopy

In recurrent ethmoidal polypi exenteration of ethmoidal cells (ethmoidectomy) should be performed through any of the three routes:

i. Intranasal, complete clearance of polypi is rarely possible.

ii. Extranasal, safe and more thorough.

iii. Transantral (Horgan's operation). Anterior ethmoidal cells cannot be reached by this method.

iv. Functional endoscopic sinus surgery (FESS).

In recurrent antrochoanal polyp, which is very rare, endoscopic removal should be combined with a Caldwell-Luc operation.

Complications and sequelae of operations for removal of polypi include:

1. Adhesions.
2. Anosmia.
3. Damage to eyeball and optic nerve.
4. Meningitis.
5. CSF rhinorrhoea due to damage to floor of anterior cranial fossa.

CEREBROSPINAL RHINORRHOEA

This is a condition where cerebrospinal fluid flows out from the nose. This may follow:

1. *Trauma:* The fracture base of the skull involving the anterior cranial fossa with the tearing off of the duramater.
2. *Spontaneous:* Rarely the malignant condition may cause erosion of the floor of the anterior cranial fossa with the result of cerebrospinal fluid leakage into the nasal cavity.

Methods of diagnosis are

1. Reservoir sign
2. *Handkerchief test:* In this condition the nose drips watery fluid. This fluid contains no mucus or albumin and the handkerchief does not become hard when it dries. This fluid contains glucose.
3. Halo sign

    β_2 transferrin in the sample (immunoelectrophoresis test):

    β_2 transferrin is the routine protein electrophoresis of serum, only one transferrin band is seen in the B1-fraction. Two electrophoretically different transferrins can be found in the electrophoresis of the CSF proteins: the β_1-fraction of normal transferrin and a second band of transferrin in the β_2-fraction. This β_2-fraction is pathognomonic of CSF.
4. Intrathecal injection of 5% fluorescein dye and its detection by nasal endoscopy
5. CT scan and CT cisternography with Iohexol dye
6. Radionuclide scan.

Treatment

Immediate

1. Systemic antibiotics.
2. Avoidance of nose blowing.
3. Avoidance of packing the nose.

Delayed

1. If traumatic—repair of the fracture base of the skull endoscopically by fascial graft.
2. Treatment of the cause.

17

Inflammation of the Nose

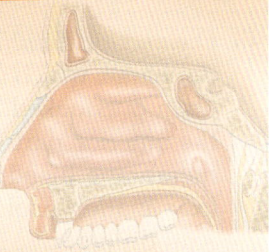

The inflammations of the nose may be acute and chronic owing to infection, allergy, and physical or chemical trauma.

INFLAMMATIONS OF EXTERNAL NOSE

The skin covering the external nose is subject to those conditions affecting the skin elsewhere.

1. Furunculosis of the vestibule of nose.
2. Non-specific nasal vestibulitis.
3. Erysipelas: It is an acute spreading *Streptococcal lymphangitis.*
4. Specific rhinitis tuberculosis and lupus vulgaris, syphilis, etc. may involve the external nose.

INFLAMMATION OF THE NASAL CAVITIES

Inflammation of the nasal mucosa is called rhinitis. Rhinitis may be acute and chronic.

Common Cold

It is supposed to be due to viral infection and an acute condition. This is usually complicated by the secondary bacterial infection.

Clinical Features

There are four distinct stages:

a. Stage of ischaemia: A burning sensation is felt in the nasopharynx. Sneezing occurs because of irritation of the nasal mucosa.
b. Stage of hyperemia: After a few hours of the first stage profuse watery nasal discharge and nasal obstruction ensue. There may be a rise in the temperature.
c. Stage of secondary infection: The discharge becomes yellow or green and thick.
d. Stage of resolution: Occurs in 5 to 10 days.

Differential Diagnosis

i. Allergic rhinitis is not associated with fever. Discharge contains plenty of eosinophils unless secondarily infected.
ii. *Influenzal rhinitis:* In this condition the constitutional symptoms are more severe.

iii. *Diphtheritic rhinitis:* It is common in children. It causes nasal obstruction and discharge, which may be bloodstained. The patient does not look ill and is very often overlooked. On examination a greyish white membrane is revealed on the anterior part of nasal septum and the adjacent parts. On removal of the membrane bleeding occurs. The diagnosis is confirmed by bacteriological examination. Isolation of the patient is essential. Antibiotics must be given. Anti-diphtheritic serum is not required to be administered.

Treatment

General
  i. Rest and warmth.
  ii. Sedation.
  iii. Antihistaminics.
  iv. Antibiotics when secondary infection is present.

Local
  i. Decongestant drops 1/2 to 1 per cent ephedrine hydrochloride in normal saline to drop into the nasal cavities. Oxymetazoline or xylometazoline drops may also be used.
  ii. Medicated steam inhalation.

Chronic Rhinitis

Chronic rhinitis may be
1. Non-specific
2. Specific

Non-specific
  i. Simple rhinitis.
  ii. Hypertrophic rhinitis.
  iii. Atrophic rhinitis.
  iv. Rhinitis sicca.
  v. Rhinitis caseosa.

Specific
  i. Tuberculosis.
  ii. Syphilis.
  iii. Lupus vulgaris.
  iv. Scleroma.
  v. Leprosy.
  v. Rhinosporidiosis.
  vi. Aspergillosis.
  vii. Actinomycosis and blastomycosis.
  viii. Moniliasis or thrush.

Atrophic Rhinitis

It is a condition in which the nasal mucosa and turbinates undergo atrophy. It is commonly found in females of the younger age group. It may or may not be associated with foetor. Atrophic rhinitis with foetor is known as ozaena.

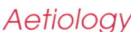

Aetiology

The aetiology is still uncertain.

The following theories have been advanced as to the cause of the disease:

1. It is the result of the local disease in one or the other of the paranasal air sinuses.
2. It is the terminal stage of a chronic purulent rhinitis
3. Hereditary factors play some role in the causation of ozaena.
4. It is due to some disturbances of the endocrine system. So the disease is very common at the age of puberty and menopause.
5. Vitamin disturbances may play a part.

The accepted view is that the disease is due to some hereditary or endocrine factor. The foetor is caused by saprophytic organisms. Poor nutrition is undoubtedly a factor in the development of the atrophic rhinitis and it is considered to be an iron deficiency disease. Recently, immunologists have considered atrophic rhinitis to be autoimmune disease.

Types

a. Primary (ozaena).
b. Secondary: Syphilis, lupus, extensive nasal surgery and gross DNS which results the unilateral atrophic rhinitis in the roomy side.

There are two types of atrophic rhinitis.

Type 1: It is characterised by endarteritis and periarteritis of the terminal arterioles which is the result of chronic infection and which might benefit from the vasodilator effect of oestrogen therapy.

Type 2: In this type, there is dilatation of the capillaries which might be made worse with oestrogen therapy. It seems likely that in the past the majority of cases were of type 1. The endothelial cell lining in dilated capillaries is having more cytoplasm than normal capillaries and showed a positive reaction for alkaline phosphatase which suggest the presence of active absorption of bone which is a feature of atrophic rhinitis.

Symptoms

1. Dryness of the nose.
2. Headache.
3. Sensation of nasal obstruction due to the formation of crusts.
4. Anosmia.
5. Epistaxis after separation of the crust.
6. A foul odour is the outstanding symptom and it may be so severe as to render the sufferer an outcast from society.

Signs

1. Widened nasal cavity.
2. The inferior turbinates are flattened and may be difficult to distinguish upon the lateral walls of the nose.
3. The greenish crusts may fill the nasal cavities.

An examination of the nasopharynx may reveal dry mucosa and crusting. The posterior wall is usually glazed because of an extension of the atrophic condition. It may be extended down to the larynx in certain cases.

Differential Diagnosis

1. Sinus suppuration.
2. Tuberculosis and Lupus.
3. Syphilis.
4. Foreign bodies or rhinolith.
5. Scleroma.

Treatment

Conservative

1. Removal of crusts by nasal douches with warm isotonic or alkaline solutions.
2. Painting of the nasal cavity with 25 per cent anhydrous glucose in glycerin. This prevents adherence of crusts and inhibits the growth of saprophytic organisms.
3. After cleansing, a spray of oestradiol in oil (0.5 ml of a solution containing 5 mg per ml) has been found beneficial. 0.25 ml is sprayed into each nostril daily. It is beneficial in type I pathology.

Promising results using tissue therapy with systemic human placental extracts gave 80% improvement in two years and sub-mucosal intranasal injection of human placental extracts produced 93.3% relief over the same period of time. Rifampicin in a dose of 600 mg orally once a day for 12 weeks has claimed to give good results.

Surgical

1. Sinus infection must be properly treated.
2. The narrowing of the nasal cavities is effected by the inward displacement of the entire lateral wall of the nose and submucous insertion of small porcelain pellets into the septum and floor of the nose.

Injections of powdered teflon in glycerin have been successfully used. The Stensen's duct is transplanted inside the nasal cavity in order to supplement the nasal secretion.

Latest development in the treatment of this disease is closure of one or both nostrils by plastic surgery. The nasal mucosa becomes normal on reopening of the nostril after a few months or years (Young's operation).

Successful results using intranasal medullary bone graft as a single long piece of bone reported to give successful results. Repeated stellate ganglion blocks have been employed with some success. Some advocate cervical sympathectomy or blockade as a first line of treatment. Bilateral closure of the nostrils was not tolerated by some patients who dislike mouth breathing and nasal voice. However, partial nostril closure leaving 3 mm hole was well tolerated and gave similar results with no recurrence of disease over a period of two years. Any further increase in the size of the hole rapidly decreases their success rate.

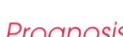

Prognosis

The prognosis regarding life is good but regarding cure is bad. The disease usually persists for years. Spontaneous cure is not unknown.

Causes of foul smelling nasal discharge

This may be unilateral or bilateral. The causes are

1. Atrophic rhinitis
2. Forgotten foreign body in the nose or rhinolith,
3. Chronic maxillary sinusitis of dental origin
4. Syphilitic rhinitis.

The most common unilateral cause in children is forgotten foreign body in the nose.

Treatment

The treatment of foul smelling nasal discharge is to treat the cause after proper investigation and diagnosis. For which please see the respective disease.

Rhinosporidiosis

This is a chronic condition caused by Rhinosporidium Seeberi or R. Kinealyi a spore-bearing parasite. It is common in Southern India, Bankura and Purulia districts in West Bengal, Srilanka and Africa. It is common in male in the younger age group. The masses appear as a slender filiform or narrow leaf like processes of a dull-pink or reddish tint and contain the spores. The surface is studded with many minute whitish spots owing to the presence of sporangia in the tissue. The growths are very friable and bleed to the touch. The mode of infection is probably by polluted dust and water from the dung of infected cows and buffaloes. Epistaxis is the main symptom with nasal discharge and partial obstruction.

Treatment

1. Surgical removal of the mass preferably with a diathermy knife.
2. Application of a 2 per cent aqueous solution of Antimony tartarate. Recurrence is very common.

The most successful treatment is wide excision with a cutting diathermy and cautery of the base of the lesions. Medical treatment in the form of local injection of depo corticosteroids into the polypoidal masses and systemic courses of amphotericine (fungizone) and dapsone may be given in addition.

Rhinoscleroma

Scleroma is a chronic granulomatous disease of the respiratory tract especially of the nose. The causative factor is *Klebsiella rhinoscleromatis* or *Frisch bacillus*. This disease is very common in northern part of our country and appears to be associated with lack of hygiene. It may occur in any age and in both sexes but young adults are mainly affected.

Pathology

The submucous tissue is infiltrated with:

  i. Mikulicz cells, i.e. large foam cells with central nucleus containing Frisch bacilli in the vacuoles of cytoplasm.
 ii. Russel bodies: These resemble plasma cells with eccentric nucleus and eosinophil staining cytoplasm.

The infiltration starts at the mucocutaneous junction and slowly progresses backwards.

Clinical Features

The disease is seen in three stages:

1. *Atrophic stage:* There is nasal obstruction, discharge, crusting and adhesion.
2. *Nodular stage:* The main symptom in this stage is nasal obstruction. Soft and red nodules may appear in the nasal cavity.
3. *Stenotic stage:* This stage comprises adhesions and cicatrization. The nasal chambers become stenosed.

Treatment

Injection of streptomycin sulphate or tetracycline for a period of about three months gives good results. The bacilli are also sensitive to chloramphenicol and polymyxin B. Steroids may be given with good results along with local and systemic antibiotics.

Excision of the lesion may be required to restore the nasal airways.

Rhinophycomycosis

It is a deep fungal infection of nose caused by *Conidiobolus coronatus*. It may present with nasal polyp and granulations. Broad-spectrum antifungal drugs like ketoconazole, an imidazole antifungal is effective. Liver function tests should be done before administration. Preferable to take in empty stomach, i.e. 1 hour before or 2 hours after food. Prolonged use of potassium iodide also helps.

Rhinocerebral Phycomycosis

It is caused by a fungus of phycomycetes or zygomycetes group. It has got an affinity to involve cerebral blood vessels. It is common in elderly diabetics and in immunosuppressive patients. It is treated with intravenous infusion of amphotericin B, surgical excision and effective control of diabetes mellitus.

Fungal Sinusitis

Fungal sinusitis can be invasive and non-invasive based on the invasion of the sinus mucosa by fungal hyphae of Aspergillus fumigatus fungus commonly. It may also be caused by *Curvularia, Conidiobolus coronatus, Candida* species, etc.

Noninvasive

  i. Mycetoma or fungal ball
 ii. Allergic fungal sinusitis (AFS)

Invasive
  i. Chronic immunocompetent and immunocompromised
  ii. Acute fulminant immunocompromised
  iii. Sclerosing
  iv. Granulomatous

Fungal Ball

It usually affects one maxillary sinus. Commonly caused by *Aspergillus fumigatus*. Fungal ball is a clay-like material studded with sporangia.

Treatment is by complete removal of the mass and improve the aeration of the affected sinus. Functional endoscopic sinus surgery (FESS) is the treatment of choice for removal of the mass through endoscopic middle meatal antrostomy (MMA).

Allergic Fungal Sinusitis (AFS)

It occurs commonly in atopic individuals. It is characterized by polyp formation and allergic mucin. There is no mucosal invasion in this type of fungal infection. The organisms are *Aspergillus*, *Bipolaris*, *Alternaria* and *Curvularia* species. It has no sex predilection. Nasal breathing difficulty and loss of smell (anosmia) are the main symptoms.

The allergic mucin contains Charcot Leyden crystals, fungal hyphae and eosinophils. Fungal hyphae require Grocott Gomori methenamine stain.

CT scan shows mucosal edema with metallic tonality (hyperdense areas).

Functional endoscopic sinus surgery (FESS) is the treatment of choice. Preoperative and postoperative prednisolone in the dose of 0.4 to 0.5 mg per kg body weight along with intranasal spray of steroids in the form of Fluticasone/ Mometasone or Budesonide, etc. are very helpful. These lines of treatment result in disappearance of sinonasal polyps and also prevent recurrence of FESS.

Prolonged use of systemic steroids in a very low dose of 0.1 mg per kg body weight, though in a very low dose, may cause osteoporosis in the long run. Therefore steroids along with systemic use of calcium should be given. In this condition antihistaminics have no role. Sinonasal douching with antifungal drugs like itraconazole in the postoperative period may reduce the recurrence.

Invasive Fungal Sinusitis (Chronic type)

The causative organisms are aspergilllus and some dermataceous fungi. The characteristic feature is the mucosal invasion.

Clinically, nasal polyposis and granulomatous inflammations are the diagnostic features. It is commonly found in the diabetic and immunocompromised individuals.

Treatment is surgical excision of the diseased tissues and proper ventilation of the sinuses. Systemic antifungals like liposomal amphotericin B are very useful with monitoring of the renal and liver functions.

18

Diseases of the Paranasal Sinuses

ACUTE SINUSITIS

Acute inflammation of the paranasal sinus mucosa is called acute sinusitis. This is almost always associated with acute inflammation of the nasal mucosa, i.e. acute rhinitis.

Maxillary sinus is most commonly involved due to two factors:

    i. Inadequate drainage of this sinus owing to the position of the ostium which is situated near the roof of its medial wall.

    ii. Relation of the upper premolar and molar teeth on to the floor of the sinus.

Involvement of the maxillary sinus is followed by the ethmoid, the frontal and the sphenoid in that order. More than one sinus may be involved at a time.

Aetiology

Predisposing Factors

The following predisposing and contributory factors are usually responsible for sinusitis:

1. Nasal, pharyngeal and dental infection.
2. Bathing in unhygienic pools and infected water.
3. Trauma, fractures of the sinus wall.
4. General diseases such as influenza, measles, whooping cough and other specific diseases in children.
5. Poor general environment like ill-ventilated housing condition, and overcrowding.
6. Lowered body resistance.
7. Undue exposure to cold.
8. Nasal obstruction due to deviation of the nasal septum, oedematous and hypertrophied turbinates, and tumours.
9. Chest diseases such as chronic bronchitis, asthma and bronchiectasis.

Exciting Factors

1. Viral infection—is likely to be most common in acute sinusitis and bacteria are the secondary invadors.
2. Bacterial infection.

Pneumococci, Streptococci, Staphylococci, *Haemophilus influenzae*, *Escherichia coli*, *Micrococcus catarrhalis*, *Bacillus pfeiffer's* and *B. Friedlander's* and *K. pneumonae* have been found in sinusitis.

The most common organism in acute sinusitis is *Pnemococcus* followed by *Streptococcus*. *E. coli* and anaerobic Streptococci are present in dental sinusitis.

Pathology

Initially there is dilatation of capillaries with increased blood supply followed by exudation of serum and outpouring of polymorphonuclear leucocytes. This is associated with redness, oedema and swelling of the mucous membrane. The oedema is due to the passage of fluid through the walls of the dilated capillaries into the tissues causing obstruction of the return of body fluids through the veins and lymphatics. The mucous glands become hypertrophied.

Clinically, the inflammation of the sinuses may be either catarrhal or suppurative. In the early stages it is usually catarrhal, with hyperaemia and mucoid discharge. With increased involvement of mucous membrane or with severe infections, the discharge becomes mucopurulent to purulent. If the sinusitis is dental in origin, it becomes suppurative from the very beginning.

The virulence and the type of organisms, together with the state of resistance of the patient decide whether in the early stages the changes are mainly catarrhal or mainly suppurative.

Clinical Features

Symptoms

General: Malaise, headache and fever in the more acute cases. Very high fever which is not usual, suggests a closed infection or a complication.

Local: Feeling of discomfort in the postnasal space, nasal obstruction, with loss of vocal resonance. There may be anosmia or cacosmia.

Nasal or postnasal discharge. Postnasal drip may be associated with an unpleasant taste.

Epistaxis is commonly associated with the acute infection of the antrum. Pain over the sinus may be referred to teeth or gum, ear and supraorbital region on the affected side.

Signs

External: There may be slight flushing of the cheek with swelling. Tenderness over the cheek in maxillary sinusitis and over the floor of the sinus in frontal sinusitis.

Anterior Rhinoscopy

General redness and swelling of the nasal mucosa are commonly associated with the sinus infection. These obscure the local signs of sinusitis.

If not associated with generalized rhinitis, localized area of red, shiny and swollen mucosa in the neighbourhood of the ostium is seen. Pus in the middle meatus is commonly seen. The middle turbinate may be found swollen.

Posterior Rhinoscopy

Pus may be seen on the upper surface of the palate or trickling down the lateral pharyngeal gutter.

Investigations

Bacteriology: Culture the organism and assess its sensitivity test.

Trasillumination: This method is used very rarely nowadays. It may be done where the X-ray facilities are not available.

X-ray examination: In routine practice occipitomental view may be adequate. The sinus may be hazy or opaque, or may show a fluid level if taken in the erect position.

CT Scan

Differential Diagnosis

1. Dental, temporomandibular, trigeminal, and herpetic or post-herpetic neuralgia.
2. Migraine.
3. Nasopharyngeal tumours.
4. Brainstem lesions: Tumours of pons and medulla, disseminated sclerosis, thrombotic lesions and syringobulbia may also set up facial pain.
5. Specific fevers: Measles, nasal diphtheria, typhoid fever, cerebrospinal meningitis, erysipelas, foreign bodies into the nose in children, rhinoliths in adults.
6. Angioneurotic oedema.
7. Insect bite.
8. Neoplasms of the sinuses.

Complications of Sinusitis

It is common during an acute exacerbation of chronic suppurative sinusitis. The infection may spread through the following routes:

1. Through the bony wall directly
2. Venous spread
3. Lymphatic spread
4. Through the perineural spaces of the olfactory nerves to the subarachnoid space.

The complications are as follows:

1. Osteomyelitis
2. Orbital cellulitis
3. Orbital abscess
4. Cavernous sinus thrombosis
5. Meningitis
6. Brain abscess
7. Extradural abscess
8. Subdural abscess

The commonest complications are orbital ones. This is associated commonly with ethmoidal sinusitis. As the ethmoidal sinuses are present at birth and expand fairly rapidly, these complications occur mostly in older children.

Treatment

Principles of treatment:

1. Treatment of infection
2. Treatment of pain
3. Establishment of proper drainage.

The treatment of acute sinusitis is mostly conservative. Minor surgical procedure like antral lavage may be required when the medical treatment for about 7 to 10 days fails to cure the patient.

1. Rest in bed in a warm, well-ventilated room and light diet.
2. Analgesics like paracetamol 0.5 g. two to three times daily.
3. Decongestive nose drop like 1/2 to 1% ephedrine saline is safe and effective.

   The patient should be taught the correct technique of instillation of nose drop in which the head should be tilted far back and a little towards the affected side to let the drops get into the middle meatus of nose.
4. Medicated steam inhalation as well as short wave diathermy for 12 to 15 days is particularly helpful.
5. Systemic suitable antibiotics in adequate doses should be given for about 7 to 10 days.

If the symptoms persist even after 7–10 days of proper treatment, antrum puncture and washout should be carried out followed by injection of penicillin and/or streptomycin solution inside the antrum.

Nasal douching should always be avoided in the acute stage owing to the risk of spreading infection.

CHRONIC MAXILLARY SINUSITIS

This usually results from a residue of an acute inflammation. It may arise in the absence of a preceeding acute process as a result of the extension of a chronic inflammation from the nasal cavity or other paranasal sinuses. Another cause of chronic maxillary sinusitis may be an infection in the root of an upper molar or premolar tooth of the respective side.

Symptoms

1. Nasal obstruction
2. Nasal discharge more or less copious. It may often be mucopurulent.
3. Headache.
4. Early weariness from mental exertion.
5. Hyposmia and sometimes, cacosmia, i.e. perception of a foul odour in the nose.

Signs

Anterior rhinoscopy reveals changes in the middle meatus, such as inflammatory changes in the mucosa and polypi, as well as a purulent or mucopurulent discharge which quickly reappears even after being wiped off with a cotton swab.

Diagnosis

The diagnosis of chronic maxillary sinusitis is based on the record of complaints and physical signs. A differential diagnosis is facilitated by other methods, such as X-ray, transillumination, CT scan, proof puncture and irrigation of the maxillary antrum.

Treatment

An effective conservative treatment of chronic maxillary sinusitis is done by irrigation of the antrum (antrum puncture and washout) with a saline solution followed by its injection with penicillin or streptomycin solutions, 200,000 to 250,0000 units in 2 or 3 ml of water.

Contraindications of antral lavage

1. A child under the age of 3 years due to proximity of orbital floor and the teeth in the small maxillary sinus.
2. In the hypoplastic maxilla with thick bony walls.
3. In acute maxillary sinusitis.
4. In the presence of trauma.

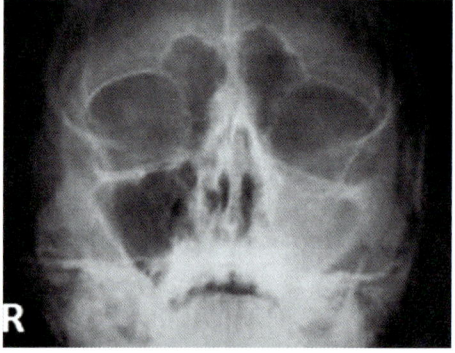

Fig. 18.1: Opacity of the left maxillary sinus

INTRANASAL ANTROSTOMY (INA)

The principle of this operation is to make an opening in the nasoantral wall of the inferior meatus by means of antrum harpoon and burr. This procedure is no longer performed nowadays. Middle meatal antrostomy (MMA) is commonly done with the help of fibreoptic rigid endoscope. This operation is preferably performed under local anaesthesia. The opening is made as far forward as possible and should be a large one. After 3 to 4 days the antrum is washed out by means of a cannula (antrum washing cannula) and Higginson's syringe. A warm sterile saline solution is usually used.

In the majority of cases, however, surgery is indicated for the removal of polypi and granulations from the sinus and to provide for a wide communication between the latter and the nasal cavity.

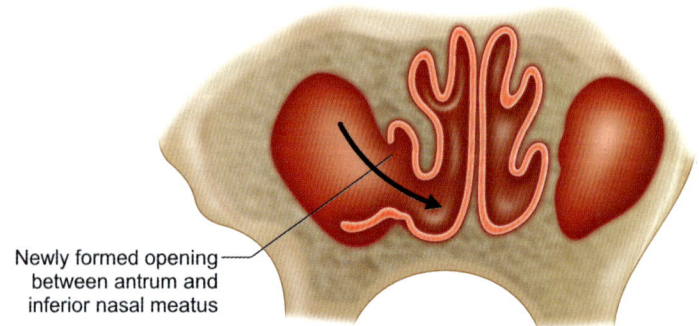

Newly formed opening between antrum and inferior nasal meatus

Fig. 18.2: Intranasal antrostomy (right)

CALDWELL-LUC OPERATION

The operation was designed to remove irreversibly damaged mucosa of the maxillary sinus and to facilitate gravitational drainage and aeration via an inferior meatal antrostomy (INA) (Fig. 18.3).

Indications

1. Chronic maxillary sinusitis.
2. Removal of foreign bodies.
3. Closure of oroantral fistula.
4. Antral dental cysts.
5. Access to the pterigomaxillary fissure, pterigopalatine fossa.
6. Removal of recurrent antrochoanal polyps.
7. Elevation and stabilization of orbital floor, fractures or removal of orbital floor in decompression.

It is not recommended as the route for biopsy of antral malignancy as it potentially opens the hitherto unaffected area to contamination.

Contraindications

It is not performed in children as it may damage the secondary dentition.

Complications

1. Pain and soft tissue swelling.
2. Haemorrhage.
3. Paraesthesia due to damage of infraorbital nerve.
4. Neuralgia.
5. Damage to the teeth and their innervation leading to alteration in dental sensation and occasional devitalization and discolouration of the tooth.
6. Oroantral fistula.

This operation is commonly performed under general anaesthesia but may also be performed under local anaesthesia. The first stage involves the incision of the

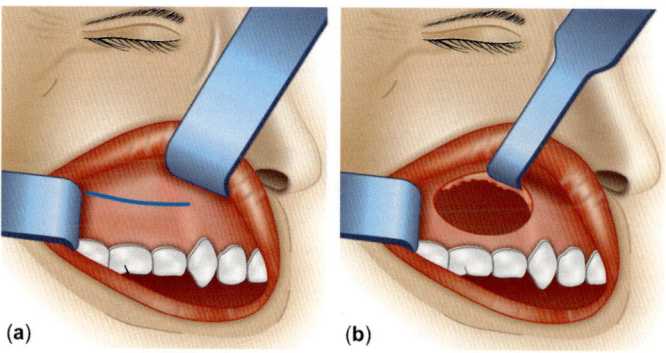

(a)   (b)

Fig. 18.3: Caldwell-Luc operation. (a) Incision in canine fossa; (b) Opening through anterior bony wall of antrum

mucosa at the gingivolabial fold. Elevation of the soft tissues exposes the canine fossa on the anterior bony wall of the antrum. The wall of the canine fossa is opened as wide as possible with a chisel and forceps. The initial cut is always made at the site of attachment of the maxillary with zygomatic process, as this will always provide access to the interior of the sinus, however small it may be. Pus and diseased mucosa are then removed from the sinus through the opening in the anterior antral wall, whereas normal mucosa is not disturbed and is left behind. Communication with the nasal cavity is established by removing part of the medial wall of the antrum in the inferior nasal meatus.

The patient is given cold liquid food for three to four days. Postoperative treatment consists in applying antiseptic douches through the newly formed nasoantral window four to five days after the operation.

Prophylaxis

Prevention of inflammatory diseases of the maxillary sinus is effected by a correct and timely treatment of both acute and chronic rhinitis and by the treatment of the upper molar teeth, which have a direct relation to these sinuses.

FUNCTIONAL ENDOSCOPIC SINUS SURGERY (FESS)

The existing concept of the surgical treatment of chronic sinusitis has drastically changed by the introduction of FESS. In this case, instead of removal of the diseased sinus mucosa, the ostium of diseased sinus is unblocked surgically. Because of the blocking of the natural ostia mainly of the ethmoidal air cells in the middle meatus, larger sinuses like maxillary and frontals are secondarily involved (Fig. 18.4). By unblocking the sinus ostia, normal drainage and ventilation of the sinus is re-established. The mucociliary transport in the paranasal sinuses always occurs towards the natural ostium.

Endoscopic Anatomy

Middle meatus is of a great interest for FESS because the frontal sinus, anterior and middle ethmoidal cells and the maxillary sinuses drain here.

Ostiomeatal Complex

The region of the middle meatus where ostium of the antrum opens with the anterior and middle ethmoidal cells is named ostiomeatal complex. Structures in the middle

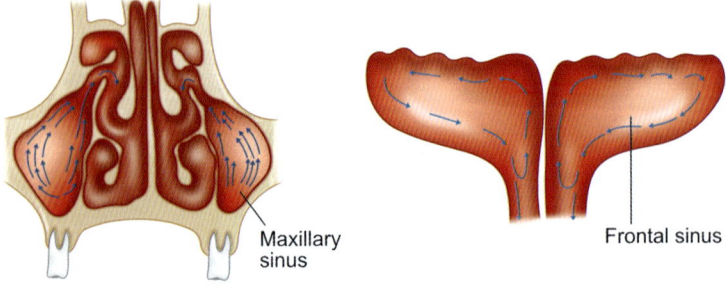

Maxillary sinus

Frontal sinus

Fig. 18.4: Mucociliary transport in the frontal and maxillary sinuses

meatus are hook-shaped uncinate process anteriorly, a semilunar groove called the Hiatus semilunaris lies behind the uncinate process, bulla ethmoidalis lies above and behind the groove and the infundibulum is the deepest part of the Hiatus semilunaris. The posteroinferior end of the infundibulum leads into the maxillary ostium. The anterosuperior end of it leads into the frontal recess where the frontonasal duct opens. Anterior to the frontal recess is the prominence of the agger nasi ridge, which overlies the anterior most ethmoidal cells, and lies on the lateral nasal wall, just in front of the anterior end of the middle turbinate. The part of the lateral nasal wall just above the inferior turbinate and anterior and posterior to the maxillary ostium is termed the anterior and the posterior fontanelles. These consist of double layer of mucosa only with no intervening bone. The ostium of the maxillary sinus lies at the posteroinferior end of the infundibulum. The bulla ethmoidalis along with its surrounding cells constitute the middle ethmoidal cells. The anterior and posterior ethmoidal arteries traverse the ethmoidal roof in the coronal plane from the orbits to the nose. These two arteries denote the upper limit of dissection. The lateral part of the roof of the ethmoid lies at a higher level. The medial part is thinner than the lateral one and slopes downwards to join the cribriform plate.

Laterally, the middle ethmoidal cells are related to the lacrimal bone and the lamina papyracea of the ethmoidal bone forms the medial wall of the orbit. Posteriorly the middle ethmoidal cells are bounded by a bony partition, which is named ground or basal lamella. The ground lamella is nothing but the bony attachment of the posterior end of the middle turbinate. The middle turbinate runs in the sagittal plane anteriorly. Its posterior end curves laterally and lies in the coronal plane (ground lamella). The posterior ethmoidal cells lie posterior to the ground lamella and are related superiorly to the dura, posteroinferiorly to the sphenoid sinus and laterally to the orbital apex and the optic nerve. Posterior ethmoidal cells vary from one to seven in number and usually open by one orifice in the superior meatus. The sphenoid sinuses lay approximately 7 cm from the anterior nasal spine. The roof of the sphenoid sinuses corresponds to the floor of the pituitary fossa. The lateral wall of the sphenoid sinus in its upper part is related to the optic nerve and posteroinferiorly the sinus is related to the internal carotid artery.

Anatomical Variations

There may be some anatomical variations, which may narrow the middle meatus hampering the mucociliary drainage. A large concha bullosa, a paradoxically curved middle turbinate with a lateral convexity, and a medially rotated uncinate process are some of the common anatomical variations. Deviation of the nasal septum, septal spur, synechiae or intranasal adhesions may cause obstruction in the ostiomeatal area and lead to complications.

Haller's cells are laterally placed middle ethmoid air cells along with floor of the orbit. These may result in narrowing of the infundibulum predisposing to maxillary sinusitis.

Onodi cells are posterior ethmoid air cells that extend posteriorly, or laterally and sometimes superior to the sphenoid sinus lying medial to the optic nerve.

To know these variations, a CT scan (axial and coronal) is of vital importance.

Indications of FESS

1. Nasal polyposis
2. Chronic Sinusitis
3. Mucoceles or pyoceles of the frontoethmoid, sphenoid or maxillary sinuses
4. Dacryocystorhinostomy (DCR).
5. Diagnosis and treatment of blowout fracture
6. Removal of a foreign body
7. Biopsy can be done by antroscopy from isolated lesions especially on the posterolateral wall
8. Cauterization of bleeding points in epistaxis
9. Closure of CSF leak
10. Vidian neurectomy
11. Optic nerve decompression
12. Orbital decompression for exophthalmos
13. Hypophysectomy
14. Surgery for choanal atresia
15. Endoscopic clipping or cautery of sphenopalatine artery

Contraindications

1. Complications associated with sinus infections such as orbital cellulitis, osteomyelitis and intracranial complications
2. Infiltrative lesions
3. A markedly stenosed frontonasal duct
4. Aggressive fungal infections like mucormycosis

Technique of FESS

Endoscopic sinus surgery is preferably done under local anaesthesia. General anaesthesia is required in children, in non-cooperative and apprehensive adults.

The patient lies supine. The surgeon stands on the right-hand side of the patient. The patient is well sedated. The nasal cavity is packed with ribbon gauze soaked in 4% xylocaine with adrenaline solution. Instruments required are:

1. Endoscopes 0°, 30° and 70° of 2.7/4 mm diameter
2. Blakesley forceps
3. Blakesley Wilde upturned forceps (biting).
4. Ostrum's reverse cutting forceps
5. Trocar and cannula of 5 mm diameter.
6. A sickle knife.
7. Optical biopsy forceps.

19

Tumours of the Nose and Paranasal Sinuses

BENIGN TUMOURS

The benign tumours are not so common. They may arise from epithelial or connective tissue.

Epithelial Tissue Origin

1. Papilloma

Papilloma mostly arises from the skin of the vestibule of the nose. This may be either single or multiple and sessile or pedunculated. Inverted papilloma—arises from the nasal sinus mucosa.

Treatment

Treatment is excision followed by cauterisation of the base of the tumour.

2. Adenoma

Adenoma is rare. This may become malignant.

Connective Tissue Origin

1. Fibroma

Fibroma is rare. Common sites of origin are turbinates and nasal septum.

2. Osteoma

Osteoma may be of three types:
   i. *Compact osteoma:* Commonly occurs in the frontal sinuses. The consistency is ivory hard. These tumours usually remain small and cause no symptoms. When enlarged they produce pain or headache by bony pressure and displacement of the eye. Obstruction of the frontonasal duct may result in empyema or mucocele of the sinus. X-ray examination reveals a densely white, well-defined mass.

   Treatment: The treatment is removal when produces symptoms.
   ii. *Cancellous osteoma:* Cancellous type commonly occurs in maxillary and ethmoidal sinuses.

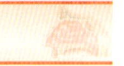

iii. *Fibrous dysplasia:* This is not a true tumour. It is the defective development of bone which is replaced by fibrous tissue. This may be of two types:

  a. Monostotic

  b. Polyostotic

The monostotic variety occurs commonly in the facial bones. The maxillary and ethmoidal bones are frequently involved. They are commonly found in younger age group and stop growing after puberty. The main symptom is deformity.

Treatment

For cosmetic reasons the affected bone may be partially removed after puberty.

3. Angioma

Angioma may be of three types:

  i. Capillary

  ii. Cavernous

  iii. Multiple telangiectasis (Osler's disease)

The commonest is capillary type, which occurs on the nasal septum and is called a "bleeding polypus of the septum". The usual symptom is epistaxis.

Treatment

Treatment is excision followed by cautery of the base.

4. Osteoclastoma

Osteoclastoma affects chiefly the ethmoidal and maxillary regions. "Egg shell crackling" is one of the important palpatory findings. X-ray examination shows "soap-bubble" appearance. Histopathological examination reveals evenly distributed giant cells in a fibrous matrix.

Treatment

Treatment is by radical excision. Other benign tumours, which are rarely found:

  i. Chondroma

  ii. Chordoma

  iii. Rhinophyma

Dentigerous Cyst (Follicular cyst)

Dentigerous cyst is defined as a cyst which envelope the whole or part of the crown of an unerupted tooth and is attached to its neck (amelocemental junction).

Clinical Features

The dentigerous cyst is a common odontogenic cyst. They occur at any age but have the highest incidence in the 3rd and 4th decades. These are much more common in men than women.

These cysts are common in the mandible than in maxilla. These most frequently involve teeth are impacted or unerupted. The majority is associated with mandibular third molar and then in decreasing frequency the maxillary canine, mandibular premolar and maxillary third molar. Rarely they may be associated with supernumerary teeth and complex or compound odontomes. Dental radiographs (OPG) taken for missing teeth or retained deciduous predecessors are usually diagnostic. They escape detected until they have enlarged sufficiently to produce expansion of the jaw. Pain is not a feature unless the cyst becomes infected.

X-rays show a well-defined radiolucency associated with the crown of an unerupted tooth. The cavity is unilocular but the erroneous multilocular effects may be produced by occasional bony trabeculations. The cysts may be related to the crown of the unerupted tooth in three ways; which can be diagnosed by X-rays.

Morphological Types of Dentigerous Cyst

1. Central type is the commonest one. It completely surrounds the crown of the tooth.
2. *Lateral type:* It projects laterally from the side of the tooth and does not completely envelop the crown.
3. *Circumferential cyst:* When the entire tooth appears enveloped by the cysts.

Treatment

Marsupialization of the cyst gives the best result. Enucleation of the tooth may lead to damage to the involved tooth. In the adult the tooth is unlikely to errupt and, therefore, enucleation together with the removal of the associated tooth is a preferred option.

Nasolabial Cyst (Nasoalveolar cyst)

It arises in the upper lip just below the alar margin of the nose. It arises from the epithelial remnants of the nasolacrimal apparatus.

Clinical Features

The age distribution ranges from 12 to 75 years with a peak incidence in the 5th decade. Over 75% of the cysts occur in women. An uncomplicated swelling is often the presenting feature. Rarely patients may complain of pain and nasal obstruction and occasionally of a poorly fitting upper denture. As the cyst enlarges, it fills up the nasolabial fold distorting nostril and producing a prominence in the floor of the nose. It can be palpated as a fluctuant swelling intra orally within the labial sulcus.

The enlarging cyst causes bone resorption of the labial surface of the maxilla and its scalloped concavity appears as radiolucency above the roots of the incisor teeth.

Treatment

The cyst lies supraperiostially. It is, therefore, best removed via a labial sulcus approach together with the periosteum.

Nasopalatine Duct (Incisive Canal) Cyst

It is the commonest of all non-odontogenic developmental cysts. It arises from epithelial remnants of the nasopalatine duct, which connects the oral and nasal cavities in the embryo.

Clinical Features

It is common in men and most commonly found in the 3rd, 4th and 5th decades of life. It may be asymptomatic. It can present as a slowly enlarging swelling in the anterior part of the palate just behind incisors. It may also be present in the midline of the upper labial sulcus. If large, a protuberance may be seen in the floor of the nose. Secondary infection may lead to pain and discharge.

On X-rays, these are well-defined ovoid or heart-shaped radiolucencies with sclerotic margins.

Treatment

The standard treatment is enucleation using a palatal flap under a local or general anaesthesia.

Radicular Inflammatory Cysts

Radicular cysts derived their epithelium from odontogenic remnants in the periodontal ligament (cell rests of malassez) and are a result of chronic inflammation. The inflammation is usually the result of pulp death and, therefore, the cysts are commonly found at the apices of the teeth (apical cysts). Radicular cysts may persist following the extraction of the offending tooth when they are called residual cysts.

Clinical Features

Radicular cysts are the commonest cystic lesion in the jaw and account for over half of all jaw cysts. The peak frequency is in the 4th decade. Approximately 60% are found in the maxilla especially associated with the anterior teeth. The majority is detected on routine radiographs of non-vital teeth. Radicular cysts are rare in deciduous teeth.

Treatment

Treatment involves removing the inflammatory source by root canal filling, apisectomy or extraction of the offending tooth and enucleation of the cyst.

Odontogenic Tumours of the Jaws

1. Benign odontogenic tumours
2. Ameloblastoma
3. Ameloblastic fibroma
4. Ameloblastic fibro dentinoma
5. Ameloblastic fibro odontoma
6. Odonto ameloblastoma
7. Adenomatoid odontogenic tumour.

Malignant Odontogenic Tumours

Carcinomas

1. Malignant ameloblastoma
2. Primary intraosseous carcinoma
3. Malignant change in odontogenic cyst.

Sarcomas

1. Ameloblastic fibrosarcoma
2. Ameloblastic fibrodentinosarcoma
3. Ameloblastic fibroodontosarcoma

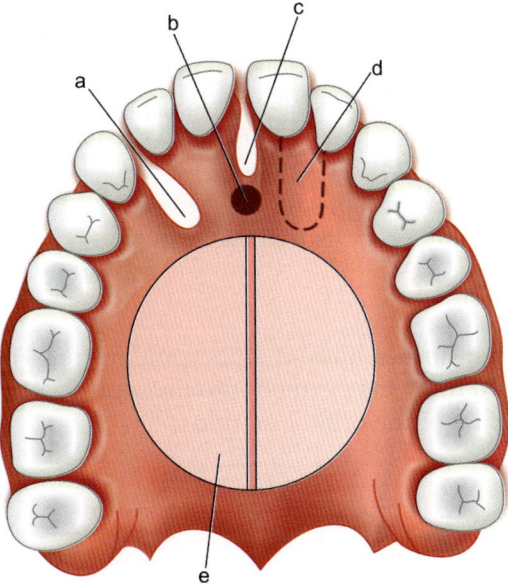

Fig. 19.1: Cysts associated with fusion of embryological elements forming the maxilla. (a) Lateral alveolar cyst, (b) nasopalatine (incisive canal) cyst, (c) median alveolar cyst, (d) nasoalveolar cyst, (e) medial palatal cyst

Cysts of the Nose and Paranasal Sinuses

Types

1. Cysts associated with fusion of embryological elements forming the maxilla.
   i. Medial group
      a. Median alveolar cyst, which separates the upper central incisor teeth.
      b. Median palatal cyst, which lies between the palatine processes of the developing maxilla.
      c. Nasopalatine cysts arising from tissue in the incisive canal or nests in the papilla palatina and present either on the palate or on the nasal floor.
   ii. Lateral group
      a. *Lateral alveolar cyst:* Sited at the line of fusion of maxillary and premaxillary elements of the palate. It gives rise to separation of canine and lateral incisor teeth.

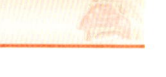

b. *Naso alveolar cysts:* Occur in the lateral half of the nasal floor, anterior to the inferior turbinate. They enlarge to splay the nostril and cause a fullness of the upper lip.

Cysts of Dental Origin

These are derived from the epithelium that has been connected with the development of the tooth concerned.

a. Primordial cyst arises from the epithelium of the enamel organ before formation of the dental tissue. The most common site is in the third molar region of the mandible.

b. *Cysts of eruption:* They arise over a tooth that has not erupted from the remains of the dental lamina. These occur in young people and may appear over a deciduous or permanent molar tooth, appearing as small bluish swellings.

c. *Dentigerous (follicular) cysts:* Usually arise from the follicle around an unerupted tooth. The tooth projects into the cavity.

d. *Dental (radicular) cysts:* Arise from epithelial remains in the periodontal membrane. These are the most common cysts that occur in jaws.

Dermoid Cysts

These are found on the surface lines of embryonic fusion. They may occur in the midline of the nose and these may extend into the septum. These may also occur at the inner and outer parts of the orbital margins.

Mucoceles of the Paranasal Sinuses

These may occur due to:

   i. Blockage of a mucous gland duct.
   ii. Cystic formation of the mucosa undergoing polyposis.
   iii. Atresia or stenosis of a sinus ostium.

Mucocele occurs most commonly in the frontal sinus.

Cherubism

It is a rare familiar multilocular cystic disease. The condition seems to regress after adolescence.

Haemorrhagic Bone Cysts

These are found in the mandible. The cause is related to an old trauma, which may have occurred several years previously. It is probable that an intraosseous haemorrhage leads to excessive osteoclastic activity, which slowly regresses leaving the cyst behind.

Differential Diagnosis

Diagnosis is from any lesion, which can produce a clearly defined radiolucent area in the bone, e.g. osteoclastoma, haemangioma, eosinophilic granuloma, myeloma.

Treatment

Complete removal or marsupialization.

Odontogenic Tumours

These tumours are derived from the cells concerned in tooth developments. They are:

1. Ameloblastoma (Adamantinoma or multilocular cyst)

This tumour does not contain enamel. It is not necessarily multiloculated and may not be cystic. It may arise from any part of the epithelium responsible for tooth formation.

Clinical Features

These occur more commonly in young adults. Mandible is more frequently affected than the maxilla. The teeth in the region of the lesion become loosened and as the tumour increases in size, it may become ulcerated. X-ray shows most commonly a multilocular cyst or a unilocular cyst. Resorption of tooth roots may be seen.

Treatment

Radical excision is necessary as these tumours are regarded as locally malignant. When the mandible is affected, partial excision may have to be followed by bone grafting.

2. Composite Odontoma

They arise from epithelial and mesenchymal parts of the tooth gum. They consist of a mixture of the dental tissues in varying degrees; some appear very nearly like normal teeth; others, at the opposite extreme consist of calcified masses or a number of toothlike structures surrounded by a capsule or cyst.

Clinical Features

These are most commonly seen in children or young adults and one or even two teeth are sometimes missing.

The smooth hard swelling is noticed in the jaw. Pain may be present with secondary infection. X-ray shows calcification, which is the most common type of odontoma. An associated cyst may also be present.

Treatment

Surgical removal.

Malignant Tumours

Epithelial Tissue Tumours

1. Carcinoma
    i. *Squamous cell carcinoma:* It is the commonest malignant tumour in the nose and paranasal sinuses. The tumour causes bony erosion and soft-tissue infiltration. Lymphatic metastasis is uncommon.
    ii. *Adenocarcinoma:* It arises from the glands of maxillary sinus mucosa.
2. Mixed salivary tumour.

Connective Tissue Tumours

1. Sarcoma
2. Melanoma
   These are rarely seen in nose and paranasal sinuses.

Metastatic Tumours

Metastatic tumours are also very rarely seen.

Clinical Features

1. Nasal obstruction—gradually increasing and usually unilateral.
2. Blood stained nasal discharge.
3. Epistaxis.
4. Swelling of the cheek, alveolar margin or palate.
5. Loosening of teeth.
6. Proptosis.
7. Epiphora.
8. Pain and headache.

Diagnosis

1. X-ray shows dense and ill-defined shadow with erosion of bone.
2. Biopsy.

Treatment

1. Irradiation.
2. Irradiation and diathermy coagulation.
3. Excision.
   Prognosis: Five-year cure rate with best possible treatment is only 35–50%.
   Carcinoma is more common in the maxillary sinus than in other sinuses. The aetiology of carcinoma of the paranasal sinuses is not known. Snuff, chronic inflammatory diseases of the sinuses and wood dust, etc. may be blamed as the etiological factors.
   These tumours are classified as follows:
1. *Ohngren's classification:* Oblique line from medial canthus to angle of mandible of the same side and a vertical line through the pupil.
2. *Lederman's classification:* Two horizontal lines, one through the floor of orbit and another through the floor of the antra. Two vertical lines through the medial canthi.
3. *American Joint Committee Classification* (AJCC) is followed widely now.

Pharynx

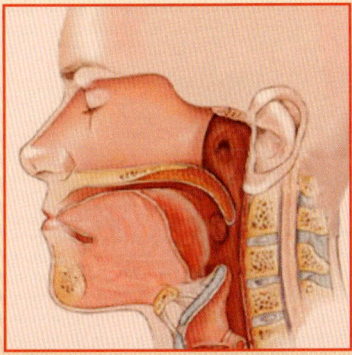

20

Anatomy of the Pharynx

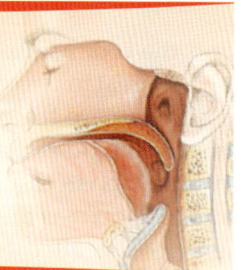

The pharynx is the uppermost part of the digestive tract. It extends from the base of the skull to the level of the sixth cervical vertebra, and the lower border of the cricoid cartilage. The lower end of the pharynx is the narrowest part of the digestive tract. The pharynx ends where oesophagus begins.

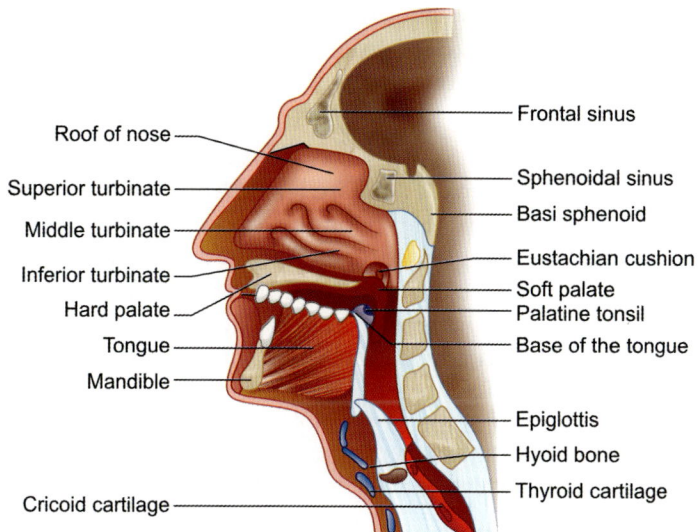

Fig. 20.1: Sagittal section of head and neck

It comprises three parts—the nasopharynx, the oropharynx and the laryngopharynx. The nasopharynx is bounded above by the basi sphenoid, below by an imaginary line at the level of the soft palate. The oropharynx is bounded above by the lower boundary of the nasopharynx and extends to the level of the tip of the epiglottis. The laryngopharynx is bounded above by the lower boundary of the oropharynx and below by a line at the level of the lower border of the cricoid cartilage (Fig. 20.1).

NASOPHARYNX

It opens anteriorly into the nasal cavity through the choana. The posterior wall of the nasopharynx arches forward into the roof. At the junction of the posterior wall and the roof a submucous collection of the lymphoid tissue is situated, called the pharyngeal tonsil or adenoids when it becomes enlarged and infected. On the lateral wall there are the openings of the eustachian tubes and are situated about 12 mm behind the posterior ends of the inferior turbinates. The eustachian tube opening is bounded posterosuperiorly by the tubal cartilage covered by the mucous membrane and is known as the eustachian cushion or the tubal elevation. Behind this elevation is a recess called fossa of Rosenmuller which is one of the common sites of the origin of the nasopharyngeal carcinoma.

OROPHARYNX

It opens anteriorly into the mouth. Its roof is formed by the soft palate, floor by the base of the tongue and lingual surface of epiglottis, lateral wall by the palatine tonsil and anterior and posterior pillars and the posterior wall is from the level of the hard palate to the hyoid bone. In its lateral walls the palatine tonsils are situated between the anterior and posterior pillars of the fauces. The anterior pillar consists of palatoglossus muscle and its covering mucosa. The posterior pillar consists of palatopharyngeus muscle and its covering mucosa. There are many small submucous collections of lymphoid tissue on the posterior wall.

LARYNGOPHARYNX

It opens anteriorly into the larynx. There are two shallow spaces present in front of the epiglottis and behind the base of the tongue, known as the valleculae. These are divided in the midline by the glossoepiglottic fold and bounded laterally by the pharyngoepiglottic folds. There are two small recesses lying on each side of the laryngeal inlet known as pyriform fossa. Each pyriform fossa is bounded medially by the arytenoid cartilage and aryepiglottic fold, laterally by the thyroid cartilage and thyrohyoid membrane. The internal division of the superior laryngeal nerve lies beneath the mucous membrane of the floor of each pyriform fossa.

STRUCTURE OF THE PHARYNX

The pharynx has four layers from outside inwards:

Buccopharyngeal Fascia

This is a thin fascia and forms the outermost covering of the pharynx. It extends anteriorly over the pterygomandibular ligament on the buccinator muscles. It is loosely attached to the prevertebral fascia posteriorly and firmly united with the pharyngobasilar fascia above the upper concave border of the superior constrictor muscle.

Muscles of the Pharynx

This coat has two layers:
a. The outer one consists of the three constrictor muscles; composed of the superior, middle and the inferior. Each is surrounded at its lower end by the upper end of the one below.
   All the constrictor muscles are inserted into the median raphe posteriorly.

Killian's Dehiscence

This is a potential gap between the oblique thyropharyngeous and transverse cricopharyngeous parts of the inferior constrictor muscle. The mucous membrane in this gap may bulge between the two parts of the inferior constrictor. It develops due to premature contraction of the transverse cricopharyngeous muscle during the second stage of deglutition. A pharyngeal pouch is caused by this neuro-muscular incoordination.

b. The inner layer consists of the three muscles composed of stylopharyngeus, palatopharyngeus, and salpingopharyngeus. The stylopharyngeus and salpingopharyngeus arise from outside the pharynx and pass in between the superior and middle constrictors to form part of the inner layer of muscular coat.

Pharyngeal Aponeurosis

It is a connective tissue coat of the pharynx between the muscular and mucosal layers. The upper part of it is thickened where the muscle is deficient and is known as pharyngobasilar fascia.

Mucous Membrane

The mucosa of the pharynx is continuous with the mucous membrane of the esophagus, larynx, mouth, nasal cavities, and eustachian tubes.

In the upper half of the nasopharynx the mucosa is of ciliated columnar epithelium. The lower half of the nasopharynx, the oropharynx and laryngopharynx are lined with stratified squamous epithelium. The junction between the nasopharynx and oropharynx is lined with transitional epithelium.

Subepithelial Lymphoid Tissue of the Pharynx

At the entrance of the pharynx there are collections of lymphoid tissue which guard the portal into the alimentary canal. This tissue situated at the entrance to the pharynx is grouped around in a circular fashion and is known as Waldeyer's lymphatic ring (Fig. 20.2). The lymphoid tissue collections of this ring have efferent but no afferent vessels. They consist of:

a. Palatine tonsils (tonsils).
b. Pharyngeal tonsils or adenoids.
c. Lingual tonsils—lie beneath the mucosa of the base of the tongue. They have the continuity with the lower ends of the palatine tonsils.
d. Tubal tonsils—lie in the fossa of Rosenmuller.
e. Lateral pharyngeal bands. These descend from the tubal tonsils behind the posterior faucial pillars.
f. Discrete nodules—lie in the posterior pharyngeal wall in the subepithelial layer.

Lymphatic Drainage of Waldeyer's Ring

This tissue drains into:
1. Tonsillar gland situated in the angle between the internal jugular and common facial veins just below and behind the angle of the mandible.

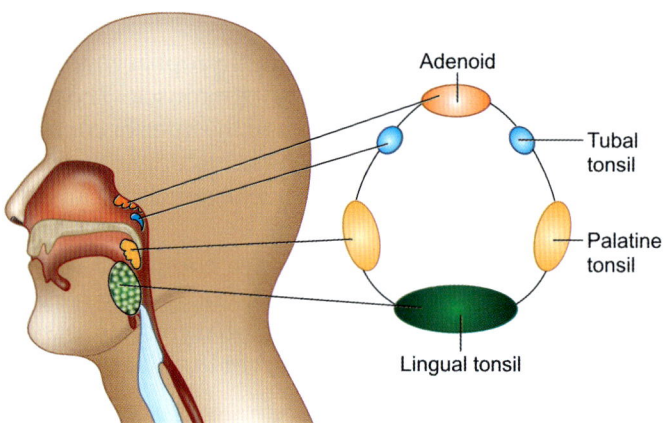

Fig. 20.2: Waldeyer's lymphatic ring

2. The adenoid glands lie below the tip of the mastoid process beneath the sternomastoid muscle and receive the lymph from the adenoids (pharyngeal tonsils).

Parapharyngeal Space

This is a potential space outside the pharynx and is triangular in cross-section. It extends from the base of the skull above to the superior mediastinum below. Infection from the surrounding structures may involve this space and its contents.

This space is bounded anteromedially by the buccopharyngeal fascia and posteromedially by the transverse processes of the cervical vertebrae covered by the prevertebral muscles and fascia. The lateral wall is formed above by the ascending ramus of the mandible in front, and parotid gland behind. In its lower part it is formed by the sternomastoid muscle, the ribbon muscles of the neck and intervening deep fascia. The contents are:

   i. Great vessels of the neck.

   ii. Ascending palatine and ascending pharyngeal arteries.

   iii. Retropharyngeal and deep cervical lymphatic glands.

   iv. The cervical sympathetic trunk and 9th, 10th, 11th and 12th cranial nerves.

Spread of Infection

The parapharyngeal space may be infected by the spread of infection from the tonsils or teeth (particularly the lower third molar). From this space the infection may spread:

1. From the base of the skull to mediastinum within the space.

2. Into the skull alongside the internal carotid artery, internal jugular vein, or the posterior cranial nerves.

3. To the paraoesophageal region and superior mediastinum.

The infection cannot spread across the midline as the median raphe of the buccopharyngeal fascia is firmly attached to the prevertebral fascia.

Retropharyngeal Space

This space lies behind the pharynx and is bounded anteriorly by the posterior pharyngeal wall and its covering buccopharyngeal fascia, posteriorly by the cervical vertebrae and their covering muscles and fascia.

Contents

1. Retropharyngeal lymph glands. They usually disappear spontaneously during the third or fourth year of life.
2. Loose areolar tissue.

Fascia and Fascial Spaces of the Neck

The localization and spread of neck space infection is dependent upon the fascial spaces. The fascia of the neck is important to surgeons, because dissection is easier, more bloodless and better controlled if it proceeds along the fascial plains rather than through them. Removal of the fascia is an important part of a radical neck dissection mainly because it surrounds those tissues which need to be removed and also because dissection along the fascia protects important structures. Fascia in the neck is called the cervical fascia which consists of two layers:

1. Superficial cervical fascia
2. Deep cervical fascia

The superficial fascia is a sheet of connective tissue encircling the neck. It is attached posteriorly to the deep fascia of the neck. Within this fascia, i.e. the superficial fascia lays the platysma muscle, a thin sheet of muscle. It is innervated by the cervical branch of the facial nerve. A potential space exists between the superficial and the deep fascia. The marginal mandibular branch of the facial nerve traverses through this space. The deep cervical fascia has three layers:

1. Superficial or investing layer
2. Middle or visceral layer
3. Deep or prevertebral fascia.

Investing layer of deep cervical fascia lies deep to the platysma. This layer of deep cervical fascia encloses the suprasternal space of burns and the supraclavicular space.

The middle or visceral layer of deep cervical fascia encircles the pharynx, larynx, esophagus, trachea, thyroid gland, strap muscles of the neck and forms the carotid sheath containing the carotid artery, internal jugular vein and vagus nerve. The carotid sheath blends with the adventitia of the aorta in the superior mediastinum, through which the infection in the neck can spread to the mediastinum. That is why it is named "Lincoln Highway" by Mosher.

The deep layer of the deep cervical fascia or the prevertebral fascia lies anterior to the prevertebral muscle and encloses the musculus longus coli, musculus longus capitis and scalene muscles.

There are five potential spaces in the neck. They are:

1. Parapharyngeal or lateral pharyngeal space
2. Retropharyngeal space

3. Parotid space
4. Submandibular space
  a. Sublingual
  b. Submaxillary
5. Masticator space

LUDWIG'S ANGINA

It is the infection of the submandibular space. Mostly it occurs due to dental infection. It is usually bilateral and involves both sublingual and submaxillary space. In extreme stages it may cause airway obstruction. Tracheostomy may be needed in severe infection with stridor. A wide decompression of the suprahyoid region is essential. The incision runs along the mandibular arch. The myelohyoid muscle is split and drained on either side of the muscle followed by placement of drainage tubes. Intravenous broad spectrum antibiotics and metronidazole should be administered along with analgesics and anti-inflammatory drugs.

SALIVATION

Salivation is a secretion of the three main pairs of salivary glands and the numerous small buccal glands. The three pairs of salivary glands are:
1. Submandibular salivary glands
2. Sublingual salivary glands
3. Parotid glands.

Afferent Impulses

These impulses arise from lingual mucosa via the 5th and 9th cranial nerves; and of the buccal mucosa via the 5th cranial nerve. They also arise from the stomach through sensory vagal endings and from the nerves of special sensations, such as the sight, taste or smell of food.

Efferent Impulses

These impulses are conveyed by fibres of the autonomic nervous system, i.e. the parasympathetic nervous system and the sympathetic nervous system. The parasympathetic fibres from the superior salivary nucleus run in the chorda tympani branch of the 7th cranial nerve and finally join the lingual branch of the 5th cranial nerve. Then they pass through the submandibular ganglion, to supply the submandibular and sublingual glands.

The fibres from the inferior salivary nucleus run to the otic ganglia, from which the post-ganglionic fibres pass to the parotid gland via the auriculotemporal nerve.

The average amount of saliva secretion is about half to one liter in 24 hours.

The saliva has certain bactericidal and coagulating properties. The average pH is about 6.5. The saliva consists of 99.42% water, 0.22% salts, mainly those of calcium phosphate and carbonate, 0.22% of organic content. Mucin is secreted by the buccal, sublingual and submandibular glands, and serous by the parotid gland. About 0.14% of the saliva is enzymes. These include ptyalin, which initiates the first stage of digestion by catalysing the hydrolysis of starches, in several stages, to maltase.

Dryness of the mouth (xerostomia) may be caused by the lesions of the salivary glands, the lesions which interrupt the central pathways of the secretory nerves, psychological disturbances, mouth breathing due to nasal obstruction and drugs.

Certain diseases such as Plummer-Vinson syndrome, uraemia, diabetes, chronic interstitial nephritis and Sjögren's syndrome associated with rheumatoid arthritis may also cause xerostomia.

An increased flow of saliva (ptyalism) may be due to the action of certain drugs, morning sickness of pregnancy, certain types of mental disorders and inflammation, foreign body or tumour of the mouth, pharynx or oesophagus.

TASTE

The end organs of taste are taste buds. They are mainly found on the tongue but also present on the hard palate, anterior faucial pillars, tonsils, posterior wall of the pharynx, epiglottis and inner surface of the cheek. The taste cells (gustatory cells) are thin fusiform cells contained in the taste buds. The hairlets of the taste cells project as delicate processes through the orifice of the taste bud (gustatory pore).

Mechanism of Taste

There are four primitive tastes:
1. Sweet
2. Sour
3. Salt
4. Bitter

These substances must be in solution to stimulate the taste cells. The tip and sides of the tongue are most sensitive to sweet and sour. The back of the tongue is most sensitive to bitter. Nerves involved in taste sensation:
1. Ninth cranial nerve from the posterior one-third of the tongue.
2. Lingual branch of 5th and chorda tympany branch of the 7th cranial nerve from the anterior two-thirds of the tongue.
3. Tenth cranial nerve from epiglottis.

TONSILS

The two palatine tonsils are commonly known as the tonsils. They are the submucous lymphoid tissue situated one in each fauce bounded anteriorly by palatoglossal arch and posteriorly by palatopharyngeal arch. They vary greatly in size and shape. The size of a normal tonsil is like that of a betel nut and the shape is oval, the long axis of which is vertical. Two-thirds of each tonsil is usually embedded in the wall of the pharynx but the variations are not uncommon.

The medial surface of the tonsils is free and is covered by mucous membrane. About 12 to 20 depressions are seen on the surfaces which are the openings of the crypts. The crypts are like test tubes with one closed end in each. These ends extend as far as its deep surface which is bounded by a firm fibrous capsule. The largest crypt lies near the upper pole of the tonsil. This is known as intratonsillar or supra-tonsillar cleft.

A fold of mucous membrane, semilunar in shape, connects the palatine arches at their junction with the soft palate. This is known as semilunar fold which forms the medial wall of the tonsillar fossa. Another fold of mucosa, triangular in shape, covers the anterior surface of the tonsil near its lower pole. This is known as triangular fold.

Relations of Tonsil

The tonsil is partly covered by anterior faucial pillar anteriorly. Posteriorly it is bounded by the posterior pillar. Medially it is free. On the surface the openings of the 12 to 20 crypts of the tonsil are seen. Laterally it is related to (from within outwards):

    i. Fibrous capsule of the tonsil
   ii. Loose areolar tissue
  iii. Paratonsillar vein
  iv. Pharyngeal aponeurosis
   v. Superior constrictor muscle
  vi. Buccopharyngeal fascia
 vii. Medial pterygoid muscle
viii.Ramus of the mandible
  ix. Masseter muscle covered by skin and subcutaneous tissue. The ninth cranial nerve and the facial artery lie outside the superior constrictor muscle (Fig. 20.3).
    The internal carotid artery lies about one inch behind and lateral to the tonsil.

Blood Supply of Tonsil

The blood supply of the tonsil is very profuse. The arteries are the following:
1. Anterior tonsillar—from dorsalis linguae, branch of lingual.
2. Posterior tonsillar—from ascending pharyngeal, branch of external carotid.
3. Superior tonsillar—from descending palatine, branch of greater palatine.
4. Inferior tonsillar—from facial.
    The veins from the tonsil form a plexus around the capsule and drain into the pharyngeal plexus.

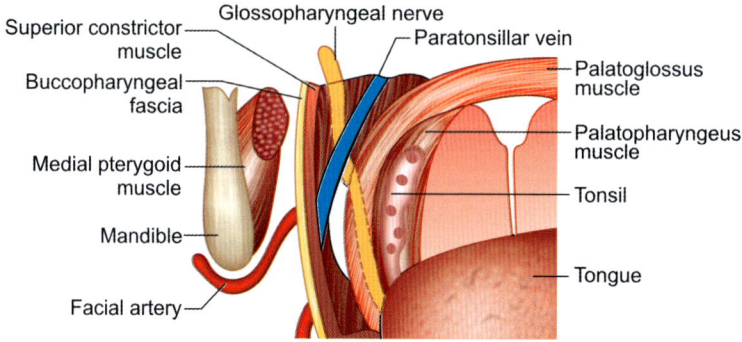

Fig. 20.3: Relations of tonsil

Nerve Supply of Tonsil

The glossopharyngeal and the trigeminal nerve carry sensation from the upper part of the tonsil through sphenopalatine ganglion.

Lymphatics of Tonsil

The lymphatics drain in the jugulodigastric gland (level II) also called tonsillar gland which lies on the carotid artery in the angle formed by the union of the common facial and the internal jugular vein.

Blood Supply of the Pharynx

Arteries

1. Ascending pharyngeal artery.
2. Ascending palatine and tonsillar branches of the facial artery.
3. Branches of the maxillary artery.
4. Dorsalis linguae, branch of the lingual artery.
5. Branches of the superior thyroid artery.

   All the arteries are branches of the external carotid artery.

Veins

The veins form a plexus which communicates above with the pterygoid venous plexus and drains into the common facial and internal jugular veins.

Nerve Supply of the Pharynx

It is derived chiefly from the pharyngeal plexus which is formed by branches of the ninth and tenth cranial nerves, together with the sympathetic fibres. The main motor element is the cranial part of the eleventh (accessory) cranial nerve, which is distributed through the pharyngeal branches of the vagus. It supplies all the muscles of the pharynx except the stylopharyngeus which is supplied by the 9th cranial nerve and the tensor palati, supplied by the 5th cranial nerve. The principal sensory nerves are the ninth and tenth cranial nerves. The nasopharynx is supplied largely by the fifth cranial nerve.

Lymphatic Drainage of the Pharynx

The vessels pass to the deep cervical glands either directly or indirectly via the retropharyngeal glands and/or paratracheal glands.

Functions of the Tonsil

The main function of the tonsils is protection in the following ways:

1. Formation of lymphocytes.
2. Formation of antibodies.
3. Acquisition of immunity to organisms entering into the mouth and nose.
4. Localization of infection.

21

Examination of the Pharynx

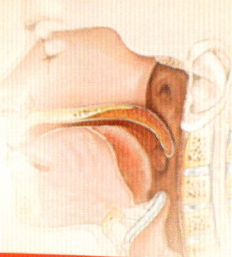

NASOPHARYNX

See examination of the nose.

OROPHARYNX

The oropharynx is examined through the open mouth with the help of a tongue depressor.

Inspection

The teeth, gum, vestibule and floor of the mouth and tongue should be examined first before inspecting the following areas of oropharynx (Fig. 21.1):

1. Anterior pillars of the fauces—for flushing, ulceration and swelling
2. Tonsils—for size, congestion, and the presence of pus, cyst and stone formation
3. Tonsillo-lingual sulcus: This is also known as the graveyard of the oral cavity and lies between the tonsil and the base of the tongue which is very often overlooked. It is an important site for the primary malignant growth.
4. Lateral pharyngeal bands for hypertrophy and congestion.
5. Posterior pharyngeal wall for hypertrophy of the lymphoid tissue, swelling, and ulceration.

   The soft palate is to be inspected for movement during phonation (Fig. 21.2).

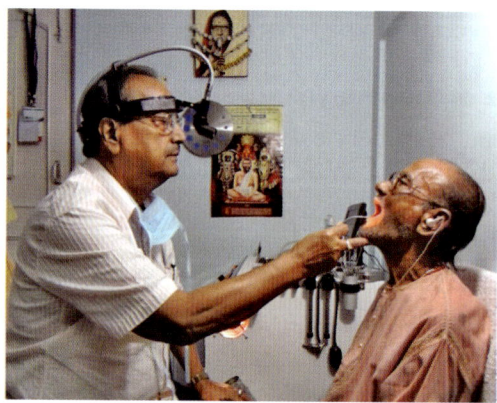

Fig. 21.1: Examination of the pharynx

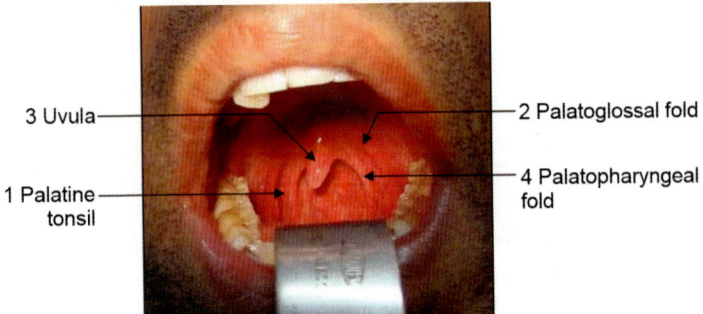

3 Uvula
2 Palatoglossal fold
1 Palatine tonsil
4 Palatopharyngeal fold

Fig. 21.2: 1. Palatine tonsil; 2. Palatoglossal fold; 3. Uvula; 4. Palatopharyngeal fold

Palpation

This is an important part of the examination to exclude malignancy especially when any swelling is present (Fig. 21.3).

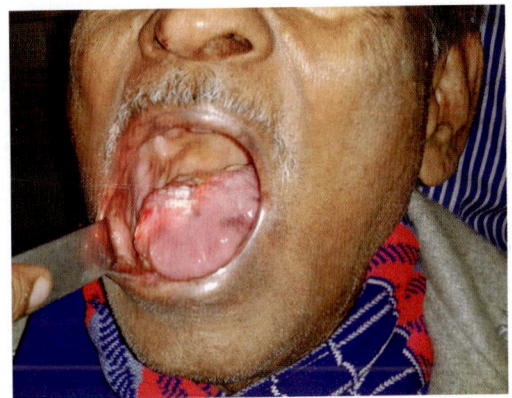

Fig. 21.3: Carcinoma right lateral border of tongue

LARYNGOPHARYNX

Laryngopharynx or hypopharynx is examined by laryngoscopy.

Laryngoscopy

a. Indirect laryngoscopy with a laryngeal mirror (vide infra).
b. Direct laryngoscopy with a laryngoscope or oesophageal speculum. The following structures must be inspected during laryngoscopy:
   1. Base of the tongue.
   2. Posterior wall of the laryngopharynx.
   3. Lateral wall of the laryngopharynx.
   4. Valleculae, one on each side of the glossoepiglottic fold.
   5. Epiglottis.
   6. Arytenoid cartilages, right and left and inter-arytenoid region.
   7. Aryepiglottic folds, right and left.

8. Pyriform fossa, one on each side of the arytenoid cartilage and aryepiglottic fold.
9. Post-cricoid region, only the uppermost portion of it can be seen by indirect laryngoscopy.

There has been a great advancement in the ability to image the human body by videoendoscopy, CT and MRI scanning. Though these investigation modalities contribute to our understanding of the normal and abnormal function of the aerodigestive tract, yet, in the case of mucosal lesions in ENT even the finest of the radiological examinations contribute a little when compared to direct visualization techniques. Advances in flexible and rigid endoscopy together with the increasing use of cameras and recording facilities require updating the earlier accounts of this subject.

The three essential functions of the healthy throat are maintenance of an airway, the ability to swallow and production of voice. Impaired performance of one of the functions of throat often causes involvement of others.

Flexible Endoscopy

Nasendoscopy/Nasolaryngoscopy

Under local anaesthesia the flexible endoscope for examination of the postnasal space, pharynx and larynx is usually performed by smaller diameter fibreoptic endoscope. The procedure may be performed at the bed side. The view with the flexible endoscope is not as good as direct laryngoscope or as clear as a mirror.

Hopkins Rod

The use of the 70° or 90° telescope allows a high resolution view of the larynx. It allows assessment of vocal cord function, high quality photography and is the ideal instrument for **videostroboscopy** of the larynx. In patients with tracheostomies, an angled telescope provides an excellent view of the trachea, carina and the anterior aspect of the glottis.

Oesophagoscopy

Flexible oesophagoscopy may be performed under local anaesthesia and sedation. It may also be performed under general anaesthesia.

Flexible endoscopy is, however, not superior to rigid instruments in the following conditions:

- The removal of foreign bodies is easier and biopsies are substantially larger with rigid scopes. Flexible endoscopes are poor at visualising the pharynx, and post-cricoid regions.
- The use of "Lugol's solution" (iodine) combined with oesophagoscopy is the best way to detect earlier oesophageal cancer. Early lesions stain vividly and may then be biopsied.

Bronchoscopy

The bronchoscopy is indicated for diagnostic and therapeutic purposes in cases of haemoptysis, suspected bronchial obstructions, obscure chest symptoms, toileting, palliation and foreign bodies. Relatively peripheral lesions can be visualized and biopsied by flexible endoscopy where the rigid endoscope cannot reach. The flexible bronchoscope is passed through nasal airway after anaesthetizing with 4% Xylocaine spray. The pharynx and vocal cords are anaesthetized through the mouth. It is helpful to provide oxygen through a cannula passed via the other nostril. Once through the cords, further xylocaine is delivered into each main bronchus through the endoscope. During the examination, aspirates should be taken for cytology and culture, using sputum traps one for each bronchus.

Neck Glands

Examination of the pharynx is not complete if the cervical lymph glands are not examined systematically.

Radiography

Sometimes, soft tissue X-ray of the laryngopharynx and nasopharynx may be helpful.

22

Principles of the Pharyngeal Surgery

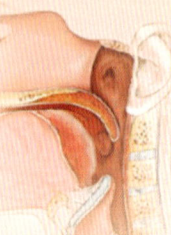

NASOPHARYNX

Removal of Adenoids

The adenoids are curetted off the roof and posterior wall of the nasopharynx by a curette with cage. Endoscopic removal with the help of a microdebrider is an excellent procedure used nowadays.

OROPHARYNX

Removal of Tonsils (Tonsillectomy)

1. Dissection Method

This method is very widely practiced nowadays. This may be performed both by local and general anaesthesia. The tonsil is pulled medially by a tonsil holding forceps after opening the mouth by Boyle Davis gag under general anaesthesia. The mucosa between the free edge of the anterior pillar and the tonsil is incised by a tonsillar knife. The capsule of the tonsil is exposed by making a niche between it and its bed. The tonsil is then separated from the fossa by a blunt dissector from above downwards. The lower pole of the tonsil (to the base of the tongue) is then severed either with Eve's tonsillar snare or by twisting with a pair of tonsillar straight haemostatic forceps.

Comparison between the dissection and the guillotine methods	
Dissection method	Guillotine method
Can be performed in all types of cases both in children and adults	Can be performed in hypertrophied tonsil with minimal peritonsillar fibrosis
Surrounding tissue trauma is minimal	Chance of injury to surrounding tissue is greater
Requires more time for dissection— prolonged anaesthesia	Requires a little time—short anaesthesia
Bleeding vessels can be ligated	Bleeding vessels cannot be ligated
Tonsillar tags are not left behind in expert hands	Even in expert hands tonsillar tags can be left behind

2. Guillotine Method

Under general anaesthesia when the child is fully relaxed, the mouth is opened widely with a Doyen's gag. The guillotine is inserted into the pharynx after depressing the tongue with the blade of it.

The lower pole and free surface of the tonsil are engaged in the fenestra of the guillotine. The tonsil is then pushed through the ring of the guillotine by pressing the anterior faucial pillar with the finger. The blade of the guillotine is closed, which passes between the tonsil and its bed. The tonsil is then removed by blunt dissection.

23

Diseases of the Pharynx

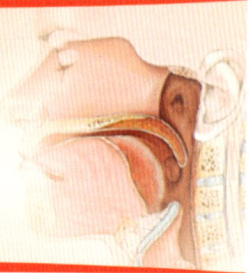

INFLAMMATION OF NASOPHARYNX

Acute Nasopharyngitis

This is generally associated with acute inflammation of the nose, paranasal sinuses or tonsils. As it sets in, dryness and sensation of warmth in the nasopharynx can be felt. Then follows pain or discomfort and a rise in temperature.

Chronic Nasopharyngitis

This can be of two types:

1. Simple

Chronic simple nasopharyngitis is usually due to extension of inflammation from the nose or oropharynx.

Remnants of adenoids predispose to this. Nasal blockage, dust and fumes, excessive smoking, alcohol and overuse of nasal drops aggravate the condition.

Clinical Features

The main symptom is irritation in the postnasal region. The mucosa becomes congested. Mucopus may also be present.

Differential Diagnosis

   i. Hypertrophied posterior ends of inferior turbinates.
  ii. Antrochoanal polyp.
 iii. Tumours of the nasopharynx.
 iv. Psychoneurosis.

Treatment

   i. The nose, paranasal sinuses, and oropharyngeal diseases should be treated first. Adenoids must be removed.
  ii. Improvement of general health.
 iii. Avoid excessive smoking, drinking alcohol, dust and fumes.
 iv. A warm alkaline nasal douche—to clean the viscid mucus.

2. Atrophic

This is generally associated with atrophic rhinitis and pharyngitis. The symptoms are negligible. Treatment of atrophic rhinitis and pharyngitis cure this condition.

Acute Non-specific Pharyngitis

Acute non-specific pharyngitis may be of three forms depending on the degree of infection:

1. Simple.
2. Suppurative.
3. Gangrenous.

The commonest organism is streptococcus haemolyticus. Sometimes non-haemolytic *Streptococcus*, *Pneumococcus*, or *Haemophilus influenzae* may also be seen. It commonly occurs in winter and rainy season and is an important early manifestation of measles, smallpox, influenza and typhoid fever.

Clinical Features

1. *Simple*
    i. Odynophagia (painful swallowing).
    ii. Otalgia (pain in the ear).
    iii. Enlarged and tender cervical glands.
    iv. Rise in temperature.
    v. Hyperaemia of the mucosa.
    vi. Complications like acute rheumatism and nephritis are not uncommon.
2. *Suppurative:* This type starts with severe pain in the throat. The temperature rises high up to even 105°F which may be associated with rigor. The patient becomes toxic with slow pulse rate. Cervical lymph glands are enlarged and tender. The soft palate and uvula may be oedematous. A soft, nonadherent membrane may be present looking like diphtheria. The inflammation may spread to the larynx, and submandibular region giving rise to oedema larynx and Ludwig's angina respectively. Septicaemia, pleurisy, pericarditis, nephritis, and meningitis may sometimes occur as a complication.
3. *Gangrenous:* This variety is not so common. It occasionally occurs in persons with lowered resistance.

Diagnosis

High fever with a relatively slow pulse rate goes against diphtheria. Bacteriological examination of throat swabs excludes diphtheria.

Exanthematous fever must be excluded.

By examination of blood for total and differential count blood, dyscrasias can be excluded.

Treatment

- Rest.
- Liquid nutritious diet.

- Analgesics and antipyretics.
- Suitable antibiotics or chemotherapy in adequate doses.
- In oedema larynx tracheostomy may be required.
- In Ludwig's angina, incision from the chin to the hyoid bone may be necessary.

Acute Membranous Pharyngitis

Vincent's Angina

This is a highly infectious and ulcerative lesion of the tonsil. It may spread to the palate and gums; it is due to two Gram-negative organisms, a fusiform bacillus and a spirochaete. Both the organisms are found together in the lesions. Nowadays it is thought to be due to virus infection though the two above-mentioned gram negative organisms are always found (Fig. 23.1).

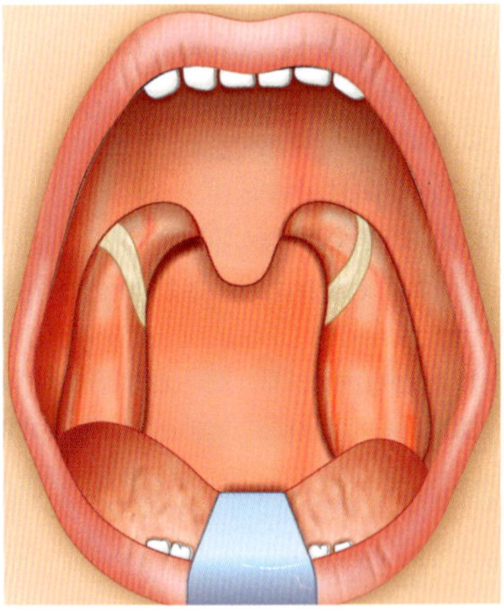

Fig. 23.1: Vincent's angina

Clinical Features

The disease appears as a sloughy grey patch. It soon ulcerates with considerable loss of tissue. The base of the ulcer is granular which readily bleeds. If the slough is removed it reforms. There may be associated cervical adenitis, odynophagia, rise in temperature and characteristic foetor.

Diagnosis

Vincent's angina may be confused with the following conditions:
  i. Diphtheria.
  ii. Acute follicular tonsillitis.
  iii. Acute streptococcal pharyngitis.
  iv. Agranulocytic angina.
  v. Thrush.
  vi. Acute lymphatic leukaemia.
  vii. Malignant growths.
  viii. Tertiary syphilis.

Treatment

1. Penicillin or erythromycin in adequate doses should be administered. Metronidazole may also be added with antibiotics with good effect.
2. The ulcer may be painted daily with liquor arsenicalis.

Acute Diphtheritic Pharyngitis

This is an acute infection of the pharynx due to Klebs-Loeffler bacillus (KLB). Children between the ages of 2 and 5 years are commonly affected.

The disease starts gradually with pain in the throat. The cervical glands are moderately enlarged and tender. The temperature is usually low (100–101 °F). The pulse rate is rapid and out of proportion. The patient looks toxic and prostrated. Examination of urine shows albumin.

The disease is characterized by the formation of a false membrane on the tonsils, soft palate and posterior wall of the pharynx. The colour of the membrane is usually grey, but it may be white, yellow or dark brown. The membrane is firmly attached to the mucosa. If it is forcibly removed, a bleeding surface is left, on which it quickly reforms. In atypical cases of diphtheria, sore throat is not associated with false membrane and in these cases it is indistinguishable from a simple sore throat. The diagnosis is confirmed by bacteriological examination of throat swab by smear technique and culture. The growth of KLB occurs in Loeffler's inspissated serum media. The typical blackish colonies usually develop by overnight incubation or within 48 hours.

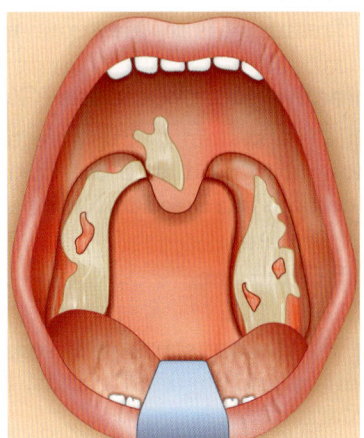

Fig. 23.2: Faucial diphtheria

Treatment

1. Isolation of the patient.
2. Absolute bed rest.
3. Antitoxin—a prophylactic dose of antitoxin (8,000 to 16,000 units) should be given before bacteriological confirmation of the disease. After confirmation, a dose of antitoxin varying from 20,000 in a mild case to 100,000 units in a severe case is injected.
4. Antibiotics like penicillin, and erythromycin, to which the organism is sensitive help to control the primary and secondary infections.

Moniliasis (Thrush)

It is one of the commonest fungus infections of the pharynx. It produces chalky white patches on the fauces, palate, gums, tongue, and buccal mucosa. The causative organism is *Candida albicans* fungus. This is commonly found in ill-nourished children.

Treatment

Well nutritious diet and painting the affected areas with one per cent aqueous solution of gentian violet are sufficient to cure the patient. Mycostatin tablet may be given with good result. Clotrimazole 1% oral paint may be used.

Herpetic Lesions of the Pharynx

Herpetic lesion is rarely found in the throat. In this a group of small vesicles appear on the soft palate or on the anterior pillars and posterior pharyngeal wall. The vesicles soon burst leaving small shallow ulcers. The ulcers may coalesce giving an appearance of a false membrane. The disease is due to a virus infection (Coxsackie-A-virus).

Treatment is by antiseptic mouth wash and one per cent gentian violet paint.

Infective Mononucleosis (Glandular fever)

This is a systemic virus infection of the younger age group (15 to 30 years). It is thought to be due to the Epstein-Barr virus. The large mononuclear cells of the blood are increased and they are atypical. The disease can be of three types:

 i. Anginal.
 ii. Glandular.
 iii. Pyrexial.

The disease starts with sore throat. The neck glands are enlarged, besides the axillary and inguinal glands. In about 50% of the cases the spleen is moderately enlarged.

The Paul-Bunnel test is diagnostic. In this the sheep red cells are agglutinated by patients' serum (serum agglutinin test). The results of this test are not so reliable. The monospot test is more dependable. In more than 50% of the cases liver function tests will show rise in the serum glutamic pyruvate transaminase (SGPT) level.

The treatment is symptomatic.

Agranulocytic Angina

It is characterized by a gross reduction of polymorphonuclear leucocytes in the blood. It causes ulceration in the pharynx. The disease is due to hypersensitivity to certain drugs, such as amidopyrine, neosalvarsan, and sulphapyridine causing bone-marrow depression. The ulcer is often situated at first on the anterior faucial pillar. The fauces, tonsils, and mouth are also rapidly involved. The white blood corpuscles are reduced to less than 2,000 per cu mm. and as such there is no inflammatory reaction.

Treatment

1. Immediate withdrawal of the suspected drug.
2. Pentanucleotide—10 ml injected intramuscularly once or thrice daily depending upon the severity of the condition, for 7–10 days.
3. Deep X-ray therapy to the long bones in small doses sometimes helps.
4. Injection of vitamin B_{12} may be given.
5. Antibiotics—broad-spectrum antibiotics should be given to combat the infection.
6. Repeated blood transfusion.

Glossopharyngeal Zoster

This has been described (Clark, 1979) in a patient who was exposed to varicella, developed vesicles on the posterior 3rd of the tongue only, with pain in the ear and rising varicella virus titres.

24
Inflammations of the Lymphoid Tissue of the Pharynx

Adenoids

Definition

The nasopharyngeal tonsil when hypertrophied so as to produce symptoms is called adenoids.

The hypertrophy of the pharyngeal tonsil may be simple or inflammatory. The inflammation may again be simple or tuberculous.

Clinical Features

The symptoms and signs may be referred to simple enlargement, and to inflammation, or to both.

Symptoms and Signs due to Hypertrophy

1. *Nasal obstruction:* Nasal obstruction leads to mouth breathing, interferes with feeding, noisy breathing and wet bubbly nose. The voice becomes nasal (Rhino-Lalia Clausa) and loses tone.
2. There is nasal discharge, partly due to obstruction of the posterior nasal apertures and partly due to chronic rhinitis secondary to infected adenoids.
3. *Deafness:* It is due to the obstruction of the eustachian tubes by the adenoids. This diminishes the volume of air entry into the middle ears and subsequent retraction of the tympanic membrane. Eustachian tubes may be inflamed after obstruction and may produce intermittent pain in the ears.

Symptoms and Signs due to Inflammation

1. The common symptoms are nasal discharge, postnasal drip and cough. On gagging a plug of mucopus is seen behind the uvula. There may be a rise in temperature.
2. Otitis media is the most serious effect. It may be of an acute or a chronic form. The eustachian tubes in infants and children are shorter, wider, and more horizontal and this facilitates the spread of infection in the middle ear.
3. The infection of the adenoid may lead to sinusitis and rhinitis.
4. The upper deep cervical glands mostly in the posterior triangles may be involved (cervical adenitis).

General Symptoms

1. Mental dullness. It may be due to deafness. The child becomes dull, shy, friendless, and lacks in concentration. The teeth are crowded and chest becomes flat.
2. Nocturnal enuresis and night terrors may be aggravated (reflex symptoms).

Diagnosis

The diagnosis is made by the following:

1. Clinical features.
2. Inspection with posterior rhinoscopic mirror reveals a lobulated mass is seen in the nasopharynx (Fig. 24.1).
3. Digital palpation—a lobulated mass with a soft rubbery feel is felt in the nasopharynx.
4. Soft tissue X-ray of the nasopharynx (Fig. 24.2).

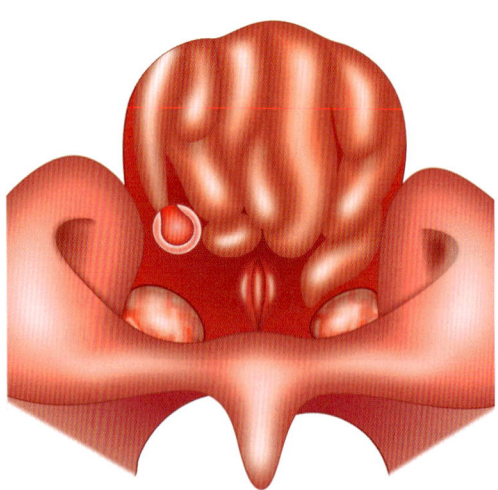

Fig. 24.1: Posterior rhinoscopic view of adenoids and eustachian cushion

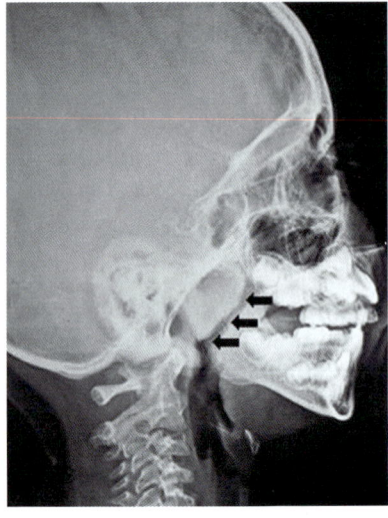

Fig. 24.2: X-ray showing enlarged adenoids

Adenoid Facies

This is a typical appearance of the face. It is developed due to obstruction of the nasal breathing during the growing period. The most common cause is enlarged adenoids. The most prominent features are:

   i. Open mouth with dried up lips.
  ii. Pinched up nose due to ill-developed alae nasi.
 iii. Absence of nasolabial furrows.
  iv. Constant rhinorrhoea.
   v. High arched palate.
  vi. Crowding of the teeth.
 vii. An underslung lower jaw and protrusion of the upper jaw. All these features together give rise to a dull idiotic and expressionless look of the child.

Differential Diagnosis

The other causes of nasal obstruction in children are:

Allergic rhinitis, foreign bodies, hypertrophied posterior ends of inferior turbinates, nasopharyngeal fibroma, deviated nasal septum, sinusitis, antrochoanal polyp, septal haematoma or abscess and Thornwald's disease.

Treatment

1. *Conservative:* When the symptoms are very slight, an operation should not be performed. Simple breathing exercises may be helpful. Non-irritant decongestant nasal drops (e.g. half to one per cent ephedrine saline) may give relief. Sinusitis and nasal allergy must be treated.
2. *Surgical:* Adenoidectomy: When the symptoms are marked, adenoids may be removed as a separate operation or during tonsillectomy. Where both the procedures are carried out, the adenoids are preferably removed first.

Adenoidectomy

Premedication

Injection of pethidine hydrochloride or barbiturates are used in a suitable dosage.

Anaesthesia

Endotracheal anaesthesia is given by nitrous oxide, oxygen, etc. The larynx is packed with a ribbon gauze to prevent the entry of blood into the trachea.

Technique

After anaesthesia and draping the Boyle-Davis gag is applied and fixed with chest piece and rod or Draffin's bipod. The adenoid curette with cage is used. The blade of the curette should be sharp for a clean removal of adenoid tissue. The patient lies on the back with a slightly flexed neck and the surgeon sits at the head end as in the dissection method of tonsillectomy. After holding the curette in the same fashion as a dagger is held, it is introduced into the mouth and passed behind the soft palate till the curette is arrested by the posterior end of the nasal septum. The curette is gently pressed downwards and then swept forwards, keeping the cutting edge in contact with the roof and posterior wall of the nasopharynx and withdrawn. The curetted adenoid tissue is held by the cage.

Finally, the surgeon passes his right index finger into the nasopharynx to be sure that all adenoid vegetations have been removed. The bleeding is fully controlled by postnasal packing. After removing the pack, the gag is taken out. The patient is quickly turned on his side, or face down, to allow the blood to escape, if any.

After Treatment

Same as tonsillectomy.

Complications

1. Incomplete removal.
2. Hypernasality.

3. Reactionary haemorrhage.
4. Secondary haemorrhage.

Obstructive Sleep Apnoea

Apnoea during sleep has been divided into obstructive, central and mixed. Obstructive apnoea is preceded by upper respiratory defects. Obstructive sleep apnoea is considered when a patient has 30 apnoeic episodes each lasting 10 seconds or more during 7 hours of sleep. During this apnoeic episodes the oxygen saturation levels in arterial blood fall. The relationship between snoring and sleep apnoea is ill-defined. Snoring is more common in elderly men and occurs in a surprisingly high proportion of the population. In obstructive sleep apnoea the patients may develop right-sided heart failure and pulmonary hypertension. The disturbed sleep with oxygen desaturation leads to daytime somnolence. Monitoring the patients during sleep with ECG, EEG, EOG, Oximetry, oral and nasal thermisters and thoraco abdominal strain gauges is necessary. Oxygen desaturation is often accompanied by bradycardia and cardiac arrhythmias eventually leading to right ventricular failure and hypertension.

Treatment

In obese patient weight reduction may help. Medical treatment includes continuous administration of oxygen at increased pressure (CPAP). Protriptyline has been shown to decrease the number of apnoeic episodes.

The most successful surgery for obstructive sleep apnoea is tracheostomy. Correction of obvious upper airway defects such as severely deviated nasal septum or removal of nasal polyp may help some patients and should be carried out before more drastic measures are undertaken. Excision of part of the soft palate and uvula (palatopharyngoplasty) has been described. The surgery involves resection of the tonsils if they are still present together with a portion of the free edge of the soft palate and uvula. In general 10–15 mm of soft palate should be resected more medially than laterally. If the tonsils are removed at the same time, suturing the anterior to the posterior pillar has been advised. The bare surface of the soft palate remaining after resection is sutured so that the mucosa of the posterior surface is brought into contact with the anterior surface. Mandibular osteotomies, hyoid bone expansion or wedge resection of the parts of the base of the tongue have, on occasions, been helpful.

25

Tonsillitis

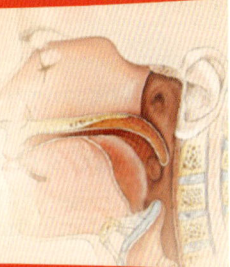

Acute Tonsillitis

The acute inflammation of the tonsils has been classified as follows:

1. Catarrhal tonsillitis: Only the mucosa is inflamed.
2. Lacunar or follicular tonsillitis: Only the crypts of the tonsils are involved. The mouths of the crypts contain pus causing spotted appearance. Sometimes the pus from the crypts coalesce, giving the appearance of a false membrane.
3. Parenchymatous tonsillitis: Here the whole tonsil is infected with marked swelling.
4. Suppurative tonsillitis
   a. Tonsillar
   b. Peritonsillar or "Quinsy"
       i. Anterior
       ii. Posterior
       iii. External

Acute Follicular Tonsillitis

Aetiology

The causes are:
   i. Predisposing
   ii. Exciting.

1. Predisposing Causes

   a. Age—common between the ages of ten and thirty.
   b. Anatomical predispositions, e.g. enlarged tonsils; adhesions of the triangular folds and anterior faucial pillars.
   c. Incomplete removal of the tonsils.
   d. Initial stage of measles and other exanthematous fevers.
   e. Drinking of infected water and milk.
   f. Overcrowding and ill ventilation of classrooms.
   g. Seasonal—common in spring and autumn and rare in summer.
   h. Postnasal drip due to suppuration in the paranasal sinuses.
   i. Impaction of foreign bodies.

2. Exciting Causes

Haemolytic streptococci are the infecting organisms in the majority of acute cases. The non-haemolytic streptococcus, staphylococcus aureus, bacillus Friedlander, pneumococcus, or micrococcus catarrhalis may also be the predominant organisms. Vincent's organisms may be an important factor. About 50% of acute tonsillitis is due to viral infection.

Clinical Features

1. Pain in the throat which radiates up to the ear. It greatly increases on swallowing (painful deglutition or odynophagia).
2. Rise in temperature-may be between 100°F and 105°F.
3. Malaise, anorexia, thirst, constipation and prostration.

The voice becomes thick and muffled. The cervical glands are enlarged and become tender. The tonsillar gland (jugulodigastric) is chiefly involved. The pulse rate is from 100 to 120, and is generally full and bounding. The tongue is coated and the breath is foetid.

The tonsils are enlarged and congested. The congested surface of the tonsils is spotted which occlude the mouth of the crypts (Fig. 25.1). In some, cases a false membrane yellowish in colour is formed which is limited only to the tonsil. This membrane can be easily separated and does not bleed from the surface on doing so.

When the parenchyma of the tonsil is more involved, the local symptoms become marked. The tonsils are greatly swollen. The mucus becomes thick and tenacious. The movement of the palate is impeded giving rise to unintelligible voice and regurgitation of swallowed fluid through nostrils.

Diagnosis

Diagnosis is not difficult. Sometimes it is difficult to distinguish follicular tonsillitis from faucial diphtheria.

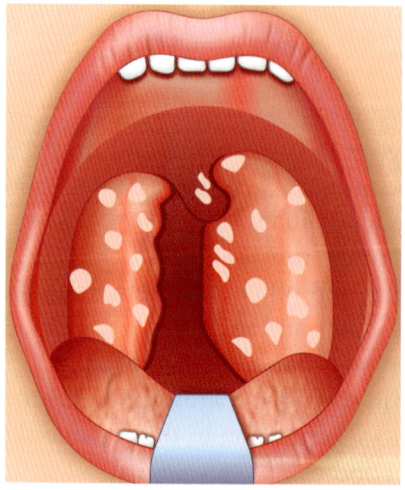

Fig. 25.1: Acute follicular tonsillitis

Differential diagnosis between acute follicular tonsillitis and faucial diphtheria		
Symptoms and signs	*Follicular tonsillitis*	*Faucial diphtheria*
Onset	Sudden	Gradual
Limitation	Limited to the tonsils which are enlarged and inflamed	Not limited to tonsils only. The palate, pillars of the fauces and other neighbouring structures are involved.
Pain and fever	More, from 100° to 104°F or more	Less, moderate fever between 99 and 100°F
Toxicity	Little or no toxicity	More
Urine	Not albuminous	Albuminous in the early stage
Trismus	Present	Nil
False membrane	Not spreading and adherent, membrane is thick and yellowish, can be easily separated, does not leave a bleeding surface, does not reform	Adherent and spreading, grayish in colour and thin, cannot easily be separated, leaves a bleeding surface and reforms in a few hours
Neck gland enlargement	Less and about the same on both sides	More marked and common on one side
Age group	Common between 10 and 30 years	2 to 10 years. Common between 2 and 5 years
Culture of membrane	No growth of Klebs-Loeffler bacillus	Growth of Klebs-Loeffler bacillus

Other diseases for differentiation are:
  i. Vincent's angina
  ii. Agranulocytic angina
  iii. Thrush
  iv. Streptococcal tonsillitis
  v. Lymphatic leukaemia
  vi. Infective mononucleosis (glandular fever).

Prognosis

Prognosis is good if not complicated.

Treatment

1. Rest in bed.
2. Paracetamol or other analgesics is very effective in mild cases.
3. Systemic antibiotics must be given in suitable dosage.
4. Antiseptic mouthwash and gargle.

Complications

1. Peritonsillar abscess (quinsy).
2. Acute retropharyngeal and parapharyngeal abscesses.

3. Oedema of the larynx.
4. Acute rheumatism.
5. Acute nephritis.
6. Subacute bacterial endocarditis.
7. Acute infection of the middle ear cleft.
8. Septicaemia.
9. Chronic tonsillitis.

Chronic Tonsillitis

Passing childhood with no attack of acute tonsillitis is rare. Suffering once or twice from acute tonsillitis a year in childhood is normal.

Chronic inflammation of the tonsils may be of two types:
1. Chronic parenchymatous tonsillitis.
2. Chronic follicular tonsillitis.

Chronic Parenchymatous Tonsillitis

This type usually follows an acute or subacute attack of tonsillitis or some of the infectious diseases, such as, measles or diphtheria. It is common in children between the ages of 4 and 15.

Clinical Features

1. Recurrent acute attack of pain in throat.
2. An irritating cough.
3. Persistent enlargement of the tonsillar glands.
4. Tonsils are markedly enlarged and may actually meet in the midline.
5. Speech may become thick, so that the child speaks as if his mouth is full.
6. Anterior pillars of the tonsils are flushed.

This condition must not be confused with the physiological enlargement of the tonsils which occurs in the childhood. The tonsils may enlarge in children twice due to physiological hyperplasia:

i. About the age of two when the child begins to play with other children.
ii. About the age of five or six when the child is at school and meets with fresh infections.

This enlargement corresponds with the development of active immunity. This is not associated with the clinical features of chronic tonsillitis and usually settles down without constitutional disturbances.

Treatment

a. Conservative
   i. Fresh air and sunlight.
   ii. A vitamin-rich diet.
   iii. A general tonic in the winter season.

b. Surgical

Tonsillectomy should be recommended if no improvement occurs with conservative treatment and if the recurrent acute attacks continue.

Chronic Follicular Tonsillitis

This is common in adults and results from repeated attacks of acute tonsillitis.

Clinical Features

1. Repeated attack of pain in throat.
2. Bad taste from the cheesy matter which collects in the crypts.
3. Unpleasant smell from the mouth (halitosis).
4. Frequent gastric upset from swallowing the septic material.
5. Systemic upsets, such as fibrositis or other rheumatic manifestations.
6. The tonsils are usually fibrotic and small.
7. Anterior pillars are flushed.
8. Cervical glands are enlarged and non-tender.
9. Pressure on the anterior pillars with a tongue depressor squeezes thin, creamy pus from the crypts.
10. Sometimes 'retention cyst' (smooth yellow swelling containing a creamy fluid and debris) is seen on the surface of the tonsil. This condition may be confused with keratosis pharynges in which the horny growths are adherent to the surface of the tonsils.

Treatment

So far no medical treatment is known which can eradicate chronic tonsillitis.

1. *Conservative:* Where surgery is contraindicated as in:
    i. Haemophilia
    ii. Active pulmonary tuberculosis
    iii. Gross hypertension
    iv. Severe diabetes
    v. Advanced age.

    In those the treatment should be in the form of suction of crypts and gurgles, a throat paint either Mandl's paint (see appendix) or resorcin with glycerine (0.3 gm of resorcin in 28.3 ml glycerine) paint.
2. *Surgical:* Tonsillectomy by dissection method in chronic tonsillitis is the only curative treatment. But the operation may be exposed to criticism because of bad selection, bad preparation, bad operation and bad postoperative management of cases.

Laser Tonsillectomy

For tonsillectomy, KTP-532 laser should be used. It reduces intraoperative bleeding.

Tonsillectomy

Indications

The indications of tonsillectomy may be classified under three headings.

A. *Local Indications*

1. An attack of peritonsillar abscess (quinsy)
2. Recurrent attacks of acute tonsillitis, more than three attacks a year
3. Chronic tonsillitis
4. Carrier state-as in carriers of *Streptococcus haemolyticus* or diphtheria bacilli
5. Persistent enlargement of tonsils producing obstruction to swallowing and breathing
6. Before the operation for cleft palate
7. Before the avulsion of the glossopharyngeal nerve for neuralgia and removal of elongated styloid process through tonsillar fossa in Eagle's syndrome
8. Early stage of malignancy of the tonsil for biopsy purpose.

B. *Focal Indications*

Where the tonsils act as septic foci, e.g.
1. Persistently enlarged neck glands for which no other cause is present
2. Tuberculosis of the cervical glands in the absence of active pulmonary lesion
3. Recurrent attacks of acute rheumatism
4. Attacks of acute glomerular nephritis
5. Infections of the conjunctiva, skin, joints and fasciae
6. Recurrent attacks of bronchitis and sinusitis associated with acute or chronic tonsillitis.

C. *General Indications*

It occurs more commonly in children.
1. General debility, failure to gain weight, and malaise.
2. For sleep apnoea syndrome when the patient is undergoing palato-pharyngoplasty.

Contraindications

1. Recent infection—for increased risk of haemorrhage.
2. Blood dyscrasias, e.g. haemophilia and leukaemia.
3. Epidemics of infectious diseases, particularly the epidemics of poliomyelitis.
4. Aneurysm of the internal carotid artery.
5. Hypertension.
6. Diabetes.
7. Active pulmonary tuberculosis.
8. Oral contraceptives for more chances of deep vein thrombosis after tonsillectomy.

Complications

1. Quinsy (peritonsillar or paratonsillar abscess).
2. Parapharyngeal abscess.
3. Intratonsillar abscess.
4. Tonsillolith.
5. Tonsillar cyst.
6. Focal infection such as rheumatic fever and glomerulonephritis.
7. Eye conditions such as episcleritis, recurrent conjunctivitis and choroiditis
8. Conditions such as psoriasis, chronic urticaria and purpura.

Technique (Tonsillectomy)

See text.

Preoperative Investigations

1. General medical check up—to exclude any chest, kidney, and liver diseases.
2. Examination of blood for Hb%, total count; differential count, erythrocytic sedimentation rate, bleeding and coagulation time, PT, APTT, platelet count.
   Total and differential count is necessary to exclude acute infections in which the leucocyte count and neutrophil polymorphs are increased. These are considerably diminished in agranulocytosis.
   ESR is increased in all chronic diseases. But here it is mainly done to exclude acute pulmonary tuberculosis in the presence of other related symptoms.
   Bleeding and coagulation time is important to exclude blood dyscrasias. Bleeding time increases in purpura and coagulation time increases in haemophilia. Normal bleeding time is 1 to 3 minutes and coagulation time is 2 to 6 minutes.
3. Examination of urine for complete analysis. Especially for sugar and albumin.

Complications of Tonsillectomy

The complications of tonsillectomy are mainly two:
1. Haemorrhage.
2. Infection.

Haemorrhage

Haemorrhage may be reactionary or secondary.
A. Reactionary haemorrhage occurs within 24 hours after operation. But commonly occurs within the first few hours and may be copious. The causes of reactionary haemorrhage are:
   i. Failure of the torn vessels to contract or retract.
   ii. Rise in blood pressure after anaesthesia.
   iii. Slipping of a ligature.

The bleeding may be arterial or venous. In the presence of fibrosis, the cut blood vessels cannot retract which is more common in cases of veins. Sometimes a clot in the tonsillar fossa keeps the cut vessel open and oozing occurs beneath the clot.

If no fresh blood is seen, there is no need to disturb the clot. The patient should be well sedated by administration of a suitable sedative drug. The case should be kept under constant watch and pulse rate should be checked after every fifteen minutes. In the presence of fresh blood oozing around the clot, it should be removed and the bleeding fossa should be pressed for a few minutes with a swab soaked in any coagulants or hydrogen peroxide. If this fails, the patient is to be reanaesthetized and the bleeding vessels must be caught and ligatured. In cases of children the second method should invariably be adopted because they will be more terrified by painful intrapharyngeal manipulations.

B. Secondary haemorrhage occurs after 24 hours and within 14 days of operation but it usually occurs between the 5th and 8th postoperative days. The cause of this is the infection in the tonsillar fossa. This type of haemorrhage is less severe than the reactionary type. Only sedation, rest in bed, and antibiotics cure majority of the cases.

If the bleeding is copious and is not controlled by the above method, the patient should be re-anaesthetized. A sterile gauze swab is inserted in the tonsillar fossa and the pillars are stitched together over the swab. The swab should be kept *in situ* for 24 hours. In this type of haemorrhage one should not try to catch hold the bleeding vessels because the tissue in the fossa becomes oedematous and friable.

Infection

Infection may be in the form of the following:
1. Cervical lymphadenitis.
2. Otitis media.
3. Parapharyngeal abscess.
4. Septicaemia.

Other complications include
1. Incomplete removal.
2. Pulmonary complications like lobar pneumonia and lung abscess. These usually follow inhalation of blood or a tooth.
3. Dental injuries.
4. Dislocation of the cervical vertebrae and prolapse of the intervertebral discs.
5. Atrophy of uvula.

Sequellae of Tonsillectomy

Recurrence of lymphoid tissue in tonsillar fossa, and extensive palatal fibrosis leading to defective speech are the important sequellae.

Postoperative Care after Tonsillectomy

1. Patient must be kept in the bed in right lateral position without a pillow until recovery of spontaneous cough reflex.
2. Watch for bleeding, pulse, respiration, vomiting and frequent swallowing movements.
3. Listen for rattling sound during breathing.

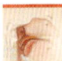

4. Four to six hours after operation sips of cold water and ice cream should be allowed to drink and kept the patient on liquid diet for 24 hours. Then onwards switch on to normal diet gradually with initial sloppy diet. Hard foods are avoided.

5. Analgesics for pain may be given.

6. A prophylactic antibiotic may be advised.

7. Antiseptic mouthwash and gargle should be encouraged from the evening or day after operation.

8. Children should be off from the school for a further period of 10 days and adults should be off from work for 3 weeks after the operation.

26

Peritonsillar, Retropharyngeal and Parapharyngeal Abscess

PERITONSILLAR ABSCESS (QUINSY)

Definition: Peritonsillar abscess or quinsy is a suppuration and collection of pus in between the tonsil capsule and the related lateral wall of the pharynx. In the majority of cases (90%), the collection of pus is in the supratonsillar region or anterosuperior to the tonsil. The collection of pus may be:

a. Anterosuperior to the tonsil, so it lies behind the anterior pillar of the fauces.

b. Behind the tonsil.

c. Lateral to the tonsil.

Aetiology

It commonly occurs in young adults between 15 and 35 years of age. It is more common in males than in females. The abscess is usually unilateral. The condition almost always follows an attack of tonsillitis especially the lacunar type. There is no relation between the size of the tonsil and the peritonsillar abscess formation. Adhesion between the tonsil and the plica semilunaris due to repeated attacks of acute tonsillitis accounts for the occurrence and recurrence of quinsies.

Clinical Features

1. Acute pain in the throat. It radiates up to the ear and behind the angle of the jaw.
2. General malaise, fever, chill, and rigor. The temperature may rise up to 104°F with increase in pulse rate.
3. Intense dysphagia so much so that the patient cannot even swallow his own saliva leading to dribbling.
4. Trismus is common due to reflex spasm of the masseter muscles.
5. Speech becomes thick and rattling due to accumulation of secretion in the pharynx.
6. The head is fixed and inclined to the affected side. The patient supports the head by the palm.
7. Breath becomes offensive (halitosis).
8. The patient becomes very anxious.
9. The tonsillar glands are swollen and tender.

10. By good illumination the tonsillar and palatal regions can be seen through the narrow opening of the jaws, which are markedly congested and oedematous. The uvula is swollen and oedematous. The tip of the uvula is seen to be pointed towards the affected side. The tonsil is pushed downwards and medially or may present the appearances of a follicular tonsillitis (Fig. 26.1).

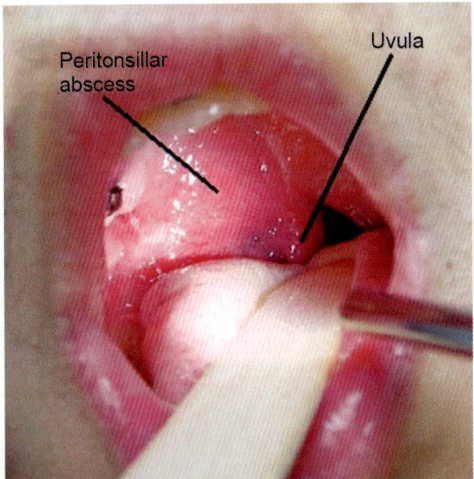

Fig. 26.1: Peritonsillar abscess on the right side

Complications

Nowadays the complications are rare. There may be parapharyngeal abscess, haemorrhage, oedema of the larynx, septicaemia and thrombosis of the internal jugular vein. Spontaneous bursting of the abscess during sleep with asphyxia and death is not uncommon.

Diagnosis

The diagnosis is not difficult after twenty-four hours of the initial symptoms. But the possibility of neoplasms of the tonsil, parapharyngeal abscess and retropharyngeal abscess should be kept in mind.

Treatment

Once an abscess has formed, incision and drainage is essential. It is best done with a guarded scalpel or bayonet-shaped sinus forceps. The site of drainage is to be determined as follows:

1. At the most prominent part of the swelling.
2. About the middle of a line drawn from the base of the uvula to the last upper molar tooth on the side of the abscess.
3. One to two cm. external to the point of interception of an imaginary horizontal line through the base of the uvula and a vertical one along the anterior faucial pillar. This is the best point for opening the quinsy.

Incision and drainage of peritonsillar abscess is commonly undertaken at the point of maximum swelling of the soft palate above the upper pole of the tonsil. The mucosa may be anaesthetized with xylocaine spray and incised with a No. 15 blade with all but the terminal 0.5–1.0 cm guarded using zinc oxide tape. A pair of sinus forceps should be introduced through the incision and opened to break down any loculi. Many surgeons have suggested that per-mucosal needle drainage of the abscess is equally efficacious, less distressing for the patients and, of course, cost effective.

Tonsillectomy, usually after 6 weeks in a patient who had a quinsy, is a common procedure to avoid recurrence. Follow-up studies on patients who have had a quinsy shows that only about 20% at the most, have a second peritonsillar abscess, so perhaps the policy of tonsillectomy after quinsy should be revised. Therefore, if the recurrence rate after quinsy is only about 20%, then abscess tonsillectomy means that many patients are having unnecessary surgery.

It is dangerous to use general anaesthesia in draining a quinsy. Carbolic acid may be used with a probe at the selected site of incision. This helps in the following ways:

1. It produces anaesthesia.
2. It marks the site of drainage.
3. It acts as an antiseptic.

After drainage of the abscess, warm antiseptic mouthwash should be given. The patient should attend the clinic regularly for check up of the opening which should be kept dilated if it tends to close up. In addition to the above treatment, one should advise suitable antibiotics for systemic disinfection, analgesics for controlling the pain, rest in bed and liquid nutritious diet (Fig. 26.2).

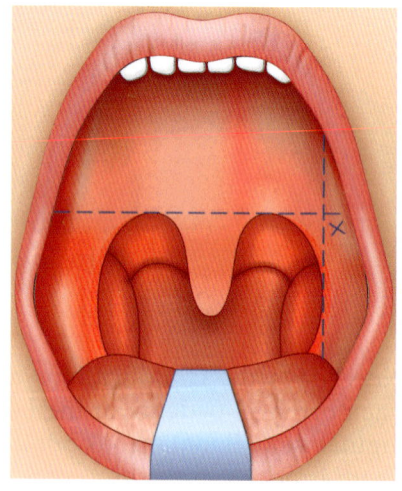

Fig. 26.2: Site for draining the peritonsillar abscess (left)

RETROPHARYNGEAL ABSCESS

Anatomy

Anatomy of the retropharyngeal spaces is important for the better understanding of the pathology of retropharyngeal abscess. The prevertebral fascia separates the visceral compartment of the neck, containing pharynx, larynx, trachea, and thyroid gland from the cervical vertebrae and prevertebral muscles. The buccopharyngeal fascia covers the sides and back of the pharynx. It is firmly attached with the prevertebral fascia at the midline of the back of the pharynx. The potential space in between the prevertebral and buccopharyngeal fascia is known as retropharyngeal space or space of Gilette. These spaces are separated from each other by the firm attachment of the two above mentioned fasciae.

In the retropharyngeal space of Gilette there are prevertebral or retropharyngeal lymph glands. These glands disappear as the child grows. This is the reason why retropharyngeal abscess is common in children (Fig. 26.3).

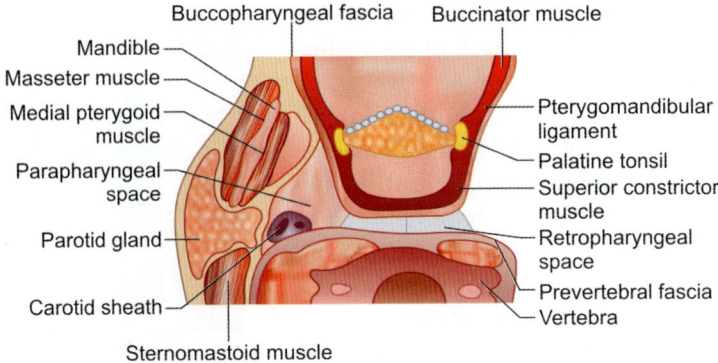

Fig. 26.3: Retropharyngeal and parapharyngeal spaces

Definition

Collection of pus behind the posterior pharyngeal wall is called retropharyngeal abscess.

Retropharyngeal abscess is of two types: acute and chronic. The acute type is more common and lies in the true retropharyngeal spaces, i.e. between the prevertebral and buccopharyngeal fascia. The chronic retropharyngeal abscess lies behind the prevertebral fascia.

1. Acute Retropharyngeal Abscess

Aetiology

The acute abscess is developed by suppuration of the retropharyngeal lymph glands. The infection reaches generally from the tonsils and adenoids. The infection occasionally may track from an acute suppurative otitis media or mastoiditis. Perforation of the posterior pharyngeal wall by foreign bodies such as fish bone or pins or needles may give rise to acute retropharyngeal abscess.

Streptococcus is the commonest organism. *Staphylococcus* and *Pneumococcus* are rarely met with.

Pathology

The retropharyngeal glands receive the lymphatics of the postnasal space, pharynx, nose, eustachian tube, and middle ear. When the infection goes via lymphatics, adenitis is the first pathological change leading to periadenitis and abscess formation. The suppuration usually occurs on one side of midline and produces swelling in the oropharynx.

Clinical Features

At least 50 per cent of the patients are under one year of age. This is common in boys than in girls. It is rare in adults.

The prominent symptoms are difficulty in breathing and suckling. The patient refuses feeds or vomits and becomes restless due to pain. There may be a croupy cough and a muffled throaty cry resembling a 'squawk' of a duck. There may be nasal obstruction if the abscess extends into the nasopharynx, stiffness of the neck or torticollis, rise in temperature, and toxoemia.

On inspection through the mouth, a lateral swelling of the posterior pharyngeal wall is seen. The pharynx is congested. On palpation the presence of fluctuation may be demonstrated in some cases.

Soft tissue X-ray of the nasopharynx may reveal the size and extent of the abscess.

Extension of inflammation may cause oedema of the larynx. The abscess may spontaneously rupture and cause aspiration and sudden death.

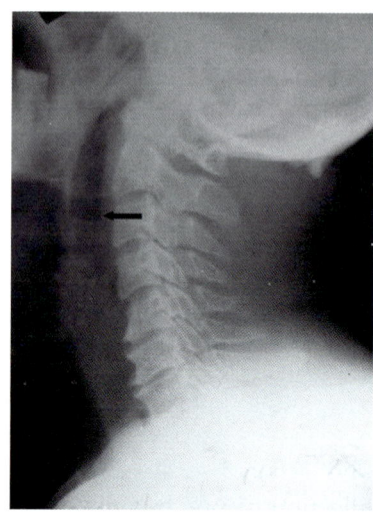

Fig. 26.4: Lateral view X-ray of the neck showing retropharyngeal abscess with fluid level in the prevertebral region

Treatment

a. Incision and drainage of the abscess: The incision is made vertically through the mouth. No anaesthesia is used.

b. Antiobiotics should be administered systemically to control infection. Tracheostomy may be required in the presence of laryngeal oedema with respiratory distress.

2. Chronic Retropharyngeal Abscess

Aetiology

Tuberculosis of the cervical vertebrae causes collection of pus behind the prevertebral fascia. It is situated in the midline. Sometimes tuberculous invasion of the deep cervical glands may cause extension of tuberculous infection to the retropharyngeal glands.

Pathology

Chronic retropharyngeal abscess is tuberculous in nature. However, osteomyelitis of the cervical vertebrae may develop as a result of pyogenic infection from the retropharyngeal region leading to chronic retropharyngeal abscess.

Clinical Features

This is common in young adults. The onset of the disease is slow. It gives rise to pharyngeal discomfort and dysphagia. On examination through the mouth a painless, fluctuating midline swelling is seen on the posterior pharyngeal wall. Cervical glands may be enlarged and painless.

X-ray of the cervical spine should be taken. Mantoux test, X-ray of the chest, and blood sedimentation rate should be done.

Treatment

The abscess is usually opened through an incision over the posterior border of the sternomastoid muscle. The dissection is carried behind the large vessels of the neck and in front of the prevertebral muscles. It is never drained through the mouth. Incision may also be made in front of the sternomastoid muscle. In addition to the above treatment, one should give a full course of antituberculous drugs and rest to the part after consultation with the orthopaedic surgeon.

Parapharyngeal Abscess

Infection and suppuration in the parapharyngeal space is called parapharyngeal abscess. As a complication of tonsillitis or quinsy, occasionally parapharyngeal abscess may develop. Sometimes, infection may spread from lower wisdom tooth and its surrounding gum and bone. Pus collects in between the superior constrictor muscle and the investing layer of deep cervical fascia (parapharyngeal space) in close proximity to the internal jugular vein and carotid arteries. It may occur at any age, but commonly occurs in adolescents and adults.

Clinical Features

1. Pain in the throat and neck.
2. Dysphagia.
3. Toxaemia with high temperature like quinsy.
4. Tender swelling in the neck below the angle of the mandible.
5. Localized infection of the tonsil or quinsy.

Complications

1. Thrombosis in the internal jugular vein.
2. Fatal massive haemorrhage due to necrosis of the wall of the vein or carotid artery.
3. Oedema of the larynx.
4. Mediastinitis.

Treatment

1. Early incision and drainage of the abscess in the neck, or through the pharynx.
2. Suitable antibiotics in adequate doses.

27 Tumours of the Pharynx

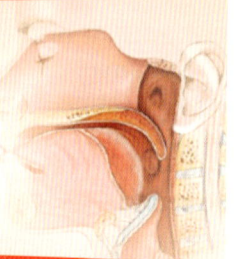

TUMOURS OF THE NASOPHARYNX

Benign Tumours

Nasopharyngeal Angiofibroma (NPA)

Nasopharyngeal angiofibroma is not so common in our country. It is a benign tumour histologically, but clinically malignant. It has a predilection for males between 10 and 25 years of age.

Modern methods of investigation and ambitious surgical procedures have focused attention on the region of the sphenopalatine foramen as the site of origin and this would most reasonably explain the subsequent behaviour of angiofibroma.

The main blood supply to angiofibroma comes by way of an enlarged maxillary artery, but other arteries, such as the ascending pharyngeal, vidian, unnamed branches of the internal carotid and rarely the vertebral, may contribute to their vascularisation.

Clinical Features

It causes progressive nasal obstruction, recurrent attacks of epistaxis and nasal voice (rhinolalia clausa). Blockage of the eustachian tubes by the extension of the growth results in conductive deafness. The tumour is pink or red in colour and the consistency is very firm. The surface is smooth and lobulated. The extension of the tumour in different directions causes:

i. Broadening of the nose with so called 'frog-face' deformity—if extends into the nasal cavities.
ii. Protrusion of the eye ball (proptosis)—if extends into the orbit.
iii. Swelling of the cheek due to extension of the tumour through the pterygopalatine fossa into the cheek.

Severe neuralgic pain appears in the later stages. Intracranial extension is not uncommon. Radiographs and CT scan will reveal the outline of the growth, its size and extension. In CT scan there will be enhancement of dye due to increased vascularity. Digital examination and biopsy should be done with due precaution for the treatment of excessive bleeding.

Stages of NPA

Stage I—the tumour is limited to the site of origin and nasopharynx
Stage II—the tumour extends into the nose and sphenoidal sinus.

Stage III—the tumour extends into the infratemporal fossa, cheek, orbits, etc.
Stage IV—the tumour extends into the cranium.

There are many other stages of NPA but this is the basic and simplest one and easy to remember.

Differential Diagnosis

Treatment is either by surgery or by radiotherapy and surgery. The tumour may be removed through transpalatal approach of Wilson. All precautions should be taken for the severe haemorrhage which occurs during removal. The larynx must be packed around an endotracheal tube. Bilateral external carotid artery ligation may help in checking the severe bleeding during removal. If available operation should be performed under hypotensive anesthesia. Radiotherapy helps in decreasing the vascularity of the tumour surgery. As the tumour is a fibroma and resistant to deep X-ray—it does not destroy it. Electrocoagulation and cryosurgery often help to eradicate these tumours. Laser surgery may be helpful in stage I. This can be excised endoscopically after embolization of the feeding blood vessels.

Other Benign Tumours

Papilloma, adenoma, mixed salivary tumours, enchondroma, exostoses, angioma and many other benign tumours may occur in the nasopharynx. They give rise to nasal obstruction, nasal discharge and epistaxis. Biopsy confirms the diagnosis. Treatment is removal and/or electrocoagulation and cryosurgery.

Malignant Tumours

Squamous Cell Carcinoma

The commonest malignant tumour of the nasopharynx is squamous-cell carcinoma. Most of them are anaplastic in nature. The commonest site is the fossa of Rosenmuller. Metastasis in the neck glands is a very common feature. It causes conductive deafness, immobility of the homolateral soft palate, and trigeminal neuralgia (Trotter's triad). The following cranial nerves may be involved:

i. Second, third and fourth cranial nerves due to orbital invasion—results exophthalmos.
ii. Sixth cranial nerve—results internal squint.
iii. Ninth, tenth and eleventh cranial nerves—result jugular foramen syndrome.

If the tumour is of proliferative in type, it causes nasal obstruction. Epistaxis is common in ulcerative type. Posterior rhinoscopy, finger palpation, and X-ray of the soft tissue nasopharynx and base of the skull, CT and MRI help in diagnosis and extent of the tumour. Confirmation is made by exfoliative cytology and biopsy.

Treatment

As most of the patients seek advice with the metastatic neck glands and most of the tumours are highly anaplastic and radio-sensitive, irradiation by supervoltage (CO60) therapy is the treatment of choice.

Cytotoxic drugs may be used along with radiotherapy.

Other Malignant Tumours

Other than squamous cell carcinoma, the most common malignant tumour is lymphoepithelioma. Sarcoma either lympho or reticulum cell types are rarely seen in younger age group. Treatment is by external irradiation.

Tumours of the Oropharynx and Lymphomas of the Head and Neck

Oropharynx is that part of the pharynx which extends from the level of the hard palate above to the hyoid bone below. For the purpose of tumour classification, the oropharynx is further subdivided into four main sites:

1. Anterior wall (glossoepiglottic area)
   a. Tongue posterior to the vallate papillae (base of tongue or posterior third)
   b. Vallecula (anterior or lingual surface of the epiglottis is included in the larynx-suprahyoid epiglottis)
2. Lateral wall
   a. Tonsil
   b. Tonsillar fossa and faucial pillars
   c. Tonsillolingual sulci
3. Posterior wall
4. Superior wall
   a. Inferior surface of soft palate
   b. Uvula

Epithelial Tumours

Benign epithelial tumours such as papillomas arise from the squamous epithelium. Malignant epithelial tumour is squamous cell carcinoma and its variant lymphoepithelioma.

Lymphoepithelioma

Lymphoma of the head and neck

   Lymphomas of the head and neck may arise in nodal or extranodal sites. Both Hodgkin's disease and non-Hodgkin's lymphoma commonly present as lymph node deposits but Hodgkin's disease is very rare in the oropharynx. Non-Hodgkin's lymphoma accounts for about 15–20% of tumours at this site most being of the B-cell type.

Salivary Gland Tumours

Salivary gland tumours account for about 5% of all tumours of the oropharynx; but this is only a very small proportion of salivary gland tumours arising in the head and neck.

Investigations

1. Fine needle aspiration cytology
2. Radiological investigation

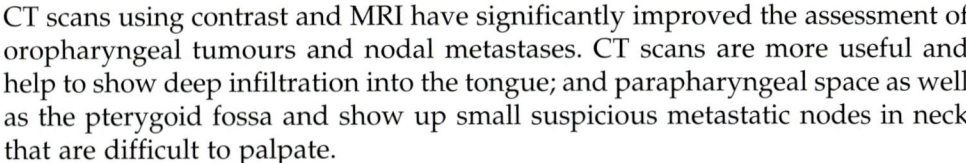

CT scans using contrast and MRI have significantly improved the assessment of oropharyngeal tumours and nodal metastases. CT scans are more useful and help to show deep infiltration into the tongue; and parapharyngeal space as well as the pterygoid fossa and show up small suspicious metastatic nodes in neck that are difficult to palpate.

3. Ultrasonic examination: It is a valuable aid in the diagnosis of lymph node enlargement. It can be as helpful as CT scans, but it has the advantage of being cheaper and more accessible for clinical evaluation in the clinic.
4. Biopsy
5. Blood investigations: This should include complete blood count, erythrocyte sedimentation rate, renal and liver function tests, plasma proteins and immunoglobulins.
6. Bone marrow aspiration and biopsy. It is essential for lymphoma staging.

Treatment

Treatment of squamous cell carcinoma
1. Radiotherapy
2. Surgery
3. Combined radiotherapy and surgery
4. Chemotherapy
5. Cryosurgery
6. Laser surgery

Treatment of Non-Hodgkin's Lymphoma

For localized lymphoma radiotherapy is curable. The use of this modality followed by chemotherapy is another approach to treatment.

Treatment of Salivary Gland Tumours

Benign salivary gland tumours are almost exclusively pleomorphic adenomas and are treated by local excision with a generous margin. Malignant tumours generally adenoid cystic carcinomas are treated by radical surgery as for squamous carcinoma. Radiotherapy has no place in the primary treatment of these diseases.

Tumours of the Hypopharynx

The hypopharynx lies below and behind the base of the tongue and behind and on each side of the larynx. It extends from the level of the hyoid bone superiorly to the lower border of the cricoid inferiorly. The three anatomical subsites are the pyriform fossa, the postcricoid area and posterior pharyngeal wall.

Benign Diseases of the Neck

1. Thyroglossal cysts. Treatment: Sistrunk operations.
2. Branchial cysts, sinuses and fistulae.
3. Neurogenous tumours: They are neurofibroma, neurilemmoma, paraganglionic tumours like carotid body tumours and glomus tumours.

4. Dermoid cysts: There are three varieties of dermoid cysts.
   a. *Epidermoid cysts:* It is the most common variety. It contains cheesy keratinous material.
   b. *True dermoid cysts:* It contains skin appendages such as hair, hair follicles, sebaceous glands and sweat glands. Dermoid cysts are either congenital or acquired. The congenital type occurs along the lines of fusion. The acquired type is due to implantation of epidermis at the time of a puncture type of injury and is often solid with areas of cystic spaces containing sebaceous material.
   c. *Teratoid cysts:* This is the rarest variety in the neck. The teratoid cysts can be lined with squamous or respiratory epithelium and contains elements formed from ectoderm, entoderm and mesoderm—nails, teeth, brain, glands, etc.

Treatment

Complete excision is carried out in all the cases.
Infective neck masses
1. Tuberculosis
2. Sarcoidosis
3. AIDS
4. Toxoplasmosis
5. Actinomycosis
6. Cat scratch disease
7. Brucellosis
8. Infectious mononucleosis

Larynx and Trachea

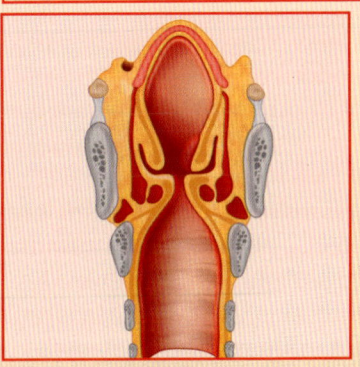

28

Anatomy of the Larynx

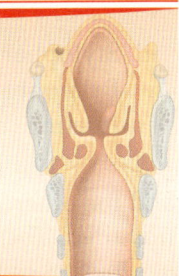

The larynx consists of cartilaginous framework. The cartilages are connected by ligaments and membranes. It is lined internally by mucous membrane and moved by muscles. It is situated in the middle of the neck and lies anterior to the lower part of the pharynx or laryngopharynx. It begins at the level of third cervical vertebra and ends at the level of sixth cervical vertebra where the trachea begins. The adult male larynx is larger than the female one. The prominence of the thyroid cartilage in male adults is called Adam's apple.

Cartilages

The cartilages of the larynx are:

Unpaired—three in number
   i. Thyroid cartilage with its two alae, which remain as a half open book. The alae are prolonged backwards. They form the superior and inferior horns.
   ii. Cricoid cartilage resembles a signet ring. It is narrow in front and broad behind.
   iii. Epiglottic cartilage looks like a thin leaf. It is attached to the posterior surface of the junction of the thyroid alae.

Paired—three in number
   i. Arytenoid cartilages: They are pyramidal in shape with three sides. The base of the pyramid is connected with the cricoid. The anterior angle of it forms the vocal process, and the lateral angle the muscular process. The medial surface is flat and forms the posterior one-third of the glottic chink. The apex of the pyramid articulates with the corniculate cartilage.
   ii. Corniculate cartilages of Santorini: They articulate with the arytenoid cartilages.
   iii. Cuneiform cartilages of Wrisberg: There is one in each aryepiglottic fold.

Muscles

Laryngeal muscles are of two types:
   i. Extrinsic
   ii. Intrinsic

Extrinsic: The muscles which have the attachment between the larynx and the neighbouring structures. They are:
   i. Sternothyroid
   ii. Thyrohyoid

iii. Stylopharyngeus

iv. Palatopharyngeus

v. Inferior constrictor

Intrinsic: The muscles that have the attachment between one laryngeal cartilage and the other. They are all paired except the transverse arytenoid muscle, which is unpaired. These muscles may be grouped as follows:

a. Openers of the glottis (abductors)

  i. Cricoarytenoideus posterior muscles.

b. Closers of the glottis (adductors)

  i. Cricoarytenoideus lateralis.

  ii. Arytenoideus transversus.

  iii. Thyroarytenoideus externa. These muscles also reduce the tension of the vocal cords during phonation.

  iv. Thyroarytenoideus interna or vocalis muscle. It is known as internal tensor muscle.

  v. Cricothyroideus: It is known as the external tensor muscle. These muscles also increase the tension of the vocal cords during phonation.

c. Closers of the laryngeal inlet

  i. Arytenoideus obliques and

  ii. Aryepiglottic muscle.

d. Openers of the laryngeal inlet

  i. Thyroepiglottic muscle.

Ligaments and Membranes

The ligaments and membranes are again of two types:

Extrinsic: These connect the cartilages of the larynx with the adjoining structures. They are:

  i. *Thyrohyoid membrane:* This is pierced on either side by:

    a. Superior laryngeal artery and vein.

    b. Internal laryngeal nerve—a branch of superior laryngeal nerve

  ii. Median and lateral thyrohyoid ligaments

  iii. Cricotracheal membrane.

  iv. Hyoepiglottic ligament.

Intrinsic: These connect the cartilages of the larynx with one another.

  The elastic membrane of the larynx: This lies beneath the laryngeal mucosa. It forms the fibrous framework of the larynx. This is divided into upper and lower parts by the laryngeal sinus of Morgagni or the ventricle of the larynx, which is a recess between the false and true vocal cords. The upper part of the elastic membrane is somewhat quadrangular and supports the aryepiglottic and ventricular folds. The lower thickened edge of this is known as ventricular ligament, which forms the false vocal cord.

  The contents of the false vocal cord or ventricular fold are:

a. Mucous membrane covering the ventricular ligament

b. Ventricular ligament

c. Upper portion of the external thyroarytenoid muscle

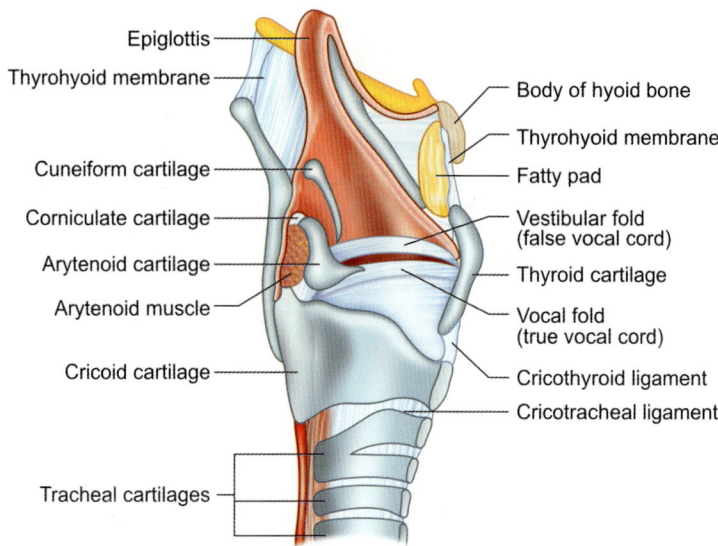

Epiglottis

Thyrohyoid membrane

Cuneiform cartilage

Corniculate cartilage

Arytenoid cartilage

Arytenoid muscle

Cricoid cartilage

Tracheal cartilages

Body of hyoid bone

Thyrohyoid membrane

Fatty pad

Vestibular fold
(false vocal cord)

Thyroid cartilage

Vocal fold
(true vocal cord)

Cricothyroid ligament

Cricotracheal ligament

Fig. 28.1: Sagittal section of larynx showing the anatomical structures

The lower part of the elastic membrane is called cricovocal membrane or conus elasticus. The lower end of it is attached to the upper border of the cricoid cartilage. The upper free edge of it is the vocal ligament, which forms the true vocal cord. The contents of the true vocal cord or vocal fold are:
a. Mucous membrane covering the vocal ligament
b. Vocal ligament.
c. Internal thyroarytenoid muscle.

Ultrastructure of the Vocal Cord

It is a multilayered structure and consists of the following layers:
  i. The mucous membrane lined by stratified squamous epithelium
 ii. Lamina propria:
      a. Superficial layer
      b. Intermediate layer
      c. Deep layer
iii. Vocalis muscle, which forms the main body of the vocal cord

Reinke's Space

It is the superficial layer of Lamina Propria of vocal cord. It consists of loose areolar substance. This is the layer that vibrates most during phonation. Oedema in this space results in fusiform swelling of the vocal cords called Reinke's edema.

The normal vocal cords appear pearly white as the covering epithelium is closely attached to the underlying vocal ligament and the blood supply is poor. The anterior part of the conus is thickened which is named
  i. Median cricothyroid ligament
 ii. The thyroepiglottic ligament
iii. The cricoarytenoid ligament.

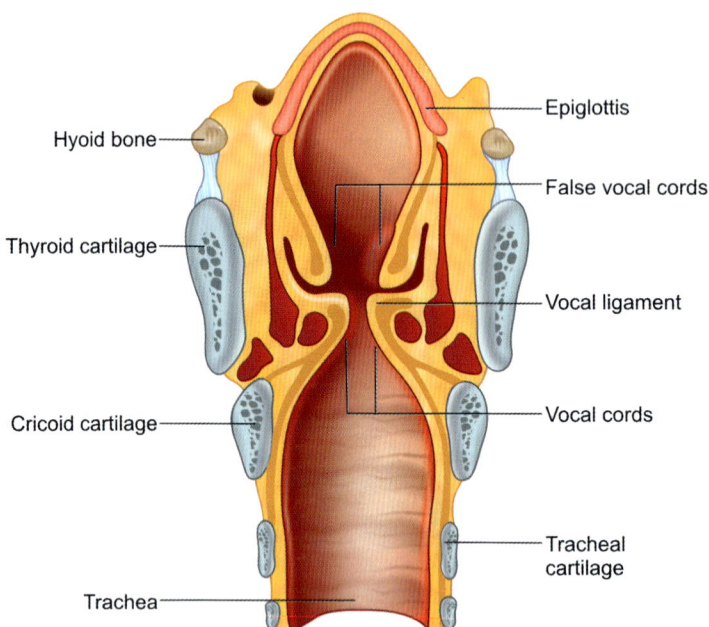

Fig. 28.2: Compartments of larynx

The cavity of the larynx extends from the inlet of the larynx to the lower border of the cricoid cartilage. The inlet of the larynx is bounded by the upper edge of the epiglottis, aryepiglottic folds, arytenoid cartilages, and interarytenoid region. The inlet of the larynx opens into the laryngopharynx. The false and true vocal cords divide the cavity of the larynx into three parts:

   i. *Vestibule:* It lies between the inlet of the larynx and the edges of the false vocal cords. It is bounded in front by the posterior surface of the epiglottis, behind by the interarytenoid region, and laterally by the inner surface of the aryepiglottic folds and upper surface of the false cords.

   ii. *Ventricle:* The space between the false cord above and the true cord below is called the ventricle of the larynx. The ascending anterior part of it is known as saccule. The mucosa of the saccule has numerous mucous glands. The secretion of these glands helps in lubricating the surface of the true cords. The interval between the true cords is named rima glottides

   iii. *Subglottic space:* It is the space between the true cords and of the cricoid cartilage.

Mucous Membrane of the Larynx

The whole laryngeal cavity is lined with ciliated columnar epithelium except the true vocal cords and the upper part of the vestibule, which are lined with stratified squamous epithelium.

There are plenty of mucous glands in the ventricles, saccule and posterior surface of the epiglottis and the margins of the aryepiglottic folds. No mucous glands are found on the free edges of the true cords.

The mucous membrane is closely attached over the true vocal cords and the posterior surface of the epiglottis. In other places it is loosely attached. That is why edema of the larynx involves the whole of it except the true cord and the posterior surface of the epiglottis.

Blood Supply

The larynx is supplied with the superior laryngeal artery, the cricothyroid artery, both of which are the branches of superior thyroid artery, and the inferior laryngeal, a branch of the inferior thyroid artery. The veins accompany the arteries.

Lymphatic Drainage of the Larynx

The lymphatic system of the larynx has been divided into two parts by the edges of the true cords:

   i. Supraglottic lymph vessels drain into the upper deep cervical glands.
   ii. Subglottic vessels drain into the prelaryngeal, pretracheal and lower deep cervical glands.
   iii. The vocal cords have practically no lymph vessels. Thus the cancer of the vocal cords does not readily spread.

Nerve Supply of the Larynx

The nerves are derived from the internal and external branches of the laryngeal, recurrent laryngeal branch of the vagus, and the sympathetic.

The sensory supply above the vocal cords is affected by the internal laryngeal nerve and that below the vocal cords by the recurrent laryngeal nerve.

Mainly the recurrent laryngeal nerve affects the motor supply. It supplies all the intrinsic muscles of the larynx except cricothyroid, which is supplied by the external laryngeal branch of superior laryngeal nerve.

The recurrent laryngeal nerve of the right side loops round the subclavian artery and that of the left side loops round the ligamentum arteriosum, close to the arch of the aorta.

Functions of the Larynx

The functions of the larynx are:

1. Protection of the lungs: This is the most important function of the larynx. Protection is given by the following mechanisms:
   i. Closure of the laryngeal inlet.
   ii. Closure of the glottis.
   iii. Cessation of respiration.
   iv. Cough reflex.
2. Respiration and regulation of air flow.
3. Fixation of the chest by closure of the false cords, which check the outlet of air, resulting in the rise of intra-thoracic and intra-abdominal pressure. This is essential during climbing, digging, defaecation, and micturition.
4. Phonation.

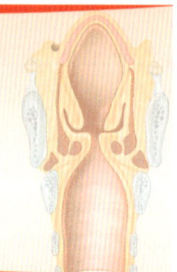

29

Examination of the Larynx

Examination of the larynx includes:
1. External examination
2. Laryngoscopy
    i. Indirect laryngoscopy with a laryngeal mirror
    ii. Microlaryngoscopy (MLS)
    iii. Direct laryngoscopy with laryngoscope under general anaesthesia
    iv. Direct laryngoscopy with
        a. Rigid (70° or 90°) fibreoptic laryngoscope (FOL)
        b. Flexible fibreoptic laryngoscope (FOL)
        c. Videolaryngoscope with camera attachment. This helps in training and documentation
3. Radiography
4. Stroboscopy
5. Cinephotography

EXTERNAL EXAMINATION

Inspection

The larynx is to be inspected from outside for any deviation of it from the midline of the neck, broadening, and movements. The normal larynx does not move during quiet respiration but it moves upwards during deglutition. In case of laryngeal obstruction, it moves upwards and downwards during expiration and inspiration respectively.

Palpation

The broadening of the larynx is felt and confirmed by palpation. Tenderness over the larynx may be elicited in acute perichondritis. When the normal larynx is being moved from side to side a grating sound is felt which disappears in postcricoid growths.

The regional lymph nodes should also be palpated.

Indirect Laryngoscopy

Indirect laryngoscopy means examination of the larynx by a laryngeal mirror. In this technique the anterior portion of the larynx with epiglottis is seen in the upper

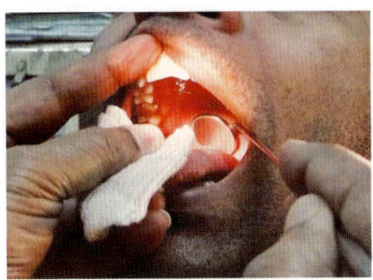

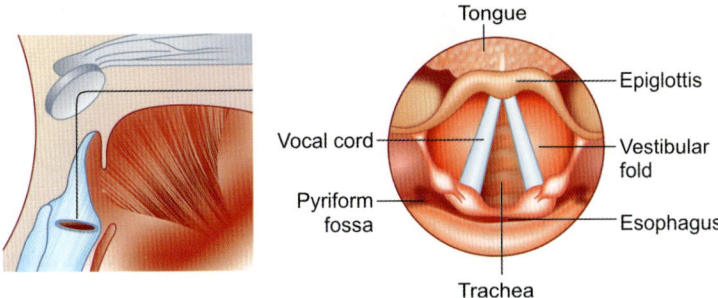

Fig. 29.1: Technique, schematic diagram and view obtained during indirect laryngoscopy

part of the mirror and the posterior portion with the arytenoids in the lower part of it (Fig. 29.1). For details of indirect laryngoscopy (*see* chapter on Instruments).

Direct Laryngoscopy

This is the examination of the larynx by a conventional direct laryngoscope, suspension laryngoscope or fibreoptic laryngoscope.

This is performed in Boyce position. In this position the patient lies with his head, neck, and part of the shoulder including half of the scapulae projecting beyond the end of the table. The occiput is raised 10 cm above the level of the table producing flexion of the neck on to the chest. The head is then extended at the atlanto-occipital joint. This position is maintained by an assistant sitting on to the right side of the patient. Bronchoscopy examination is also done in this position of the patient.

Laryngoscope is inserted viewing sequentially the uvula, epiglottis and arytenoids until its tip lies a few millimeters above the anterior commissure. Backward, upward, and rightward pressure (BURP) by an assistant helps in viewing the larynx in many patients (Fig. 29.2).

This examination is necessary both for diagnostic and therapeutic purposes such as:

a. Examination of the larynx in young children.
b. When the view of the larynx is unsatisfactory by indirect laryngoscopy in adults.
c. For removal of a foreign body or a small benign tumour from the larynx, or for taking a tissue for biopsy.

The direct laryngoscopy is contraindicated in the diseases of the cervical spine.

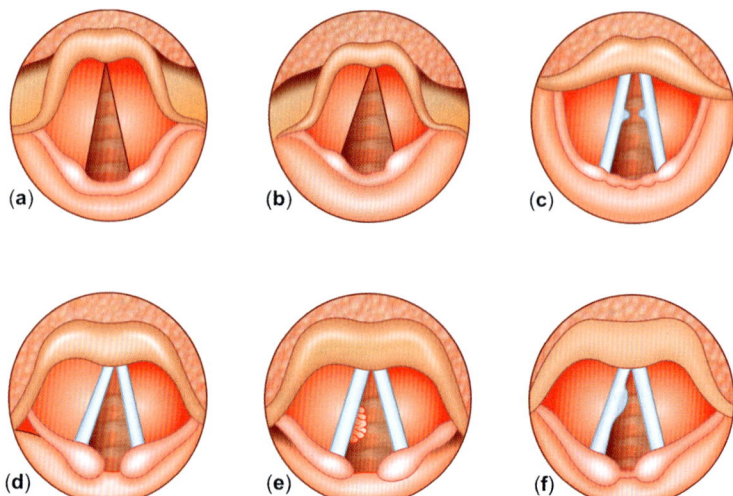

Fig. 29.2: Different types of laryngeal pathology. (a) Acute simple laryngitis; (b) Submucus haemorrhage of the vocal cords; (c) Singer's nodules, (d) Fibroma of right vocal cord; (e) Subglottic (right) carcinoma; (f) Carcinoma of right vocal cord

Microlaryngoscopy

Kleinsasser (1965) introduced microscopic examination and treatment of laryngeal lesions the advantage of which is now available in most of the ENT departments equipped with operative microscope and microlaryngeal instruments. For microlaryngoscopy a 400 mm objective on the operative microscope is required for adults and 275 mm objective for children instead of the 200 mm, one used in ear surgery. It can be comfortably carried out under general anaesthesia with a 6 to 7 mm size nasotracheal tube in adults with normal and controlled respiration. This helps in accurate surgical manipulations within the larynx.

Fibreoptic Laryngoscopy

This is one of the recent methods of examination of the larynx especially when it is not visualized by indirect laryngoscopy due to overhanging epiglottis. Usual direct laryngoscopy may be avoided by the introduction of this technique. What is done here is to pass a small fibreoptic bundle (a flexible laryngoscope) into the larynx through the nose. The laryngeal surface of the epiglottis and the anterior commissure may be examined properly by this technique.

Stroboscopy

Vibrations of the vocal cords during phonation are so rapid that one cannot follow it during indirect laryngoscopy. An interrupted source of light is used during indirect laryngoscopy causing an apparent slowing down of the vibrations of the vocal cords during phonation (optical illusion).

If the frequency of the note uttered corresponds exactly with the frequency of the flashes of interrupted light, the same phase of the vocal cord movement will be illuminated by each flash and the cords will appear to be motionless. It helps to follow and analyse the vocal cord vibration during phonation and faults of voice production. It is called stroboscopic examination of the larynx.

This is done with an instrument called Stroboscope. This is attached with the flexible or rigid fibreoptic laryngoscope. The machine emits flashes of light, which can be adjusted. When the emitted flashes of light at a fixed frequency are synchronized with the movement of the vocal cords, it appears that the vocal cord movements are considerably slowed down. It helps to identify the tumours of the vocal cord limited to the mucosa only, to assess the vocal cord mobility in patients with hoarseness and also the mucosal waves of the vocal cords.

Stroboscopy is generally performed with video equipment for instant replay and frame-by-frame analysis (video stroboscopy). Parameters to measure are symmetry, amplitude, speed and phase difference of waves compared on the two cords.

Radiography of Larynx

The radiological examination of the larynx is carried out to establish the clinical impression of a new growth and to determine the extent of it. The following X-rays help:

   i. Soft-tissue X-ray of the larynx (lateral view),
   ii. Laryngogram—anteroposterior and lateral view X-rays of the larynx and hypopharynx are taken after dropping about 10 cc of dionosil or any suitable contrast media into the cavity of the larynx with a special laryngeal syringe.
iii. Tomography.
iv. CT scan.

Hoarseness of Voice

Hoarse literally means rough and harsh in sound. Hoarseness is one of the important symptoms of the laryngeal diseases—especially when the vocal cords are involved. Causes of hoarseness of voice may be classified as follows:

A. Congenital

1. *Web of the larynx:* Laryngeal web may also be acquired by accidental or surgical trauma.
2. *Cysts*
   a. Cystic hygroma
   b. Dermoid cyst
   c. Branchial cyst
3. *Tumours*
   a. Lipoma
   b. Fibroma
   c. Leiomyoma
   d. Chondroma
   e. Haemangioma

B. *Acquired*

1. *Traumatic*

   i. Compression injuries by blows and strangulations,

   ii. Inhaled foreign body

   iii. Anaesthetic intubation injury

   iv. Acute submucosal haemorrhage in the vocal cord by coughing, shouting, weight lifting, etc.

2. *Inflammatory*

   a. Acute

      1. Non-specific

         i. Acute simple infective laryngitis

         ii. Inhalation of irritating fumes and gases including tobacco smoking

         iii. Acute laryngotracheobronchitis

         iv. Oedema of the larynx

      2. Specific

         i. Diphtheritic laryngitis

   b. Chronic

      1. Non-specific

         i. Chronic simple laryngitis

         ii. Chronic atrophic laryngitis

         iii. Nodular laryngitis (Singer's nodule or vocal nodule)

         iv. Chronic hypertrophic laryngitis (pachydermia laryngis)

         v. Hyperkeratosis of the larynx

         vi. Laryngeal polyp

         vii. Arthritis of the cricoarytenoid joints

      2. Specific

         i. Tubercular laryngitis

         ii. Syphilitic laryngitis

         iii. Leprosy of the larynx

         iv. Scleroma of the larynx

3. *Neoplastic*

   a. Benign

      1. Papilloma

         i. Juvenile (multiple)

         ii. Adult (single)

      2. Fibroma

      3. Chondroma

4. Angioma
5. Lipoma
6. Myoma
   i. Leiomyoma
   ii. Rhabdomyoma
b. Malignant:
   1. Squamous cell carcinoma (common)
   2. Sarcoma (rare)
4. *Paralytic*
   1. Unilateral or bilateral complete paralysis of vocal cord due to organic diseases involving the motor laryngeal nerve.
   2. Functional aphonia due to hysterical changes.
5. *Miscellaneous*
   1. Cyst
   2. Prolapse of the ventricle of the larynx
   3. Laryngocele.

Sulcus Vocalis

Sulcus vocalis is a disease of the vocal cords where a furrow develops along the upper medial edge of the true vocal cords. The patients present to the clinician with complain of hoarseness. Sulcus vocalis are of three types:
- Type I (physiological): Sulcus confined to the superficial layer of the lamina propria
- Type II (sulcus vergenture): Sulcus penetrating the superficial layer and approximating the intermediate and deep layer
- Type III (sulcus vocalis): Sulcus penetrating the intermediate and deep layer and exhibiting a pouch-like configuration.

Treatment

Injection of fat and collagen usually gives good results in type I and II varieties but the effects may be temporary. Excision of the sulcus and fat, fascia or collagen implantation are also being practiced by some surgeons. Type III sulcus is usually difficult to treat permanently.

Laryngeal Stridor

Stridor may be defined as a noise or sound produced during respiration. It is due to obstruction to the passage of air into or out of the lower respiratory tract.

Types

i. Inspiratory—the obstructive factor is in the larynx
ii. Expiratory—due to bronchial obstruction.
iii. Both inspiratory and expiratory—the obstruction lies usually in trachea.

Causes

The causes of stridor may be classified in Table 29.1.

Table 29.1: Classification of causes of stridor

		Congenital			Acquired
Site	*Functional*		*Organic*		Foreign body
		Supraglottic	*Glottic*	*Subglottic*	infection, e.g.
Larynx	Paralysis	Congenital Laryngeal Stridor (laryngo- malacia) Cysts Tumours	Web Tumours	Tumours Congenital subglottic stenosis	acute epiglottitis, acute laryngitis, acute laryngotracheo- bronchitis Diphtheria
Trachea	Vascular anomaly	Congenital tracheal stenosis Absent tracheal rings			Foreign body infection
Bronchus	Asthma				Foreign body infection

Clinical Approach to the Stridulous Child

Careful history taking followed by clinical examination is vital. The duration of the noise should first be noted. History of eating peanuts or with small articles is important. If the child develops the symptom after getting up from sleep, it indicates inflammatory stridor. If it is present since birth with normal cry, it is likely to be due to laryngomalacia.

Examinations

    i. Note the type of stridor.
    ii. In inspiratory type the sound will be of musical croupy quality. Bronchial obstruction will cause wheezy sound during expiration. A gruff tone during expiration may be heard in tracheal obstruction.
    iii. Turn the child into prone position, notice if the stridor disappears. If it does not disappear, it suggests that the cause of stridor lies in the surrounding structures as in laryngomalacia rather than in the lumen of the larynx or trachea.
    iv. Direct laryngoscopy and bronchoscopy should then be done.

Treatment

1. A stridulous child should be hospitalized.
2. Clinical and radiological examinations are done.
3. Endoscopic examination of the larynx (direct laryngoscopy) is done.
4. Oxygen and humidification are provided with.
5. When a cause is found, the appropriate treatment is instituted as follows:
    i. Aspiration of crusts or pus from the tracheobronchial tree.
    ii. Antibiotics with or without steroids in the case of infection.
    iii. Endotracheal intubation or tracheostomy should be done if the obstruction is severe to assist respiration.
    iv. Foreign bodies must be immediately removed.
    v. Tumours like multiple papilloma should be excised.

30

Inflammations of the Larynx

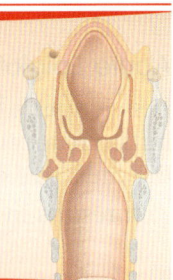

Acute Simple Laryngitis

The acute simple laryngitis is an acute superficial inflammation of the mucosa of the larynx.

Aetiology

The factors responsible are the following:
Nasal obstruction, sinusitis, overuse of the voice in the presence of a mild catarrh, inhalation of irritating fumes, tobacco smoke and trauma due to vocal abuse, intubation of endotracheal tube and endoscopic manipulation.

Clinical Features

The predominant symptom is hoarseness of voice or a complete loss of voice. Pain and irritation in the throat with difficulty in deglutition are usually present. A dry and irritating cough is a frequent associate. There may be rise in temperature and malaise.

On examination of the larynx the whole mucosa is seen to be hyperaemic and oedematous. The surface of the vocal cords may be covered with mucopurulent secretion. The secretion may become purulent in severe forms with the development of perichondritis. Sometimes in influenza or after exposure to irritating gases, there are opaque coatings on the anterior part of vocal cords and laryngeal inlet. This condition is especially named "corditis fibrinosa".

Treatment

A. Local
    i. Voice rest is an important advice to be given.
    ii. Inhalation of medicated steam (Tr. Benzoin Co. and Menthol) by means of a suitable inhaler helps.
    iii. Antiseptic and mild local anaesthetic lozenges are soothing.
    iv. A cough linctus helps in controlling the irritating cough.
    v. Smoking should be prohibited.
B. General
    i. Rest in bed if the general symptoms are severe with rise in temperature.
    ii. A suitable antibiotic in adequate doses should be administered if the temperature is markedly high.

Acute Epiglottis

It is a special form of acute laryngitis in which the epiglottis is affected by inflammatory changes. It commonly occurs in children with oedema of the epiglottis, the causative organism is *H. influenzae*.

It results in dyspnoea and odynophagia (painful swallowing).

Treatment

1. Antibiotics in high doses
2. Steroids in the form of prednisolone or betamethasone
3. Tracheostomy may be urgently needed.

Acute Laryngotracheobronchitis

Infants and young children are commonly affected. Haemolytic *streptococcus* is the usual causative organism, but it may be caused by a virus.

It causes dry croupy cough and hoarseness following an attack of cold or influenza with a high rise in temperature. From involvement of trachea and bronchi, dyspnoea and cyanosis may be present. The characteristic findings are tenacious exudation, crusting, and oedema of the larynx. Collapse of the lung may develop due to occlusion of the bronchi.

Treatment

1. Rest in bed.
2. Systemic antibiotics and steroids must be immediately started.
3. Inspired air should be humidified.
4. Oxygen.
5. Oral or intravenous fluid.
6. Endotracheal intubation or tracheostomy may be required.
7. Secretions may require to be removed by bronchoscopy through tracheostomy.

Oedema of the Larynx

Oedema of the laryngeal mucosa may be of two types.
1. Non-inflammatory
2. Inflammatory

1. Non-inflammatory Oedema

This may be due to:
  i. Nephritis.
  ii. Cardiac disease.
  iii. Intrathoracic diseases causing venous stasis in the neck.
  iv. Angioneurotic oedema.
  v. Idiosyncracy to drugs, e.g. antibiotics, iodine and aspirin

2. Inflammatory Oedema

This may be:

a. *Primary:* In this cases, oedema occurs in the larynx which was previously normal and is due to acute septic laryngitis, e.g. streptococcal or diphtheritic laryngitis and the spreading of oedema in the neighbouring structures such as peritonsillar abscess and Ludwig's angina.

b. *Secondary:* It means oedema in the larynx which was previously diseased. It is due to tuberculosis, syphilis and cancer.

Clinical Features

The patient complains of hoarseness of voice, and difficulty in breathing. On examination, the colour of the oedematous mucosa is seen pale in noninflammatory type while it is red in inflammatory type. The oedema is marked on the arytenoids; aryepiglottic folds, and false vocal cords. The true vocal cords are not usually involved. In children oedema may also involve the subglottic mucosa.

Treatment

The causes responsible for oedema must be treated along with the treatment of complications in the larynx.

In mild cases rest in propped-up position, sucking of ice and application of ice over the neck may be helpful. Xylocaine and adrenaline solution (1% xylocaine and 0.1% adrenaline in equal quantities) may be sprayed into the larynx with reduction of edema.

Tracheostomy or laryngofissure may be required if the dyspnoea becomes severe.

In the inflammatory type, in addition to the above-mentioned treatment, appropriate antibiotics and chemotherapeutics should be administered in suitable doses.

Laryngeal Diphtheria

Laryngeal diphtheria is commonly due to an extension of faucial diphtheria in children. It may involve the larynx primarily and in such cases it is difficult to diagnose. Infection is owing to diphtheria bacilli.

Clinical Features

The disease starts insidiously with hoarseness and cough followed by inspiratory stridor (noisy respiration). The temperature is usually low. Pulse becomes rapid and thready. The condition may lead to complete laryngeal obstruction owing to diphtheritic membrane and asphyxial death if not treated promptly.

The diagnosis is confirmed by identification of diphtheria bacilli (KLB) in laryngeal swab examination by smear technique and culture.

Treatment

Antitoxin in the doses of 20,000 to 1,00,000 units should be given as soon as the condition is suspected to be a diphtheritic infection. Antibiotics should be given to control the infection.

Tracheostomy should be performed during early signs of laryngeal obstruction.

Chronic Laryngitis (Non-specific)

Repeated attacks of acute laryngitis results in chronicity. The causes are the same as acute laryngitis, e.g. overuse of voice, excessive smoking, infection in nose, sinuses, and tonsils.

Clinical Features

Hoarseness of voice, which becomes worse in the morning, is a prominent symptom. Cough with expectoration of mucus blobs and a desire to clear the throat are frequently present.

On examination the changes seen in the larynx may be classified in the three following types:

1. Hyperemic
2. Hypertrophic
3. Atrophic

The involvement of the larynx in all types is bilaterally symmetrical.

Differential Diagnosis

    i. Tuberculosis of the larynx
    ii. Cancer of the larynx

Treatment

1. Rest to the voice.
2. Avoid smoking and dusty atmosphere.
3. Inhalations and sprays of medicated steam (Tr. Benzoin Co., Menthol and oil of pine) are of value.
4. The infections in the tonsils, nose and sinuses should be properly treated.

Vocal Nodules

This is a localized chronic hypertrophic laryngitis also known as singer's nodules, commonly found in females rather than in males. This is due to the abuse of voice and occurs in the junction of the anterior and middle thirds of the vocal cords which, is the site of maximum friction. The condition is almost always bilateral.

These patients present with the history of hoarseness and vocal fatigue. Laryngoscopically the nodules appear smooth and white. Satisfactory result is obtained only by absolute voice rest for a few weeks provided the nodules are small. If the nodules persist in spite of the vocal rest and are sufficiently large in size, they should be removed by direct laryngoscopy preferably under operative microscope (microlaryngoscopy). The nose sinuses and

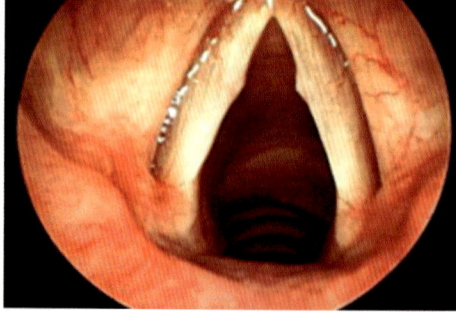

Fig. 30.1: Singer's nodules

pharynx should be treated for recurrent affections. Speech therapy helps to re-educate voice production.

Reinke's Oedema

The accumulation of fluid under the epithelium of the true vocal cords involving the superficial layer of the lamina propria is called Reinke's oedema.

Allergy, infection and especially local irritants like tobacco is one of the major culprits. Chronic sinusitis has also been implicated.

Treatment

All known causative factors especially smoking should first be eliminated. Surgery consists of microsurgical removal of strips of vocal cord mucosa by micro-laryngoscopy. After the procedure, absolute vocal rest is advocated for 1 week. Speech therapy is instituted after 2–3 weeks and is continued as long as it is felt to be beneficial.

Leucoplakia of the Larynx

This condition is characterized by epithelial hyperplasia of vocal cords. It is supposed to be due to chronic irritation and smoking. This is a rare disease and commonly found in males.

The patients come with the history of progressive hoarseness. Laryngoscopically it appears as white raised patches either on one or both vocal cords. The mobility of the cords remains normal.

Leucoplakia is definitely a precancerous condition. Therefore it is kept under constant supervision and the cancerous development may be diagnosed early by cytology and biopsy.

The preliminary treatment includes prohibition of smoking and removal of septic foci in the nose, sinuses, throat, and mouth. To prevent epithelial hyperplasia vitamin-A may be given. If the condition persists even after proper conservative treatment, laryngofissure and removal of the effected cord should be done.

Tuberculosis of the Larynx (Laryngeal phthisis)

Aetiology

Tuberculous infection in the larynx is almost always secondary to a pulmonary lesion. Primary lesion also is not uncommon. Infections are mostly through sputum. Both sexes are affected commonly between 20 and 40 years of age.

Pathology

The tubercle bacillus infects the intact laryngeal mucosa of the posterior third of the larynx by infected sputum, which lies in the interarytenoid region. Small round-cell infiltration then occurs in the submucosal layer. Nodules appear in the beginning on the surface, which caseate and lead to ulceration. Gradually masses of granulation tissue and cellular swelling (a pseudooedema) develop. Cellular swelling involves the epiglottis, aryepiglottic folds, arytenoids, and ventricular bands. Ultimately, there is perichondritis and cartilage necrosis, together with the oedema.

Clinical Features

1. Weakness of the voice due to myasthenia of the phonatory muscles is the first symptom.
2. Hoarseness of the voice.
3. Cough.
4. Pain on swallowing (odynophagia).
5. Referred pain in the ear.
6. Laryngoscopy will reveal slight impairment of abduction due to myositis. Congestion of one vocal cord or ulceration of the edge of the cord ('mouse-nibbled'), granulation in the interarytenoid region or vocal process of the arytenoid cartilage are the common findings in tuberculous lesion. There may be oedema of the ventricular mucosa resembling a prolapse. 'Turban larynx' due to pseudooedema of the epiglottis and arytenoids, perichondritis and cartilage necrosis cause erosion of the epiglottis, laryngeal stenosis, or vocal cord fixation from ankylosis of the cricoarytenoid joint. Right vocal cord paralysis may occur from apical pulmonary tuberculosis with thickening of the pleura.

Diagnosis

The disease must be differentiated from syphilis or carcinoma. Chest X-ray must be taken. Sputum examination will usually contain tubercle bacilli. Biopsy is essential in suspected cases of cancer.

Prognosis

It depends on early diagnosis and treatment, which may completely cure the patient.

Treatment

Local
1. Absolute voice rest and complete rest in bed.
2. Smoking should be stopped.
3. Insufflation of an analgesic powder (orthoform and benzocaine) or chewing of analgesic and antiseptic lozenges help in reducing pain on swallowing.
4. Diathermy coagulation of an exposed ulcer and galvanocautery of the granulations may give relief.
5. Superior laryngeal nerve may be blocked by infiltration with novocaine and alcohol.
6. Tracheostomy may be helpful in late cases.

General
1. Injection of streptomycin sulphate in suitable doses for a prolonged period (1 gm daily in adults).
2. Para-aminosalicylic acid (PAS) orally 10 to 12 gm daily in divided doses in adults.
3. Isoniazid orally 300 mg daily in divided doses.
4. Ethambutol and/or rifampicin are also used in combination with other antitubercular drugs.
5. Thoracoplasty and collapse therapy may be necessary.

Laryngocele

It can be external laryngocele and internal laryngocele.

Soft tissue X-ray of the neck (anterposterior and lateral view) shows pocket in the neck. The lateral view shows the dilated ventricle of larynx with large area of air sac above the glottis. The diagnosis is laryngocele (Fig. 30.2).

Treatment

Laryngoceles discovered radiologically and that are confined within the larynx require no treatment.

Internal laryngoceles may be uncapped and marsupialised which will stop recurrence. If recur, then they should be excised with the approach used for the external laryngocele.

An infected laryngocele should be aspirated and treated with antibiotics. When infection has subsided, formal excision should be carried out.

The best operation for a laryngocele aims at excising the saccule at its neck. This is found by removing the upper half of one thyroid ala, or fracturing it downwards and replacing it. Once access to the supraglottis is obtained, it is an easy matter to follow the neck of the laryngocele down as far as possible. The neck is transected and closed in layers and oversewn. If the thyroid ala is not replaced, then the thyroid perichondrium is sewn into the area. Recurrence after this operation is extremely rare.

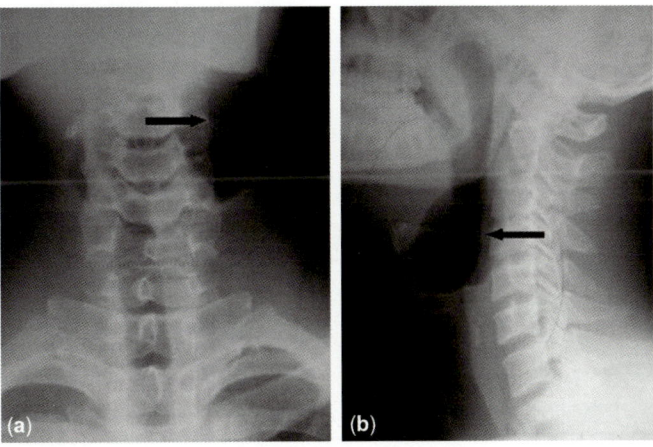

Fig. 30.2: X-ray of laryngocele. (a) AP view; (b) Lateral view

Laryngopharyngeal Reflux Disease

Laryngopharyngeal reflux refers to backward flow of gastric contents into pharynx through the sphincters of the esophagus. Some people have abnormal retrograde flow of stomach contents through the lower esophageal sphincter into the esophagus, which is known as Gastroesophageal reflux disease (GERD). If the reflux occurs through the upper esophageal sphincter into the pharynx, it is known as Laryngopharyngeal reflux disease (LPRD). Patients of GERD usually suffer from nocturnal reflux, while LPRD patients experience upright daytime reflux and symptoms. Common symptoms of LPRD are hoarseness, chronic cough, frequent throat clearing, pain or lump sensation in throat, problems while swallowing, bad or bitter taste in mouth, asthma like symptoms, etc. The clinician diagnoses LPRD by the presence of congested arytenoids, interarytenoid region and vocal folds; swellings, ulcers or granulomas of the vocal cords, thick strands of mucus and edema of the false cords. LPRD may be associated with hiatus hernia. Rarely LPRD has been attributed to carcinoma larynx also. A 24 hours ambulatory dual probe pH monitoring is the gold standard for diagnosing LPRD. The mainstay of treatment for LPRD is lifestyle modification; vocal hygiene and medications with proton pump inhibitors and H_2 blockers.

31

Tumours of the Larynx

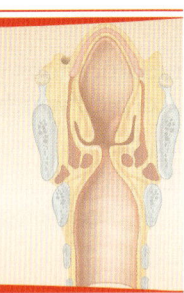

BENIGN TUMOURS

Benign tumours of the larynx are more frequently seen than the malignant tumours. Papilloma and fibroma are common amongst all other benign tumours. Intubation granuloma, chondroma, adenoma, lipoma, angioma, and myoma are rarely come across. The cysts like retention cysts, and rarely branchial or dermoid cysts also occur in the larynx. Laryngocele is a rare condition due to dilatation of the saccule of the larynx. This was once thought to occur in glassblowers and players of wind instruments but was proved to be false. This occurs in persons in whom residue of air sac persists in the ventricle of larynx as it remains in lower animals.

Papilloma

Papilloma of the larynx may be single and multiple. The single type occurs commonly in adults, whereas the multiple types occur commonly in infants and young children. A virus has been blamed as the causative factor of the latter. The single type arises usually from the anterior commissure and the anterior half of the vocal cords. This type may turn towards malignant change. The multiple types arise usually from the vocal and ventricular bands. Hoarseness is present in both the varieties. Dyspnoea is common in the multiple types due to obstruction by the papillomas. Treatment in both types consists of removal under direct laryngoscopy. In the multiple types the process is to be repeated for several times with suction and diathermy of each papilloma. Laser surgery is more promising. Cryosurgery is disappointing and tracheostomy may be needed if associated with dyspnoea.

Fibroma

Fibroma of the larynx usually arises from the vocal cords. It may be from the epiglottis, aryepiglottic folds, ventricular bands and the interarytenoid region. These appear as reddish mass with smooth surface. Treatment lies in removal under direct laryngoscopy preferably under operative microscope.

MALIGNANT TUMOURS

Malignant Tumours of Larynx

Krishaber (1879) classification of the cancer larynx as intrinsic and extrinsic still holds good as regards pathological and therapeutic viewpoints. Some minor modifications of Krishaber's classification have recently been made and widely accepted which is as follows:

Regions	Sites
Larynx	
Supraglottic	Posterior surface of the infrahyoid portion of epiglottis
	Ventricular band
	Ventricles and arytenoids
Glottic	Vocal cords (the margin and upper surface of the cord) and anterior and posterior commissures
Subglottic	Walls of the subglottis and under surface of the cord
Marginal zone	Tip of the epiglottis (suprahyoid) and aryepiglottic folds
Laryngopharynx (hypopharynx)	Pyriform fossa postcricoid area and posterior pharyngeal wall

But in some literatures marginal zone sites are included within intralaryngeal carcinoma and classified as supraglottic variety.

The so-called extrinsic type is not true growths of the larynx because they arise from the hypopharynx or outside the larynx, e.g. pyriform fossae, postcricoid area, and the posterior pharyngeal wall.

TNM CLASSIFICATION

This is the latest accepted classification of the malignant tumours of the larynx. Here TNM stand for primary tumour, regional lymph nodes and distant metastasis respectively.

T. Primary tumour

Tx   Tumour that cannot be assessed by rules.

T0   No evidence of primary tumour.

Ts   Carcinoma in situ.

T1   Tumour confined to one anatomical site within the larynx.

T2   Tumour confined to one anatomical region within the larynx.

T3   Tumour extending beyond one anatomical region but confined within the larynx.

T4   Tumour extending beyond the larynx.

N. Lymph node involvement

Nx   Nodes cannot be assessed.

N0   No palpable lymph node.

N1   One palpable homolateral mobile (3 cm or less in diameter).

N2   One or more palpable homolateral node (more than 3 cm and less than 6 cm in diameter).

N2a One palpable homolateral node more than 3 cm but less than 6 cm in diameter.

N2b Multiple palpable homolateral nodes, none more than 6 cm in diameter.

N2c Contralateral nodes or bilateral nodes, none more than 6 cm.

N3   Big homolateral node(s), bilateral nodes or contralateral nodes.

N3a Homolateral palpable node(s), more than 6 cm in diameter.
N3b Bilateral palpable nodes more than 6 cm.

M. Distant metastasis

Mx   Metastasis is not assessed.
M0   No distant metastasis.
M1   Distant metastasis.

Thus the stage classification of the malignant tumours of the larynx may be grouped as follows:

Stage I	T1, N0, M0
Stage II	T2, N0, M0
Stage III	T3, N0, M0
	T1 or T2 or T3, N1, M0
Stage IV	T4, N0 or N1, M0
	Any T, N2 or N3, M0
	Any T, any N, M1

Mode of Spread

The spread of cancer to lymph nodes is dependent upon normal anatomical pathways. In general the site of a metastasis in the neck is from the site of the primary tumour (Fig. 31.1). The factors, which affect the rate of metastasis, are as follows:
1. Site of the primary tumour
2. Size of the primary tumour

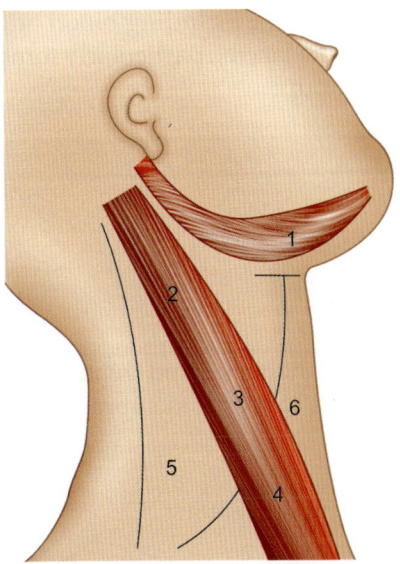

Fig. 31.1: The location of cervical lymph node groups commonly affected by metastases from specific primary sites. 1 and 2 Cancer larynx, anterior floor of mouth, lip, anterior two-thirds of tongue, gums and mucosa of cheek, 3. nasopharynx, 4. nasopharynx, oral cavity, pharynx or larynx, 5 and 6. thyroid, nasopharynx

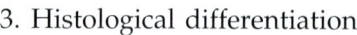

3. Histological differentiation
4. Host factors

The patient's immunological response of the disease to the tumour is of vital importance in the spread and prognosis of head and neck cancer.

The malignant tumours of the larynx spread by continuity, lymph, and blood-stream. Lymph node metastasis is very commonly seen in supraglottic tumours (40 per cent), not so common in subglottic tumours (15 per cent), and very rare in glottic tumours (4 per cent).

Symptoms

The earliest symptom of glottic cancer is hoarseness. Hoarseness persisting for more than two weeks without improvement needs laryngeal examination and treatment by an ENT specialist. The early symptom of supraglottic tumours is some sticky sensation in the throat. Other symptoms are increased expectoration, thickness of the voice and irritable cough.

The early symptoms of subglottic tumours are voice change and dyspnoea on exertion. The late symptoms are dyspnoea, dysphagia, loss of appetite, cachexia, halitosis, haemorrhage and otalgia. These will depend on the site, directions of spread and complications of the tumour.

Diagnosis

Diagnosis is made after consideration of
1. Symptoms.
2. Examination of the pharynx and larynx by both indirect and direct methods.
3. Examination of the neck.
4. General examination of the patient including blood and sputum examination.
5. Radiological examination of the larynx, particularly tomography and CT scanning assist in delineating the tumour.
6. Exfoliative cytology.
7. Biopsy.

Differential Diagnosis

1. Tuberculosis
2. Syphilis
3. Benign tumours

   Prognosis: It depends on early diagnosis and treatment. As a whole the prognosis is good in glottic cancer and bad to worse in supraglottic and subglottic cancer.

Treatment

Treatment depends on the following factors:
   i. Site of the tumour
   ii. Extent of the tumour
   iii. Histological character
   iv. Occupation of the patient
   v. Physical and mental fitness of the patient

vi. Facilities available

vii. Skill of the surgeon

Three main types of therapy are available

  i. Radiotherapy

  ii. Surgery

  iii. Chemotherapy

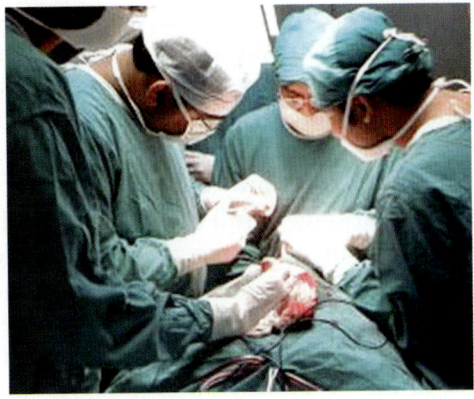

Fig. 31.2: Laryngectomy operation in progress

The modern trend in the treatment of early tumours is more conservative with preservation of voice. In advanced tumours it is more radical including block dissection of the neck.

The choice of the treatment in the beginning is irradiation by either linear acceleration or Co60. A curative dose should be given.

If the tumour extends beyond the limits of the larynx, e.g. subglottic extension and fixation of the vocal cord where radiotherapy should be given with or without chemotherapeutic agents like cyclophosphamide, methotrexate, 5-fluorouracil. Bleomycin and methotrexate act synergistically when administered with radiotherapy (Fig. 31.2).

Unknown Primary Tumour

One of the practices, which tend to provoke head and neck surgeons into criticism of their general surgical colleagues, is open biopsy of neck nodes. The general surgeon goes straight to biopsy where the patient presents with a lymph node in the neck as a primary complaint without investigating the patient for a primary tumour. It is not a good medicine to biopsy a neck node without a thorough search for a possible primary tumour (Fig. 31.3). Thus when the patient presents with a

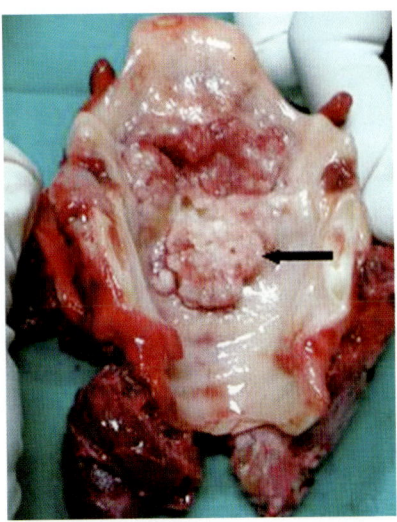

Fig. 31.3: Postlaryngectomy specimen showing transglottic carcinoma

palpable mass in the neck, which is suggestive of metastatic cancer in a cervical node, the patient should be investigated by history, clinical examination (general, physical and detailed otolaryngological examination) and a chest radiograph. Detailed radiological examination should only be performed in the presence of suggestive history or examination, i.e. dysphagia, dyspepsia, etc. Fine needle aspiration biopsy may be very helpful.

The next stage is full examination of the upper respiratory and elementary tracts and biopsy of suspicious areas, or if none is present, biopsy of the nasopharynx at least. Some would remove the tonsil on the side of the lesion. If all these investigations are negative, probably the correct course of action is to prepare the patient for neck dissection. Postoperative radiation should almost certainly be given to the neck and to the nasopharynx, oropharynx and hypopharynx. However, an alternative form of treatment is not to treat the patient by primary surgery, but to irradiate the neck and likely sites of primary tumours. There is a little difference in survival of the patients treated with radiotherapy, surgery or combined therapy. If the node is small, then excisional biopsy and radiotherapy may be appropriate. If the node is much larger, then perhaps, primary neck dissection and postoperative radiotherapy is the correct course of action. Either way cure rates of the order of 25–40% are usual.

32

Paralysis of
the Larynx

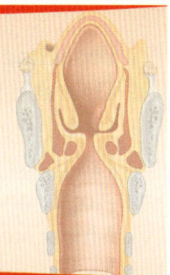

It may be of the following types:

A. Organic
  1. Motor (unilateral/bilateral)
     a. *Incomplete:* Only abductor muscles are paralysed
     b. *Complete:* Both adductor and abductor muscles are paralysed
  2. Sensory (unilateral/bilateral)
B. Functional: Only adductor muscles are paralysed and it is almost invariably bilateral.

Motor Paralysis

The motor paralysis may be of two types. They are:
1. Abductor paralysis
2. Adductor paralysis

When only one group of muscles, either abductors or adductors is paralysed, then it is incomplete paralysis, which may be unilateral or bilateral. When both the groups of muscles are paralyzed, then it is called complete paralysis, which again may be unilateral or bilateral. However, Semon's law helps in distinguishing the two types of paralysis.

Semon's Law

"In all progressive organic lesions of the centers and trunks of motor laryngeal nerves, the fibres supplying the abductors of the vocal cords become involved much earlier than do the adductors. When the paralysis is confined to the adductors of the vocal cords, it is almost invariably bilateral and is due to functional change in the central nervous system."

Aetiology of Motor Paralysis

The causes of motor paralysis may be:
1. Central (bulbar lesions), e.g. haemorrhage in the medulla; locomotor ataxia; disseminated sclerosis; tumours of the base of the brain.
2. Peripheral (lesions involving the recurrent laryngeal nerve). The left recurrent laryngeal nerve is more commonly affected than the right. This is due to its longer course. The common causes of left nerve paralysis are:

  i. Bronchogenic and oesophageal carcinoma.
 ii. Operations for the removal of goitre.
iii. Peripheral neuritis due to virus infections or diphtheria or lead poisoning.
 iv. Enlarged thyroid glands or carcinoma of the thyroid.
  v. Aortic aneurysm.
 vi. Mitral stenosis.
vii. Mediastinal tumours and enlarged lymph nodes.

The common causes of right nerve paralysis are:
  i. Aneurysm of the innominate or right subclavian arteries.
 ii. Thickened pleura over the apex of the right lung.
iii. Cancer of the oesophagus.
 iv. Operations for the removal of goitre.
  v. Peripheral neuritis as mentioned above.
 vi. Enlarged or carcinoma of the thyroid.

In about 30 to 50 per cent of all cases, the causes could not be determined (idiopathic).

Clinical Features

In the incomplete unilateral recurrent laryngeal nerve paralysis where only the adductors are involved, the voice and respiration remain unaffected. The affected vocal cord remains fixed in the median position.

If the condition progresses further leading to complete paralysis where both abductors and adductors are involved, the affected vocal cord remains fixed in the paramedian position, e.g. midway between the median and cadaveric position (Fig. 32.1). This position is maintained by the action of cricothyroid muscle, which is supplied by superior laryngeal branch of the vagus nerve. The patient becomes hoarse till the normal cord compensates to close the glottic space.

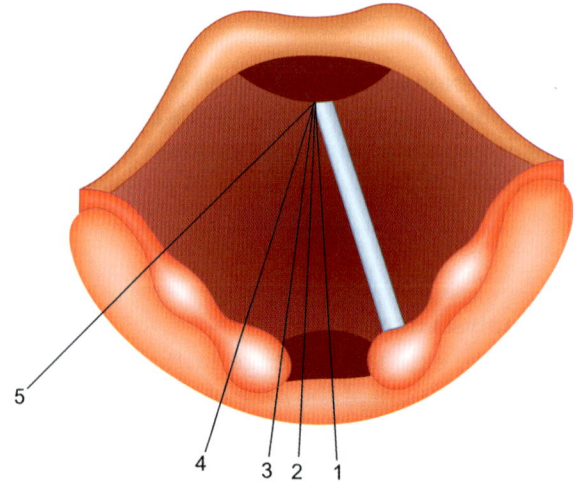

Fig. 32.1: Distance of vocal cords from median plane in mm. 1. Median, 2. paramedian (3.5 mm), 3. cadaveric (7 mm), 4. gentle abduction (13.5 mm), 5. full abduction (19 mm)

In the incomplete bilateral recurrent laryngeal nerve paralysis or bilateral abductor paralysis the voice remains unchanged. But the respiration is affected giving rise to dyspnoea and cyanosis. The vocal cords remain fixed in the median position.

In the complete paralysis of the recurrent laryngeal nerves the patient becomes hoarse, as the cords remain fixed in the paramedian position during phonation. Respiration remains unaffected at rest but embarrassed on exertion.

In the superior laryngeal nerve paralysis which is almost always associated with the paralysis of the recurrent laryngeal nerve, the voice becomes hoarse in unilateral cases and almost lost in bilateral cases. Owing to the loss of sensation of the larynx above the vocal cords, the patients become asphyxiated by inhalation of food, especially in bilateral cases. The cords become wavy and remain fixed in cadaveric position, e.g. between the median position and the position of quiet respiration. The position is attained owing to the paralysis of all the intrinsic muscles of the larynx.

Treatment

In unilateral paralysis the treatment is to remove the cause, otherwise no treatment is required.

In **bilateral abductor paralysis** with difficulty in respiration, tracheostomy is to be performed first with subsequent treatment of the causes. If the condition persists for more than six months and if the patient does not make his living by the use of his voice, operation should be performed. Three types of operations are usually done:

i. Excision of the vocal cord.

ii. Transplantation of the vocal cord (Woodman's operation).

iii. Mobilization and outward fixation of the arytenoids.

Adductor Paralysis

According to Semon's law, the primary adductor paralysis is always bilateral and is caused by functional changes.

It is commonly found in young females and emotionally unbalanced individuals. The patient suddenly becomes aphonic (functional aphonia). On indirect laryngoscopy the cords are seen in the abducted position on phonation. Sometimes they lie in the median position without any voice production. These patients cough normally and the abducted cords are seen in the position of adduction during coughing.

Treatment is by persuasion and removal of underlying psychological cause. Faradic stimulation sometimes gives better results. Light hypnosis may be used.

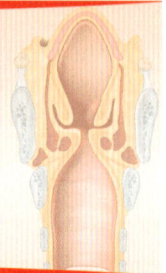

33

Tracheostomy

Tracheostomy is an operation by which an opening is made on the anterior wall of the trachea mainly for the purpose of respiration. Tracheostomy or a simple incision, is an exposure of the tracheal lumen temporarily for the treatment of a tumour or a stenosis.

Functions of Tracheostomy

1. It bypasses and relieves the upper respiratory obstruction.
2. It helps in removing the excess bronchial secretion and instillation of drugs.
3. It diminishes the dead space and thus improves the respiratory efficiency.
4. It decreases the airway resistance.
5. It permits insertion of a cuffed tracheostomy or intratracheal tube and helps to apply positive-pressure respiration and prevention of aspiration of saliva, etc.

Indications of Tracheostomy

I. Obstruction of the respiratory airway.

This may be due to intrinsic or extrinsic causes.

A. *Intrinsic*
   i. Congenital: Laryngeal web and stenosis. Bilateral choanal atresia.
   ii. Traumatic: Inhalation of steam and irritating fumes. Foreign bodies and swallowing of corrosives.
   iii. Inflammatory: Laryngeal diphtheria, tuberculosis and syphilis.
   iv. Neoplastic: Laryngeal papillomatosis, other benign tumours and malignant tumours of the larynx, pharynx, and base of the tongue.
   v. Paralytic: Bilateral incomplete (abductor) paralysis. After thyroidectomy, bulbar palsies.
   vi. Miscellaneous: Angioneurotic oedema, haemophilia.

B. *Extrinsic*
   i. Traumatic: Blows on larynx, gunshot injury or cut-throat wounds.
   ii. Inflammatory: Ludwig's angina.
   iii. Neoplastic: Carcinoma of the thyroid gland; metastatic neck glands.

II. As a precautionary measure wherever asphyxia is anticipated (elective)
   i. Removal of multiple papilloma of the larynx.
   ii. Laryngofissure.

iii. Operation on the face, jaws, and total glossectomy.

iv. Block dissection of the neck glands.

Any major operation in the mouth, pharynx and the larynx always constitutes a danger to the airway, both as a direct result of the surgical trauma and by the physiological disturbance of the swallowing mechanism.

III. Mechanical respiratory insufficiency.

i. Comatose conditions.

ii. Cerebrovascular accidents.

iii. Head and chest injuries.

iv. Barbiturate poisoning.

v. Chronic obstructive pulmonary disease (COPD)

IV. Interference with the nervous pathways.

i. Poliomyelitis.

ii. Polyneuritis.

ii. Lesion of the cervical cord.

V. Lesions of the neuromuscular junction.

i. Myasthenia gravis.

ii. Overdosage of muscle relaxants.

iii. Tetanus

Types of Tracheostomy

1. Temporary tracheostomy:
    i. Elective as in acute epiglottitis, or recoverable coma, or as a safety measure in head and neck surgery.
    ii. Emergency.
2. Permanent tracheostomy. As in total laryngectomy.

Surgical Anatomy

The trachea is situated exactly in the midline of the neck. The upper part is superficial and can be easily palpated. The suprasternal part is much deeply situated and can be felt only by deep palpation. The trachea is covered by skin, subcutaneous tissue, and deep fascia. The isthmus of the thyroid gland lies in relation to the second, third and fourth tracheal rings in between the two layers of deep fascia. The branches of the anterior jugular vein are encountered superficially. The sternohyoid and sternothyroid muscles (ribbon muscles of the neck) overlap the sides of the trachea, but they do not come up to the midline of the neck. No arteries of importance are present in front of it.

The opening made in the trachea above the isthmus is called a high tracheostomy and that below the isthmus a low tracheostomy. The opening made behind the isthmus is called midtracheostomy.

Anaesthesia: In adults the operation may be performed under a local anaesthetic. General anaesthesia is preferred in children. In case of acute emergency, tracheostomy may require to be performed even without any anaesthesia.

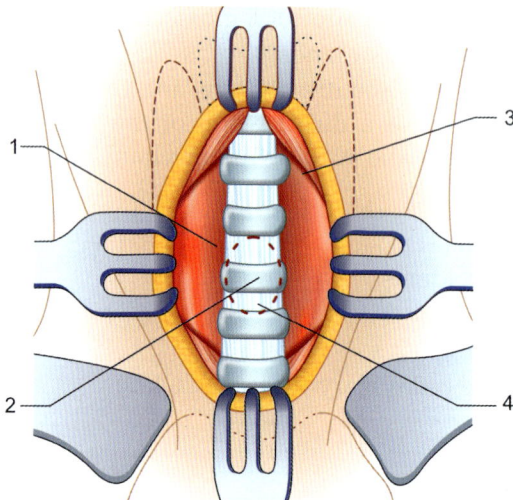

Fig. 33.1: Tracheostomy: 1. Isthmus of thyroid gland divided and ligated, 2. third ring of trachea, 3. sternothyroid muscle retracted, 4. site of incision in trachea

For local anaesthesia 1 to 2% xylocaine or lignocaine in adrenaline (1 in 100,000) should be injected under the skin along the line of incision and by the side of the trachea.

Position of the Patient

The patient lies in the supine position with a small cushion under the shoulder. This produces extension of the neck.

Operation

I. *Emergency Tracheostomy*

Steps

The trachea is fixed in the midline of the neck by the middle finger and thumb of the left hand.

An incision is given in the midline from the thyroid notch to the suprasternal notch. This cuts the skin and superficial fascia. The trachea is felt by the left index finger and steadied. The knife is slid down the side of the left index finger and the trachea is incised. A tracheal dilator is quickly introduced through the tracheal incision and dialated to allow entry of the tracheostomy tube. Attention is not given to the amount of bleeding which stops after the introduction of the tube.

If it does not stop, the bleeding vessels should be ligated and the wound above is stitched loosely to avoid surgical emphysema.

II. *Elective Tracheostomy*

The incision is the same as mentioned in emergency tracheostomy or transverse (or collar) incision is given about 2 cm below the cricoid cartilage.

The skin and superficial fascia are cut. A transverse cut of the pretracheal fascia is made just below the cricoid cartilage. The isthmus of the thyroid is retracted by a blunt hook or it is cut in between and ligated. Then the first three or four rings come into view. After a careful haemostasis, the trachea is fixed by passing a sharp hook below the cricoid cartilage. The trachea is punctured below the fourth ring exactly in the midline. A circular disc of tracheal wall at the level of third and fourth tracheal rings is cut out. In children a vertical incision is used and no cartilage is removed. Injection of a few drops of 4% xylocaine into the trachea, before opening it, minimizes the spasmodic cough. The tracheal incision is temporarily closed with the left index finger and then allowed the air to enter slowly to prevent sudden apnoea. The tracheal opening may be sutured with the skin edges before introducing the tracheal tube.

The circular opening made in the trachea by removing a small portion from each cut edge helps in the following ways:

i. Easy introduction of the tracheal tube
ii. Makes subsequent nursing simpler
iii. Prevent necrosis of the tracheal rings.

The tracheal tube is introduced as follows:

The outer tube is introduced first after being held by the right hand and presented tracheostomy horizontally from the far side of the neck. The convexity of the tube is kept forward. If the Fuller's bivalved tube is used, a tracheal dilator is not required. Otherwise, a dilator will have to be used. The tape attached to the outer tube is fastened around the neck after flexing the head to release the neck muscles. Then the inner tube is inserted.

Choice of Tracheostomy

The choice of tracheostomy in acute emergencies is the 'mid' operation. Because third, and fourth rings are conveniently situated except that they lie behind the isthmus of the thyroid gland. This operation can be more easily performed than the low tracheostomy. 'High' operation has the risk of injuring the cricoid cartilage followed by stenosis of the larynx and the site of laryngeal disease causing obstruction may be very close to the site of operation. 'Low' operation may encounter anterior jugular vein and its branches, inferior thyroid veins and thyroidea ima, innominate artery and the thymus in infants. Hence low tracheostomy operation is dangerous than the other types.

Aftercare

The important aftercare is the maintenance of a clear airway. The patient should be in a propped-up position and encouraged to move about freely. During first 48 hours secretions should be removed half-hourly and thereafter every 1 or 2 hours. The inner tube should be removed for cleaning after every four hours. The tracheostomy tube should not be disturbed for the first 2 to 3 days. After that the whole tube should be replaced by a sterile tube every day. If a tracheostomy tube with an inflatable cuff is used, the cuff should be deflated every half an hour to prevent ischaemic necrosis of the tracheal wall with which it is in contact. The moist sterile swab round the tube should be changed as soon as it becomes soiled for humidification of inspired air. The excess of secretion should be removed by suction with a soft catheter passed through the tracheostomy tube. Physiotherapy to improve the respiratory efficiency is also important.

Decannulation

If the tracheostomy tube remains for a long period, the patient forgets to breathe through the normal airway. It then becomes highly difficult to educate the patient to breathe without a tracheostomy tube. The method for decannulation is to insert tubes of progressively smaller diameter. In this way the patient is made to breathe gradually through the normal airway.

Postoperative Complications

1. Bronchopneumonia.
2. Mediastinal emphysema.
3. Pneumothorax.
4. Mediastinitis.
5. Necrosis of the anterior tracheal wall owing to the pressure of a malshaped metal tube.
6. Tracheo-oesophageal fistula.
7. Blockage of tracheostomy tube.
8. Difficult decannulation.

Phonosurgery

Phonosurgery is designed to improve or restore the voice. It was popularized by Hans von Laden in the late 1950s.

Phonosurgery can be internal or external. The external laryngeal surgery or thyroplasty is also known as laryngeal framework surgery.

Internal laryngeal surgery: It is required for vocal nodules, cysts, sulcus vocalis, multiple papillomas, spastic dysphonia, etc.

External laryngeal surgery: After development of this procedure by Isshiki in 1980s, the laryngeal framework surgery or thyroplasty has gained popularity.

Type I thyroplasty is medial positioning of the vocal cord done for chronic *adductor* paralysis.

Type II thyroplasty produces lateralization of vocal cord in chronic *abductor* paralysis.

Type III is performed to shorten the vocal cord.

Type IV for lengthening the vocal cord.

Surgeries for bilateral abductor paralysis of vocal cords are:

    i. King in 1939 described an extra-laryngeal surgery to move the vocal cord and the arytenoid laterally and fix it to the omohyoid muscle and the thyroid ala.
    ii. Woodman in 1946 modified the procedure of King by excising the arytenoid and suturing the vocal process to the inferior cornua of the thyroid cartilage.
    iii. Thornell in 1949 described endolaryngeal arytenoidectomy which can now be carried out bloodlessly using CO_2 LASER.
    iv. Cordectomy, cordotomy, cordoplasty, etc. are done with CO_2 LASER through endoscopy or videoendoscopy techniques with satisfactory result.
    v. Isshiki type II procedure.

Oesophagus

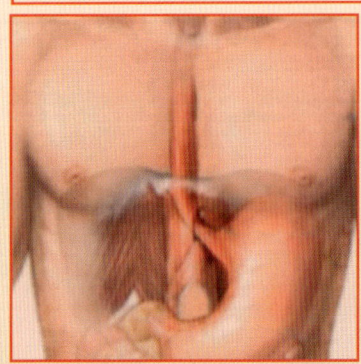

34

Anatomy of the Oesophagus

The oesophagus is a thin muscular tube. Its length in adults is 10 inches or 25 cm. It begins where the pharynx ends, at the level of the lower border of the cricoid cartilage or of the 6th cervical vertebra and ends at the level of the 11th thoracic vertebra. The wall of the oesophagus is composed of three coats:

1. Muscular
2. Submucous
3. Mucous.

It is also covered with fibrous tissue by which it is loosely attached to the surrounding structures. Its wall is thin and lacks the protective covering, i.e. peritoneum. It can be divided in three parts, e.g. cervical, thoracic and abdominal. The blood supply is from:

i. The inferior thyroid artery, in the cervical part.
ii. The descending thoracic aorta, in the thoracic part.
iii. The left gastric artery in the abdominal part.

The nerve supply is derived from the vagus (parasympathetic) and sympathetic.

There are four constrictions in the oesophagus (Fig. 34.1). They are:

i. At the beginning of the oesophagus, i.e. at the level of the 6th cervical vertebra or 6 inches from the upper incisor teeth.
ii. At the crossing of the aorta opposite the 4th thoracic vertebra or 10 inches from the upper incisor teeth.
iii. At the level of the 5th thoracic vertebra where the bronchus crosses the oesophagus or 11 inches from the upper incisor teeth.
iv. At the level of the 10th thoracic vertebra where it passes through the diaphragm or 16 inches from the upper incisor teeth.

Examination

The esophagus may be examined in the following ways:

1. A barium X-ray of the oesophagus
2. Endoscopy (oesophagoscopy).
   a. Oesophageal speculum: It is used for the upper end or the thoracic oesophagus.
   b. Oesophagoscope: For the whole length of the oesophagus, which may be rigid or flexible type of oesophagoscope with fibreoptic illumination.

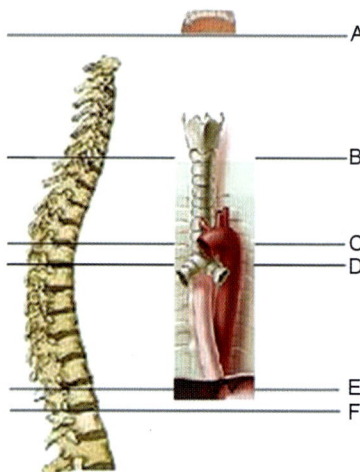

Fig. 34.1: Normal constrictions of the esophagus in relation to the vertebrae and incisor teeth. A. incisor line, B. cricoid line (C6): 15 cm from incisors, C. sternal angle (T4): 25 cm from incisors, D. left bronchus (T5): 27.5 cm from incisors, E. xiphisternal line (T10): 40 cm from incisors, F. level of cardia

Mechanism of Deglutition

After mastication, food is carried to the stomach by an orderly sequence of coordinated movements of the muscles of the mouth, pharynx and oesophagus. There are three uninterrupted stages of swallowing of deglutition. Except the oral stage, which is voluntary, other two stages occur reflexly. The afferent nerves are maxillary division of the Vth, IXth and Xth cranial nerves. The deglutition centre is situated in the medulla near the nucleus of the vagus nerve. The efferent fibres pass in the Xth and XIth nerves mainly and also in the XIIth cranial nerves.

1. *Oral stage:* It is a voluntary stage. The bolus of food is pushed backwards after mastication into the oropharynx from the mouth in between the anterior faucial pillars. The posterior pillars contract closing the oropharyngeal isthmus at the end of this stage, thereby preventing return of food towards the mouth.
2. *Pharyngeal stage:* This stage is a reflex one and carries food through the oropharynx, which is common to the digestive and respiratory systems. The reflex contraction of the constrictor muscles pushes food through the cricopharyngeal sphincter, which relaxes reflexly at this stage.
3. *Oesophageal stage:* This is also a reflex stage. Peristaltic movement of the oesophagus carries the food downwards. In erect position gravity also assists to move the food down.

Dysphagia

Dysphagia means difficulty with swallowing which is a symptom of various diseases of the mouth, tongue, pharynx and oesophagus. Hence, a thorough investigation is necessary to find out the cause of dysphagia. Carcinoma of the oesophagus is one of the common causes of dysphagia and a disease with a grave prognosis. However, many causes are non-malignant conditions. Painful swallowing is termed odynphagia or odynophagia. It is also included in the broad term—dysphagia. The causes of dysphagia are as follows:

1. Mouth: Stomatitis, cleft palate and paralysis of the soft palate.
2. Tongue: Tuberculosis, dyspeptic and carcinomatous ulcerations.
3. Pharynx: Tonsillitis.
    Peritonsillar abscess (quinsy)
        Retropharyngeal abscess
        Foreign body impactions
        Malignant growth, etc.
4. Oesophagus:
    a. In the lumen: Foreign body (coin, dentures, etc.)
    b. In the wall:
        1. Benign strictures
            i. Traumatic
            ii. Corrosive injury
            iii. Reflux oesophagitis
        2. Malignant strictures (carcinoma oesophagus)
        3. Benign tumours
        4. Paterson-Brown Kelly syndrome
        5. Achalasia (cardiospasm)
        6. Bulbar paralysis
        7. Tetanus
        8. Myasthenia gravis
        9. Scleroderma
        10. Globus hystericus
    c. Outside the wall:
        1. Pharyngeal pouch
        2. Inflammatory and malignant diseases of the thyroid gland
        3. Retrosternal thyroid
        4. Mediastinal lymphadenopathy and tumours
        5. Aortic aneurysm
        6. Dilatation of the heart
        7. Pericardial effusion
        8. Paraoesophageal hiatus hernia
        9. Dysphagia lusoria
        10. Gross cervical spondylosis with large anterior osteophytes.

Investigation

Diagnosis of a case of dysphagia may be established after consideration of the history, radiological and endoscopic findings. Certain special tests may be helpful, such as exfoliative cytology, cineradiography and manometry.

History

Age: 20–40 years—suggests cardiospasm
　　　Menopause—suggests Paterson-Kelly syndrome
　　　50–70 years—suggests carcinoma oesophagus
Sex: Paterson-Brown Kelly syndrome occurs almost always in females.

Past History

a. Anaemia, glossitis and stomatitis in a female suggest Plummer-Vinson syndrome or Paterson-Brown Kelly syndrome.
b. Corrosive swallowing and instrumentation suggest benign stricture.
c. Poliomyelitis or diphtheria suggest oesophageal paralysis.
d. Psychiatric disorders may suggest globus hystericus.

Symptoms

Dysphagia
a. Sudden onset suggests foreign body or acute oesophagitis.
b. Slow onset suggests carcinoma oesophagus, cardiospasm, and stricture formation.
c. Difficulty in swallowing solids initially is typical of carcinoma and stricture of the oesophagus, while fluids may be obstructed initially in cardiospasm.

Pain
Difficulty in swallowing with retrosternal pain suggests reflux or peptic oesophagitis.

Regurgitation
Suggests cardiospasm.

Signs

In majority of the patients with history of dysphagia clinical examination reveals nothing. However, weight loss, palpable neck glands, hepatomegaly or ascites may help in diagnosing a case of carcinoma oesophagus.

Special Tests

Barium swallow X-ray and oesophagoscopy are mostly helpful.

35

Diseases of the Oesophagus

Congenital Atresia of the Oesophagus

Congenital atresia occurs due to developmental abnormalities of the lateral septa between the primitive oesophagus and trachea and in the recanalization of the obliterated primitive oesophagus. The main types are:

a. Atresia in the oesophagus without any connection with trachea. Stomach does not contain gas (simple atresia).

b. Blind upper end. Lower end is connected with trachea or a bronchus. This type is more common (Tracheo-oesophageal fistula). Stomach contains gas.

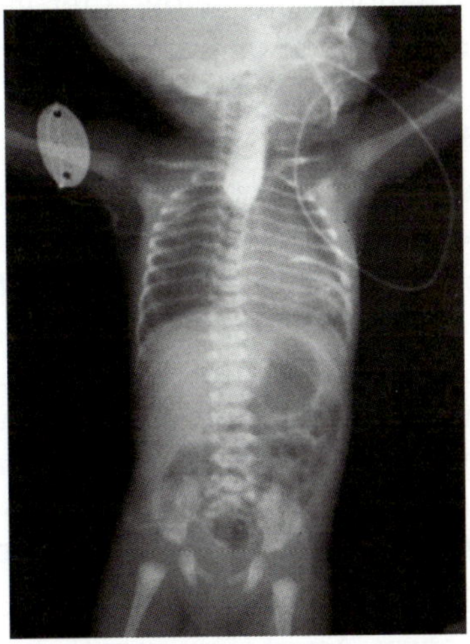

Fig. 35.1: Tracheo-oesophageal fistula with gas in stomach in a newborn baby (1 day old)

Clinical Features

1. Regurgitation of food.
2. Coughing, choking and asphyxia.

Diagnosis

1. By passing a soft catheter, which fails to enter the stomach.
2. By X-ray of the oesophagus after introducing iodized oil. In case of fistula, air is present in the stomach.

Treatment

1. Transthoracic closure of fistula with end-to-end anastomosis must be immediately performed in atresia with tracheo-oesophageal fistula.
2. In atresia without fistula, a gastrostomy should be performed.

Congenital Stricture

It may rarely occur:
1. At the cricopharyngeal sphincter, where there may be a wave, fold or narrowing.

2. In the thoracic oesophagus, usually in the lower third. A smooth pinhole size lumen is seen with considerable dilatation above.

Clinical Features

Dysphagia, more common in the adult life. These patients accommodate themselves to a small swallow throughout life.

Treatment

1. Dilatation with bougies from above is usually successful.
2. Dilatation from below after gastrostomy may be indicated in some cases.
3. Transcervical or transthoracic resection is sometimes necessary.

Diverticulum

It can be rarely congenital and usually acquired.

Congenital diverticula are usually small and situated near the lower end of the oesophagus. They are of Pulsion type.

Acquired diverticulum is a traction pouch. It usually occurs at the level of the bifurcation of the trachea. It usually occurs in the tuberculosis of the tracheo-bronchial lymph nodes. It is generally symptomless. There may be a vague dyspepsia or dysphagia. It can occur at any age.

Corrosive Burns of the Oesophagus

Swallowing of strong acids or alkalis either accidental (children) or suicidal cause this injury. Apart from mouth and pharynx the middle third of the oesophagus is very commonly involved. It may also cause oedema of the larynx. It may cause multiple stricture of the oesophagus if the muscle coat is also involved in addition to the mucous and submucous layers.

Treatment

1. Neutralize the acid or alkali.
2. Pass a nasogastric feeding tube.
3. Prednisolone 60 mg per day in a divided dose for a week, then to taper down the dose over a period of 3 to 4 weeks.
4. Systemic antibiotics in adequate doses.
5. Oesophagoscopy should be done after 3 to 4 weeks.

If a stricture has formed, dilatation under direct vision should be started.

Achalasia Cardia (Cardiospasm)

It is due to a defect in the Auerbach's myenteric plexus (intramural vagal supply). The tone of the oesophageal muscle is lost due to a lack of integrated parasympathetic stimulation and gets dilated. The cardiac sphincter also fails to relax which acts as a stricture. The patient of the younger age group (20 to 40 years) presents with history of intermittent attacks of retrosternal or epigastric fullness after meals, dysphagia to liquids and regurgitation of food. In spite of all these features the

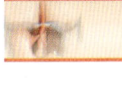
patient rarely loses weight and becomes cachectic. Diagnosis is made by barium swallow X-ray of esophagus and confirmed by oesophagoscopy. Barium X-ray shows dilatation of the oesophagus above the level of diaphragm. The site of obstruction of the oesophagus at the level of diaphragm does not show any irregularity or filling defect. Normal gas bubble in the fundus of the stomach is absent as the oesophagus never empties adequately (Fig. 35.2).

Treatment

1. Oesophageal lavage.
2. Dilatation of the lower end of the oesophagus under direct vision with gum elastic bougies. The patient himself may dilate repeatedly by Hurst's mercury bougie.

Fig. 35.2: Fusiform dialation of the oesophagus with constriction at the level of diaphragm (cardiospasm)

3. Inhalation of amyl or octyl nitrate before meals. Anticholinergics like probanthine, belladona group of drugs given one hour before meals may allow comfortable swallowing,
4. Heller's operation: In this the cardiac sphincter is incised down to the mucosa. (cf. Ramstedt's operation for congenital pyloric stenosis).

Benign Stricture of the Oesophagus

Benign stricture may follow the swallowing of caustics (strong acids alkalis) or may result from ulceration following injury by a foreign body. The commonest site of stenosis following the swallowing of caustics is the middle third of the oesophagus. The stricture may be multiple. Symptoms include difficulty in swallowing, regurgitation of food and cough. Barium swallow X-ray of the oesophagus shows considerable narrowing of it with maintenance of regularity all through its walls.

Diagnosis is confirmed by oesophagoscopy.

Treatment

The treatment is frequent dilatation for a prolonged period by bougies (either gum elastic or metallic) under direct vision.

If this fails, surgery in the form of resection anastomosis should be recommended.

Foreign Body in the Oesophagus

Unlike inhaled foreign body, which is most commonly met with in children, swallowed foreign body is frequently found in adults.

Common Foreign Body

In children—coins or small disc-shaped or irregular play things.

In adult—fish bones, meat bones, unchewed meat may cause obstruction in older people especially so if the patient is odentulous.

Improper preparation of food, hasty eating and drinking, permitting children to play while eating, and talking with food in the mouth, giving foods such as peanut to children who do not have the proper molar teeth to chew them, improper supervision of small children playing in the vicinity of infants are responsible for the impaction of foreign body in the throat, oesophagus and tracheobronchial tree. Careful supervision may prevent foreign body ingestion.

Patients or parents give history of initial choking and gagging. There may be a subjective feeling of "something" foreign in the throat, which may be constant or more often present on the act of swallowing. There may be substernal or epigastric pain that sometimes extends to the back. Flat objects such as coins, most often lie in the coronal plane. Disc-shaped objects are most often found just below the cricopharyngeus in the cervical oesophagus. This is thought to be due to the increased retention by the circular fibres of the oesophagus once the coin has dropped below the slit-shaped lumen of the cricopharyngeus at its point of attachment to the cricoid cartilage.

The powerful inferior constrictor, by its swallowing movement, forces the foreign body into the upper end of the oesophagus where there is nothing but peristalsis to send them downwards. However, this peristalsis is relatively weak as applied to a rather large foreign body in this region.

The most common foreign bodies in the oesophagus are the coins, which are frequently seen in children. The second place is held by fish and meat bones and dentures, which are common in adults.

The common site of impaction is the hypopharynx or just below it (Fig. 35.3).

Symptoms and Signs

    i. Stabbing retrosternal pain.

   ii. Dysphagia—may be extreme at times.

 iii. Pooling of saliva in the pyriform fossae.

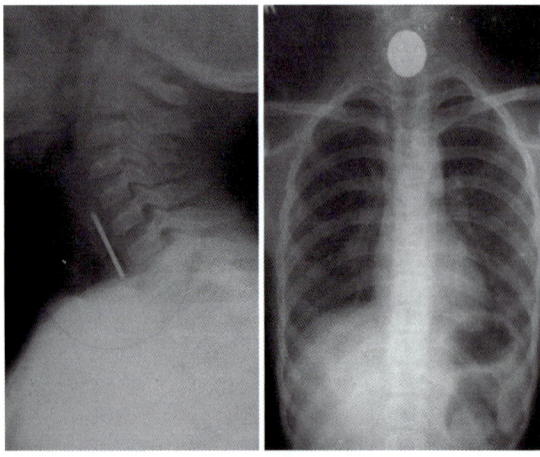

Fig. 35.3: Foreign body oesophagus (lateral and AP views)

In case of hypopharyngeal foreign body there may be hoarseness and difficulty in breathing. The difficulty in breathing may be due to:

a. Swelling of the laryngeal mucosa

b. Compression of the trachea by the foreign body in the oesophagus.

iv. A passive movement of the larynx causes the patient pain.

v. In cases of paraoesophageal abscess there may be localised swelling in the supraclavicular region.

Diagnosis

1. Plain X-ray of the oesophagus in PA view. To establish the diagnosis of the presence of a foreign body and to decide upon the process of removal, X-rays provide invaluable assistance. The ingested object may lodge anywhere between the base of the skull and the floor of the perineum, which should be X-rayed in one plate. Many foreign body are radiopaque. So plain X-rays are helpful in majority of the cases.

   Lateral X-ray of the neck is one of the most useful single film available to the endoscopist. The coin will appear as opaque object lying in coronal plane in AP. view, whereas the rim of the coin is visible in lateral view.

   The fish bones may be translucent. This may be localised by an X-ray taken after swallowing a small pledget of cotton wool soaked in barium.

2. Oesophagoscopy or hypopharyngoscopy by oesophageal speculum.

Treatment

Endoscopic removal. The dental plates may be required to be cut with shears before removal. The coins and other larger foreign bodies are removed with endoscopic forceps under oesophagoscopy. These foreign bodies do not pass through the oesophagoscope or oesophageal speculum. Therefore these types of foreign bodies should be caught with an endoscopic forceps and then removed along with the oesophagoscope. (The foreign body, the forceps and oesophagoscope all together.)

Complications

If the foreign body is not removed or if there is injury to the oesophagus during removal, the following complications may result:

i. Paraoesophageal emphysema, cellulitis or abscess in the neck.

ii. Mediastinal emphysema, mediastinitis, or mediastinal abscess.

iii. Tracheal compression.

iv. Perforation of the aorta.

v. Tracheo-oesophageal fistula.

vi. Benign stricture of the oesophagus.

Paterson-Brown Kelly Syndrome (Plummer-Vinson syndrome)

This syndrome consists of gradually increasing dysphagia to solids and hypochromic microcytic anaemia with certain changes in the epithelium. Aetiology is not known. The serum iron is lowered in all cases and iron binding capacity becomes high. It commonly occurs in females in the menopausal stage. The mucosa of the mouth, tongue, pharynx and oesophagus becomes atrophic resulting in glossitis, angular stomatitis, koilonychia, pruritus and brittle nails. At the cricopharyngeal region folds or webs of mucosa may develop, as a result of chronic inflammation (chronic pharyngo-oesophagitis) and hyperkeratinization along with spasm of the cricopharyngeus muscle. In about 50 per cent of these patients, carcinoma of the upper end of oesophagus may develop.

Barium swallow X-ray of the oesophagus may show a filling defect at the upper end with dilatation of the hypopharynx.

Oesophagoscopy may reveal a web or stricture at the upper end of the oesophagus.

Treatment

Large doses of iron and vitamin A in the form of antioxident and B complex should be administered to combat anaemia and mucosal changes respectively.

The patient is to be kept under close observation to exclude early malignant changes. A check on the course of the disease during follow up should always be by means of the serum iron rather than the haemoglobin.

Hiatus Hernia

Hiatus hernia may be congenital and acquired. It is difficult to differentiate between the two.

Types

1. *Sliding:* In this type the cardiac part of the stomach and oesophagus enter into the thorax through the oesophageal opening in the diaphragm. It occurs in middle aged and elderly persons. Causes: Increased abdominal pressure in obesity, constipation and compression of the abdominal wall by trauma.
2. *Paraoesophageal:* The fundus of the stomach enters into the thorax alongside the oesophagus. The cardia retains its normal position.

Symptoms

1. Heartburn and pain due to reflux of the acid into the oesophagus, which aggravate in lying position. These are common in sliding type due to ineffective cardiac sphincter.
2. Bleeding due to oesophagitis in sliding hernia, or due to peptic ulcer in the thoracic stomach in paraoesophageal hernia.
3. Dyspnoea due to distension after meals.

Diagnosis

Carcinoma must be excluded by:
1. Barium swallow X-ray of the oesophagus; and
2. Oesophagoscopy.

Treatment

1. Weight reduction.
2. Alkalies by mouth.
3. Sleeping in propped up position.
4. Surgical repair of the diaphragm with replacement of the stomach in the abdomen.

Carcinoma of the Oesophagus

The great majority of the oesophageal malignancies are squamous-cell carcinoma. They may be of any grade from highly differentiated to undifferentiated forms. The growth may be of ulcerative, proliferative or infiltrative type. There may be adenocarcinoma in the lower end of the oesophagus, which is radio-insensitive.

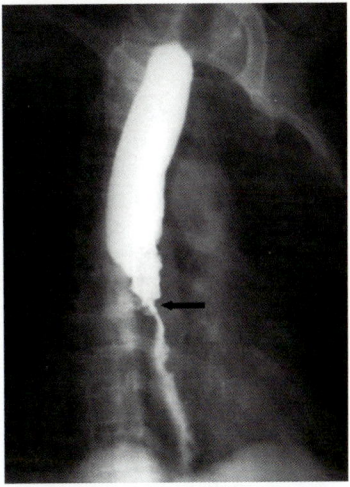

Fig. 35.4: Barium swallow X-ray oesophagus showing irregular filling defect in the lower third of the oesophagus

The patient complains of vague discomfort behind the sternum in the early stage. This is followed by marked dysphagia, at first with solids, which progressively increases until complete obstruction occurs with dysphagia to liquids. The patient becomes emaciated to a great extent. The diagnosis is made by barium swallow X-ray of the oesophagus, which is confirmed by biopsy (Fig. 35.4).

Treatment

As the great majority of the patients turn up in very advanced stage with absolute dysphagia, the preliminary treatment should be gastrostomy to regain or maintain nutrition. Basically the treatment depends on the following factors:

   i. Site of the growth.
  ii. Nature and extent of the growth.
 iii. Pathological character of the growth.
 iv. Mental and physical state of the patient.
  v. Skill and experience of the surgeon.
 vi. Facilities available.

The main forms of treatment are surgery and deep X-ray therapy.

In the advanced stage palliative radiotherapy is the treatment of choice either by cobalt (Co60) therapy or by linear accelerator.

Intubation with a Souttar's tube helps in relieving the obstruction in the growth of the middle or lower third of the oesophagus. If the Souttar's tube fails, the Mousseau-Barbin technique may be tried.

The surgical treatment is basically the excision of the growth and anastomosis of the cut ends of the oesophagus with the stomach or intestine.

Prognosis

Prognosis is grave. The majority of the patients die in 6 months if not treated. Even if treated with the best possible methods many patients die within 2 years.

Instruments

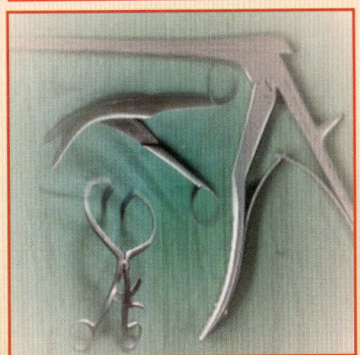

36

Ear Instruments

1. Otoscope (Electrical)

It is self-illuminating. This instrument like Siegel's speculum must also have an aural speculum with it, otherwise it is incomplete.

This is used for examining minute perforations of the tympanic membrane and other structures in canal wall. It is also used to look for honeycombing of the tympanic membrane in otosclerosis.

2. Aural Speculum (Toynbee's)

It is used for examination of the external ear and the tympanic membrane. It is also essential during myringotomy operation and certain other ear operations. During the use of the aural speculum one has to pull the pinna upwards, backwards and laterally in adults and downwards and laterally in children. Introduce the speculum inside the auditory canal up to the junction of the cartilage and bone. Pushing the speculum beyond the cartilaginous meatus becomes painful as the bony meatal skin is highly sensitive. The colour and landmarks of a normal tympanic membrane are important to note. The colour is pearly white. The landmarks are the following:

   i. Short process of malleus.
  ii. Handle of malleus.
 iii. Cone of light in the anteroinferior quadrant of the tympanic membrane.
  iv. Anterior and posterior malleolar folds.

3. Tuning Fork (Hartmann's)

It is used to determine the type of deafness, i.e. the quality of deafness (qualitative test). For details of deafness and different types of tuning fork tests see text.

4. Aural Metallic Syringe

This instrument has three rings with which it can be manipulated by one hand. The other hand is to be engaged for the purpose of pulling the pinna in the directions—the same as in the use of aural speculum. This is used for removing an unimpacted foreign body from the ear canal and dried discharge of chronic suppurative otitis media.

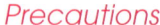

Precautions

The following precautions are to be taken during syringing:

i. The patient must sit comfortably (if stands, he might fall down owing to vasovagal attack).

ii. Water should be at body temperature. If it is too hot or too cold, there may be vertigo owing to vestibular irritation or vasovagal attack due to irritation of the auricular branch of vagus.

iii. The nozzle of the instrument should not be introduced inside the lumen of the external ear canal as it will obstruct the way of the returning fluid and as such wax or foreign body.

iv. The jet of the fluid should not be very forceful; if so, there is the possibility of the tympanic membrane being damaged.

v. The jet of the fluid should be directed towards the wall of the ear canal (preferably towards the roof).

vi. In the case of removing a foreign body a chink or a gap must be found or made out in between it and the wall of the external auditory canal.

5. Eustachian Catheter (Kramer's)

(Commonly confused with antrum washing cannula).

The ring near the base of the catheter is to guide the direction of the tip. The tip of this instrument is open (cf. Antrum washing cannula). It is use of eustachian catheter:

It is used for eustachian catheterization for diagnostic and therapeutic purposes. Two other accessories are necessary during the use of this instrument:

i. Auscultation tube,

ii. Politzer's bag.

• Diagnostic use

When the instrument is used to know the patency of the eustachian tube.

• Therapeutic use

a. To remove blockage of the eustachian tube.

b. In some cases, for medication in the middle ear.

Method of Catheterization

Pass the instrument with its tip touching the floor of the nose, into the nasal cavity. Push it along the floor of the nose backwards till it touches the posterior wall of the nasopharynx. Rotate the instrument medially up to 90°, pull the catheter forward till it hinges against the free margin of the nasal septum. Then rotate it laterally up to 180°. The catheter now enters in the opening of the pharyngotympanic tube. The Politzer's bag is then attached to the outer end of the eustachian catheter. The two ends of the auscultation tube with eartips are fitted, one in the patient's ear to be inflated and the other in the examiner's ear. Air is now pushed by the Politzer's bag into the middle ear through the catheter. The sound passing through the tube is heard by the examiner through the auscultation tube.

Types of Sound Heard

   i. Normal: Blowing sound indicates patent eustachian tube
  ii. Abnormal
     a. Bubbling sound: It indicates catarrh of middle ear and eustachian tube
     b. Whistling sound: It indicates partial stenosis or blockage of eustachian tube
  No sound indicates either complete obstruction of the eustachian tube or failed catheterization.

6. Seigel's Pneumatic Speculum

This instrument like otoscope has got one lens for magnification. When the attached speculum is fitted in the ear canal, it makes an air-tight chamber. Thus the mobility of the tympanic membrane may be tested by pressing the rubber bulb attached to the instrument. The uses of this instrument are:

   i. To test the movement of the tympanic membrane (mobility).
  ii. To see the magnified view of the minute perforation (magnification).
 iii. To push the medicines (ear drops) inside the middle ear in the treatment of chronic suppurative otitis media (medication).

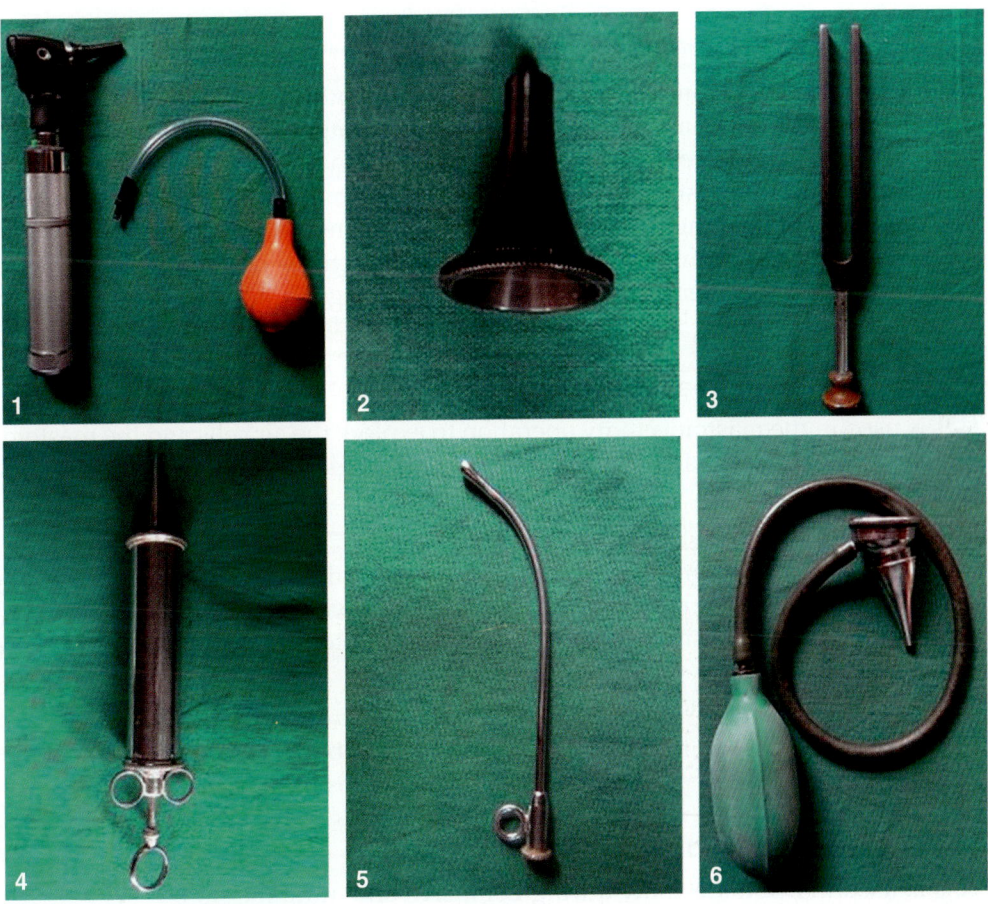

iv. To perform the fistula test for vestibular function and to know the pathological fistulous connection between the middle and inner ears. For details of fistula test *see* text.

7. Self-Retaining Haemostatic Mastoid Retractor

It is used in both cortical and radical mastoidectomy operations and in thyrotomy or laryngofissure surgery. Jansen's type of retractor is commonly used. Mollison's and Plester's retractors may also be used.

The retractor is applied after elevating the periosteum on either side of the incision in mastoidectomy operations.

No assistant is required to hold this instrument after application. That is why it is called self retaining.

By exerting lateral pressure with the two blades on the incision line, it causes haemostasis.

The skin, superficial fascia, a few fibres of the temporalis muscle above, sternomastoid muscle (only in the lower part of incision) and periosteum are retracted by this instrument.

8a. Mollison's and 8b. Plester's Retractors

9. Mastoid Gouge (Jenkin's)

It is used in mastoidectomy operation (cortical and radical) to explore the mastoid antrum and the mastoid air cells. The groove of the gouge faces the site of operation during its use. The surgeon must have a good grip on the instrument. To prevent injury to the important structures such as sigmoid sinus posteriorly, the temporal lobe of brain with meninges superiorly and the facial nerve anteriorly, the surgeon should place the instrument parallel to these structures during gouging. This instrument should be very sharp. The larger size gouge should be used whenever possible.

10. MacEwen's Cell Seeker with Scoop

This is used in the mastoidectomy operation to explore the air cells and the mastoid antrum with the seeker and to scoop out the pathological cells with the scoop.

11. Myringotome (Dagget's)

It is used in myringotomy which means incision of the tympanic membrane for better drainage of pus from the middle ear. It is always better to be performed under general anaesthesia. For details about myringotomy see text.

12. Aural Snare (Ballance's)

This is the smallest of all the snares used in ENT operation. Its function is to cut the pedicle of the aural polyp. The number "0" steel wire is used in this snare.

13. Lempert's End-aural Speculum

This is used in mastoidectomy during Lempert's end-aural incision.

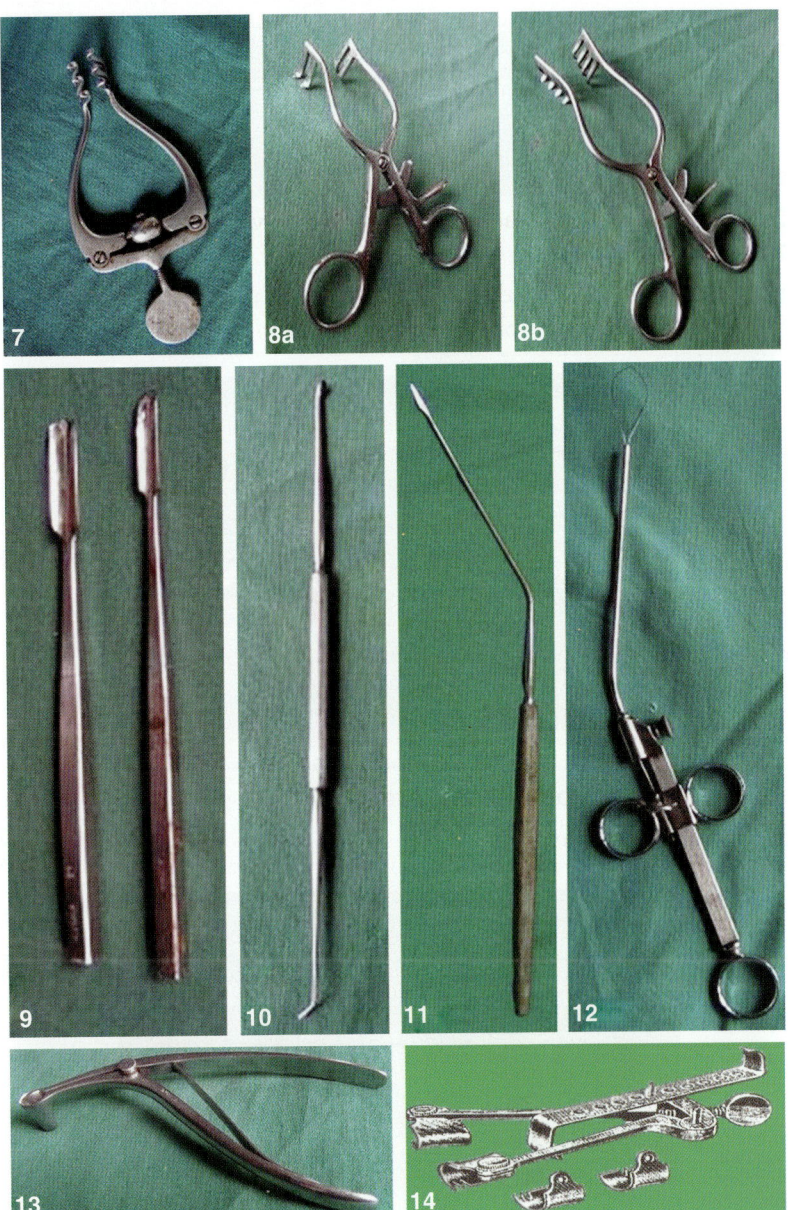

14. End-aural Retractor with the Third Blade (Lempert's)

This instrument is used to retract the incision lines in the mastoidectomy operation through end-aural route. The third blade is used to retract the temporal muscle and fascia away from the field of operation.

MICRO-EAR SURGERY INSTRUMENTS

1. Zollner's Suction Tube with Detachable Tips

Used in the microsurgery of the ear like stapedectomy and tympanoplasty.

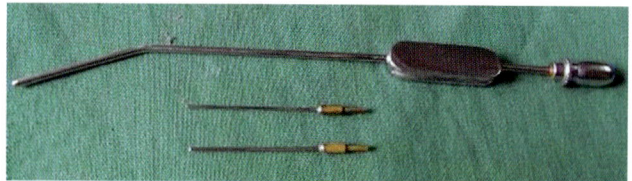

2. Crocodile Aural Forceps

Round cup jaws of Angell James used in tympanoplasty operations. It may be of oval cup jaws as used by John Shea in microsurgery of the ear.

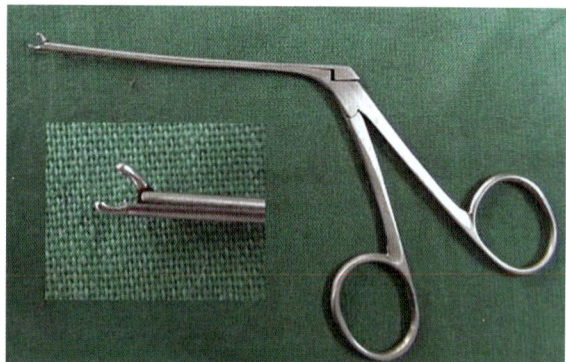

3. Crocodile Aural Forceps with Serrated Jaw

Used in microsurgery of the ear.

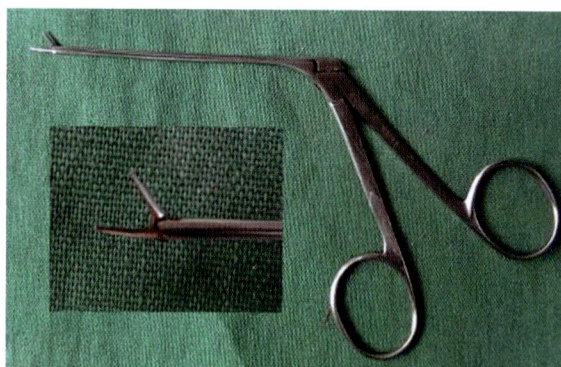

4. Sickle Knife (Lempert's)

Used to cut the stapedius tendon in stapedectomy operation. Also used for preparing the meatal flap in mastoidectomy operation.

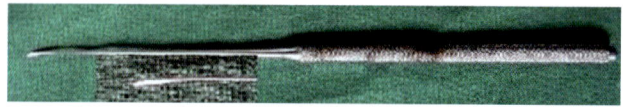

5. Small Meatal Knife (Lempert's)

Used in stapedectomy and tympanoplasty operations for endaural incision of Rosen. It is also useful to elevate the circular layer of tympanic membrane in onlay graft tympanoplasty.

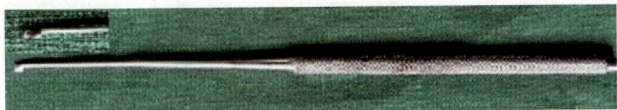

6. Fuller's Forceps

Used for holding and introducing Teflon piston in stapedectomy operation.

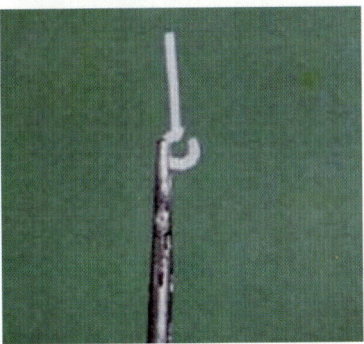

7. Shea's Teflon Piston

Used in stapedectomy operation. Available in 3 sizes: 4, 4.5 and 5 cm in length and standard shaft of 0.8 mm and slim shaft of 0.5 and 0.6 mm in diameter.

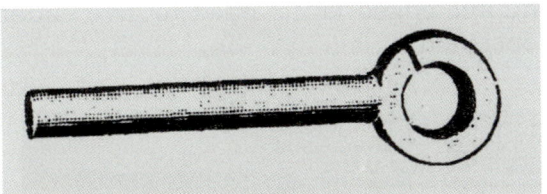

8. Wire closing Forceps (McGee's) with Crocodile Jaw

Used to close the wire prosthesis in stapedectomy operation.

Shea's Stapedectomy Instrument Set

1. Anterior crurotomy knife: Used to cut the anterior crus of the stapes.
2. Straight sharp needle used in micro-ear surgery. Specially used for making the fenestra on footplate of the stapes in stapedectomy operation.
3. Pick, right angled: Slightly blunt used to remove the pieces of foot plate of the stapes.

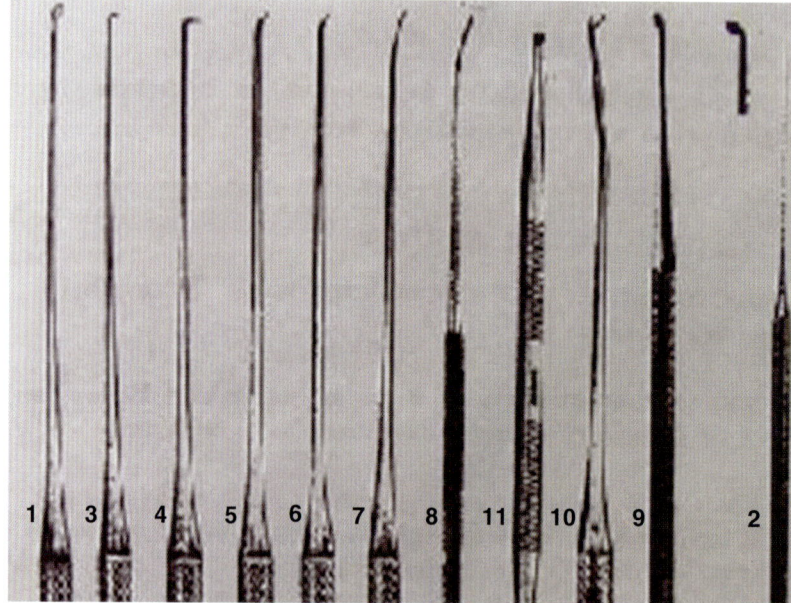

4. Fenestra hook: 90° angle.

5. Do: 45° angle

6. Do: 25° angle

Used to make the opening in the footplate of the stapes.

7. Pick sharp: Used to make the initial opening in the footplate of stapes and for manipulation of the graft.

8. Elevator: Used to elevate and/or repose the tympanomeatal flap.

9. Curette: Used to remove the posterosuperior bony overhang for exposure of the long process of the incus and stapes with stapedius tendon.

10. Oval-shaped double edged knife: Used to give endomeatal incision in stapedectomy operation.

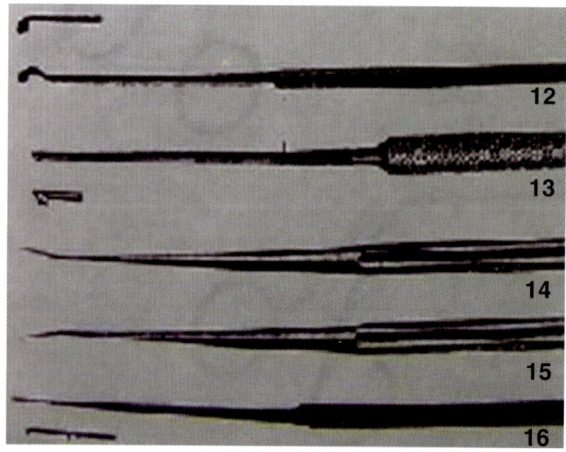

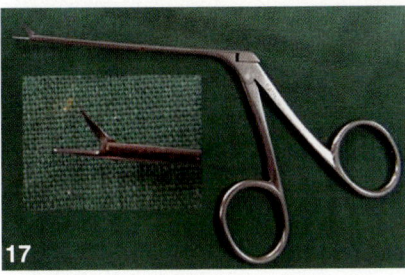 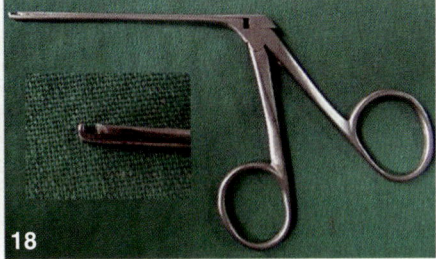

11. House curette: Straight, double ended, 7 inch long used to remove the postero-superior bony rim.
12. Rosen's oval scoop: Straight. Four sizes are available, e.g. 000, 00, 0 and 1.
13. Oval-window fenestrator: Retrograde, used in stapedectomy operation to make the fenestra on the foot plate of the stapes. It should not be introduced inside the vestibule for more than 0.5 mm. If it is pushed in for more than 0.5 to 0.75 mm, there is a chance to cause injury to the membranous labyrinth.
14. Simson Hall's vein graft hook-right: It is used to place and manipulate the vein graft over the fenestra in the foot plate of the stapes in stapedectomy operation.
15. Do: Left.
16. Shea's Teflon piston depth gauge: It is used to measure the appropriate length of the Teflon piston in stapedectomy operation.
17. Microaural scissors used in sectioning the stapedius tendon in stapedectomy operation for otosclerosis. It may also be used for dissecting the fibrous strands, etc. in tympanoplasty operation.
18. House malleus nippers used in cutting the neck of malleus for removal of its head in myringomalleo stapediopexy operation.

37

Nasal Instruments

1. Thudicum Nasal Speculum

This is used for examination of the anterior part of the nasal cavity (anterior rhinoscopy). Structures seen are:

   i. Anterior part of the floor of the nasal cavity.

   ii. Anterior and lower part of the medial wall of the nasal cavity that is septum.

   iii. Anterior part of the lateral wall of the nasal cavity where middle and inferior turbinates and meati are seen.

During introduction the blades of the speculum are to be kept closed. After examination of the nasal cavity, the speculum is to be removed keeping the blades open.

The middle meatus and the Little's area are the two important sites to be observed along with other structures.

Middle meatus is important because the anterior group of the paranasal sinuses, i.e. maxillary, frontal and anterior ethmoidal sinuses drain here. If there is infection in any of these sinuses, discharge will be visible in this meatus either without any postural test or after postural test. Therefore, the examination of the nose is not complete if the middle meatus is not seen. The posterior group of the paranasal sinuses (posterior ethmoidal and sphenoidal) drain in the superior meatus either directly (posterior ethmoidal) or indirectly (sphenoidal). The nasolacrimal duct drains in the inferior meatus.

The Little's area is important because it is the commonest site of epistaxis owing to excessive vascularity. Slightest trauma in this area may cause severe bleeding and the commonest type of trauma is nose-picking.

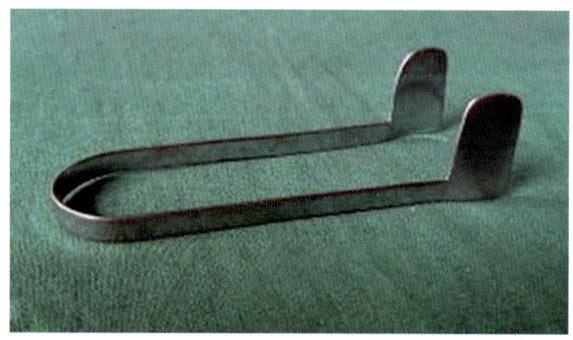

The following blood vessels anastomose in the Little's area and account for the high vascularity:

i. Septal branch of the sphenopalatine artery (the artery of epistaxis).

ii. Septal branch of the greater palatine artery.

iii. Septal branch of the anterior ethmoidal artery.

iv. Septal branch of the superior labial artery.

The olfactory area or dangerous area of the nose is described in detail in the text.

2. Posterior Rhinoscopic Mirror (St. Clair Thomson's)

Rhinoscopy: Rhino-nose, scopy-examination. Used for examination of the posterior part of the nose and the nasopharynx (posterior rhinoscopy).

Technique of Posterior Rhinoscopy

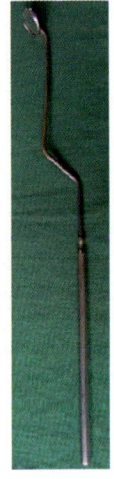

Warm the mirror to avoid condensation of moisture. Ask the patient to open the mouth. Depress the ant. 2/3 of the tongue with the tongue depressor and pass the mirror, after making sure that it is not too hot, into the oropharynx placing it in between the uvula and the posterior pharyngeal wall. Take care not to touch the latter. Ask the patient to breathe through the nose so that the soft palate falls down and the nasopharynx becomes more spacious. This helps in better examination of the parts. Structures seen are:

i. Posterior free margin of the nasal septum.

ii. Posterior nasal apertures or choanae.

iii. Superior, middle and inferior turbinates.

iv. Superior and middle meati.

v. Adenoids in cases of children (normally persist up to 14 years of age) situated at the middle of the junction of roof and posterior wall of the nasopharynx.

vi. Pharyngeal openings of the pharyngotympanic tubes, one on each lateral wall of the nasopharynx at a level of the posterior end of the inferior turbinate.

vii. Fossa of Rosenmuller: A recess just behind the cushion of each eustachian (pharyngotympanic) tube.

3. Antrum Washing Cannula (Rose's)

The function of the ring near the proximal end of the instrument is to guide the direction of its tip during use. This is used for giving wash to the maxillary antrum on the 4th to 6th postoperative day of intranasal antrostomy (INA). The tip of the instrument is introduced into the maxillary antrum through the artificial opening made during INA operation. The site of this opening is in the inferior meatus. The Higginson's syringe is then attached to the outer end of the cannula; the other end of the syringe is being dipped in the warm sterile normal saline in a tumbler. Water is now pushed into the maxillary antrum till the colour of the returning fluid collecting in tray is the same as that in the tumbler (no anesthesia is required for this procedure).

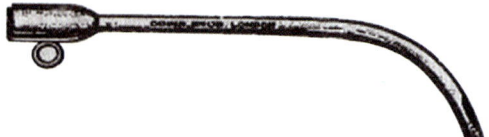

The washing fluid returns via the artificial opening through which the cannula is introduced inside the antrum.

4. Nasal Foreign Body Hook

This is used for removal of foreign body from the nose. The hook is to be passed above and beyond the foreign body and then pulled out. The baby must be fixed well during this procedure and usually does not require any anaesthesia. Sometimes removal under general anaesthesia becomes essential. During removal under general anaesthesia the posterior nasal aperture of the same side should be closed by a finger. This precaution is to be taken to prevent the foreign body dropping accidentally into the lower respiratory tract and causing asphyxia and death.

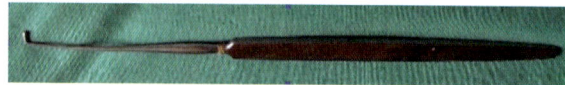

5. Antral Harpoon (Tilley's)

This is used for making an artificial opening in the inferior meatus of the naso-antral wall in intra nasal antrostomy operation.

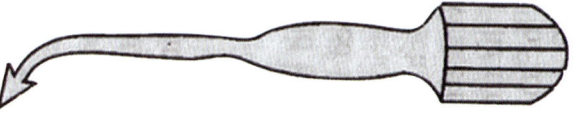

6. Antral Rosette Burr (Tilley's)

This is used for enlarging and smoothening the margin of the artificial opening made by the harpoon in INA. The harpoon has a pointed tip, whereas the rosette burr has a ball-like expansion at its tip with teeth on it like a drill.

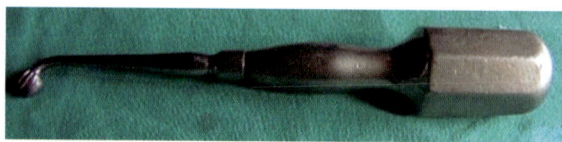

7. Antral Trocar and Canula (Tilley-Lichtwitz)

This is used for washing the maxillary antrum in cases of chronic and subacute maxillary sinusitis for either diagnostic or therapeutic purposes.

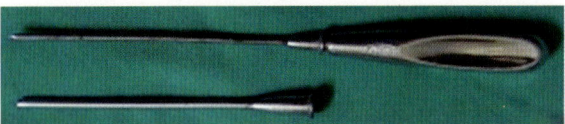

Diagnostic: To confirm the clinical and radiological diagnosis of chronic maxillary sinusitis.

Therapeutic: To give antral lavage in maxillary sinusitis. Usually 6–8 lavages are given twice in a week.

Local anaesthesia of the site of puncture should be done with a piece of gauze or swab soaked in 4% xylocaine introduced into the nasal cavity and inferior meatus. A puncture is made in the inferior meatus just below the attachment of the inferior turbinate, half an inch behind the anterior end of it. That site is chosen because it is the weakest part of the nasoantral wall and can be easily perforated. Take out the trocar after puncture keeping the cannula in situ. The fluid contents of the antrum, (if any) will come out through the cannula or be washed out with the help of Higginson's syringe by sterile normal saline. The returning fluid can be collected and examined so as to detect the presence of pus which should be sent for culture and sensitivity test for pyogenic organisms.

In therapeutic purposes repeated lavage is given bi-weekly for 3 weeks. The washing fluid, unlike the wash given by the antrum washing cannula after I.N.A. operation, returns through the natural ostium in the middle meatus. Sometimes the fluid may not return through the cannula if it enters into a cyst or if the tip of the cannula is blocked by any pathological structure. In that situation another puncture is to be made by the side of the original puncture.

The direction of the tip of the trocar during puncture should be towards the outer canthus of the ipsilateral eye or towards the upper border of the pinna. If it is directed more horizontally the cheek might be injured; if more vertically, the orbit might be damaged; if more posteriorly, the pterygoid venous plexus is liable to be injured which will cause profuse haemorrhage and swelling in the submandibular region.

It is contraindicated in fracture of the maxilla and in acute sinusitis.

8. Freer's Elevator

This is used in submucous resection of the septum (SMR) or septoplasty operation done for deviated nasal septum for elevating the mucoperichondrium.

9. Long-bladed Nasal Speculum (St. Clair Thomson's)

This is used to keep the elevated mucoperichondrium of either side away from the bare septum during its removal in SMR operation.

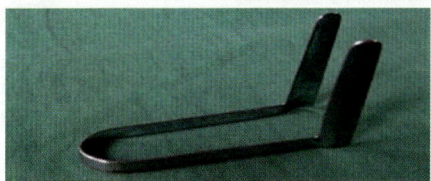

10. Ballenger's Swivel Cartilage Knife

This is used to cut a quadrangular piece of cartilage of the septum in SMR operation.

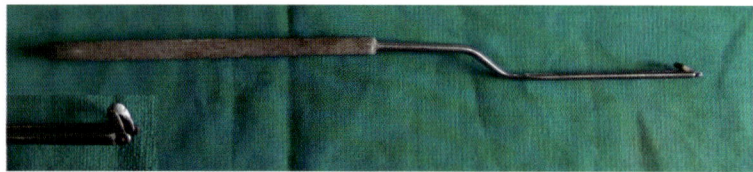

11. Luc's Forceps

Use:

  i. Originally used in Caldwell-Luc's operation which is indicated in certain cases of chronic maxillary sinusitis, antrochoanal polyp, biopsy from antral growth, etc.
  ii. In submucous resection (SMR) of nasal septum for removing the deviated nasal septum in piecemeal after the elevation of mucoperichondrial and mucoperiosteal flaps.
  iii. For taking tissue for biopsy from oral cavity and oropharynx.
  iv. In intranasal antrostomy (INA) operation. After making the artificial opening with the harpoon some surgeons enlarge it by removing the bony spicules from its margin.
  v. For holding the tonsil in dissection method of tonsillectomy (Negus).

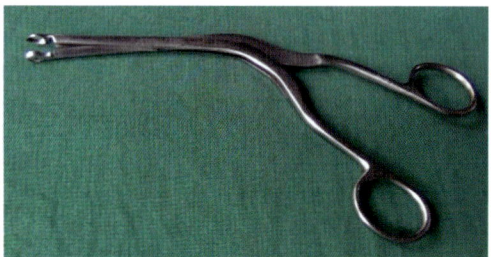

12. Negus' modification of Glegg's Nasal Snare

The site of the nasal snare is in between the tonsillar and the aural snare. Its use is to crush and avulse the nasal polyp from its base. The number '1' steel wire is used in this snare.

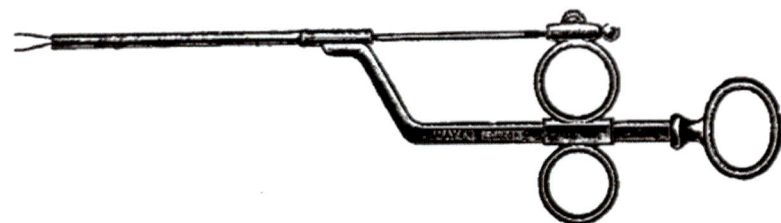

13. Bayonet Shaped Bone Gouge (Killian's)

This is used to cut the bony thickening or spurs along the maxillary crest. The bayonet shape is designed to avoid the obstruction of the field of vision. The V-shaped or fish tailed end of the gouge of **Tilley's** variety is more suitable than the rounded variety because this type of gouge does not slip.

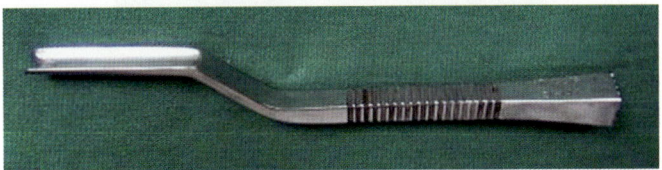

14(a). Cottle's Upper Lateral Cartilage Retractor

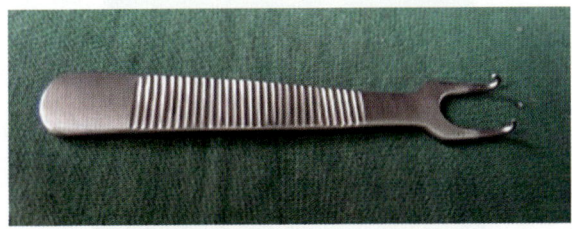

14(b). Alar Retractor for Rhinoplasty

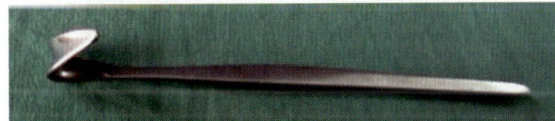

NASAL INSTRUMENTS

1. Jansen Middleton's septum cutting forceps, double action. Used in SMR operation to remove the bony portion of the deviated nasal septum.

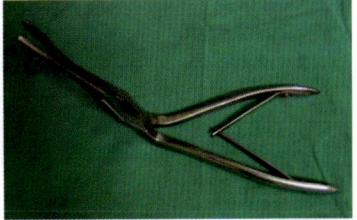

2. Beckmann's turbinectomy scissors, for middle turbinate

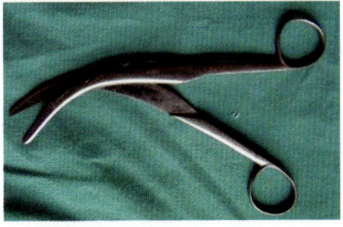

3. Asch's septum forceps used to straighten the fresh traumatic fracture and dislocation of the septum.

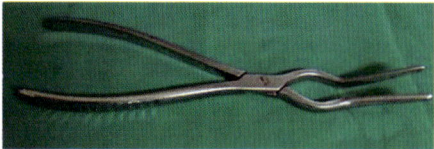

4. Walsham's redressing forceps, right used to correct the fracture displacement of the nasal bone on the right side.

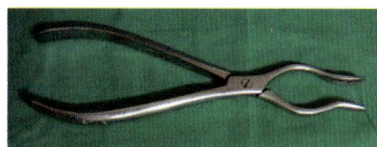

5. Grunwald's nasal turbinate forceps with narrow punch jaws used for excision of small tumours and to take tissue for biopsy from the nasal turbinates and cavities.

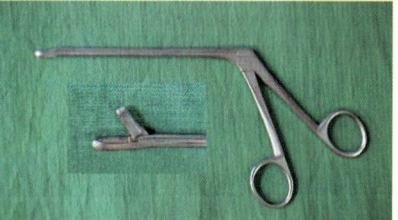

6. Ostrum's antrum punch forceps backward cutting. For nasoantral wall used to remove the bone for enlarging the opening in the inferior antrostomy meatus in intranasal antrostomy or middle meatal.

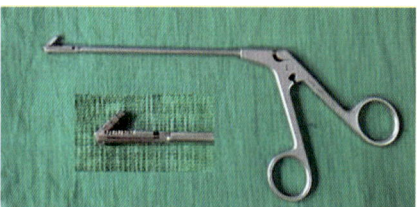

7. Killian's nasal speculum used in septoplasty and SMR operation; may also be used for median rhinoscopy.

Instruments used in FESS

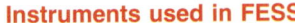

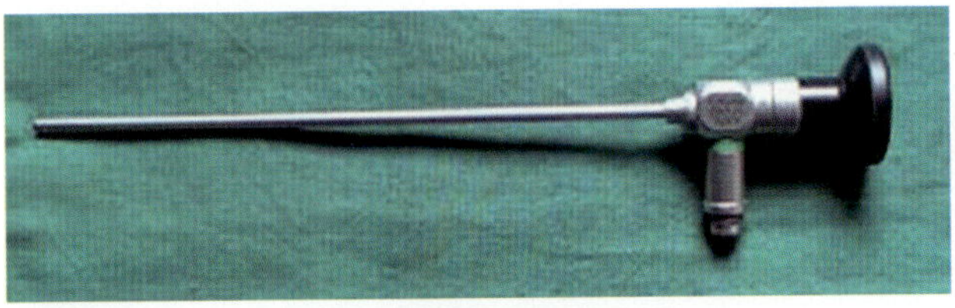

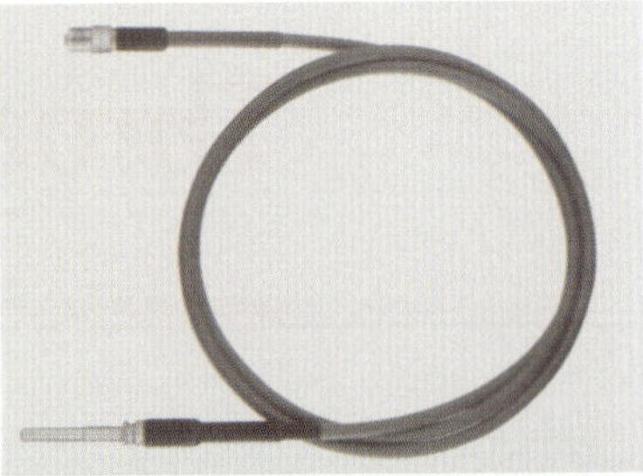

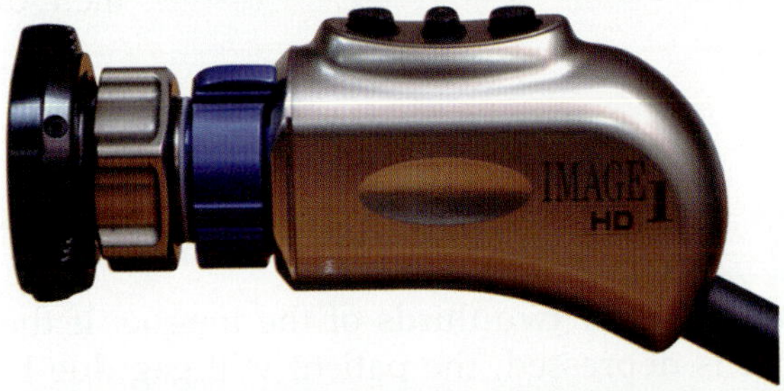

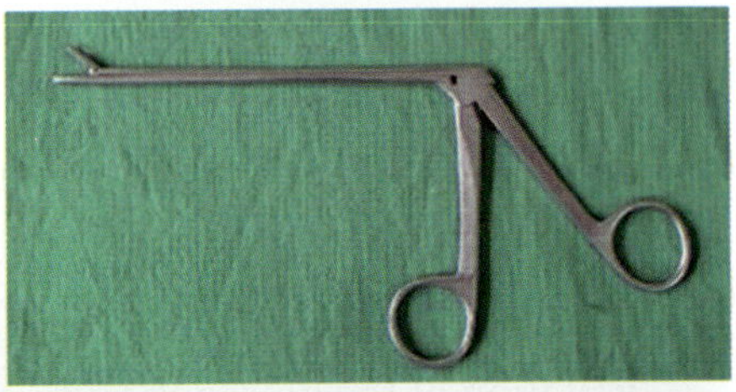

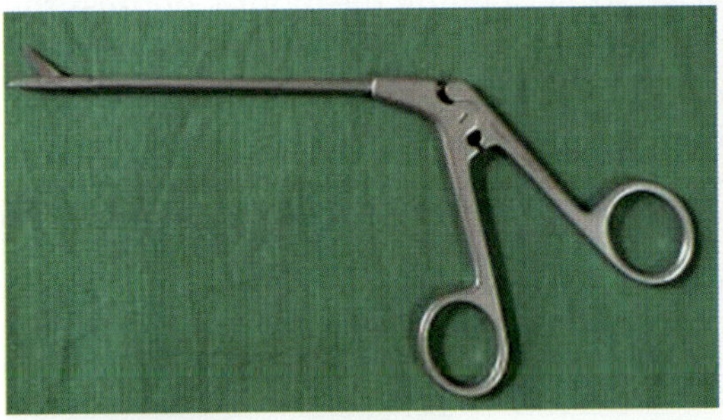

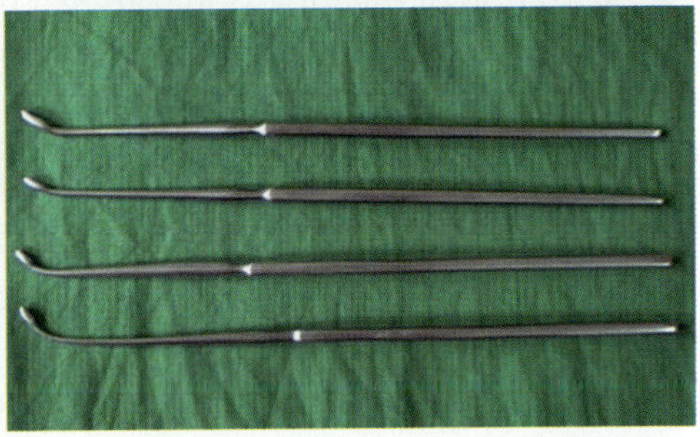

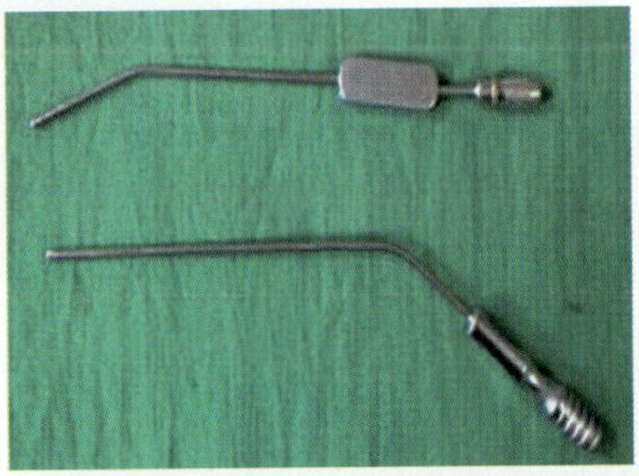

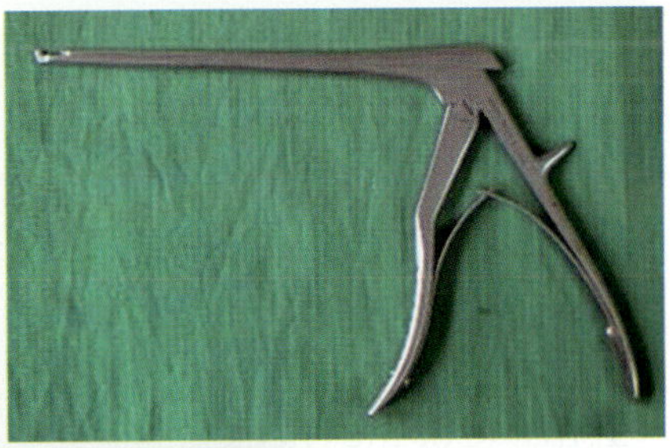

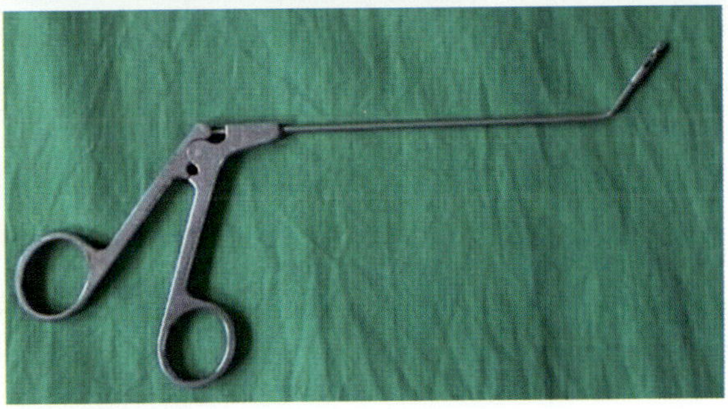

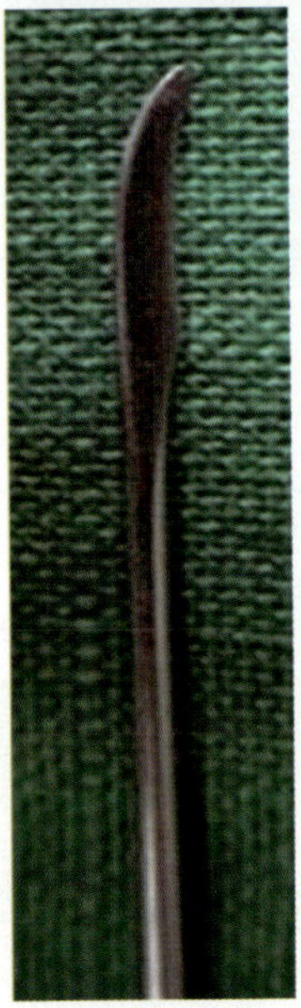

38

Throat Instruments

1. Tongue Depressor (Lack's)

It has two parts:

i. A holding part which has a bend at the lower end. Its purpose is to hold the instrument.

ii. A depressing part to depress the anterior two-thirds of the tongue. If the posterior one-third of the tongue is depressed, the patient will gag due to irritation of the glossopharyngeal nerve. After opening the mouth, depress the anterior two-thirds of the tongue with the depressing part and ask him to say "Ah" so that the soft palate is raised like a curtain which will facilitate better examination. Palatal paralysis is excluded by noticing this movement of the soft palate.

Use

1. For examination of the following structures:

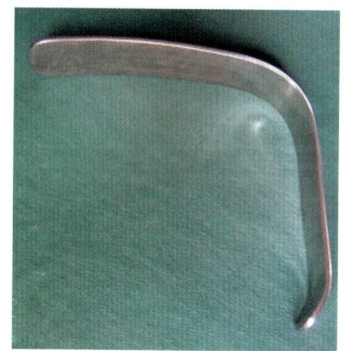

i. Palatine tonsils with their pillars

ii. Tonsillolingual sulcus (graveyard of the oral cavity)

iii. Posterior pharyngeal wall (oropharynx)

iv. Uvula

v. Soft palate

vi. Hard palate

vii. Tongue anterior two-thirds

viii. Teeth

ix. Gum

x. Inside of the cheeks

xi. Examination of the nasopharynx with the help of posterior rhinoscopic mirror.

2. i. Minor operative procedures like removal of fish bone from tonsils;

ii. Drainage of peritonsillar abscess and

iii. Removal of tonsils by dissection method under local anaesthesia.

2. Laryngeal Mirror

This instrument is usually confused with the posterior rhinoscopic mirror. A mirror with a straight handle is laryngeal mirror. A mirror with a bent handle is posterior rhinoscopic mirror.

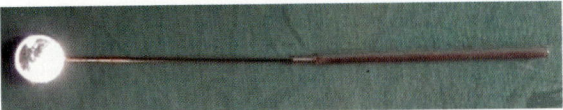

Use: For indirect laryngoscopy. Indirect because of visualization of the laryngeal image on the mirror. Parts seen from above downwards are:

 i. Base of the tongue
 ii. Vallecula: One on each side of the glossoepiglottic fold
 iii. Epiglottis
 iv. Arytenoid cartilages
 v. Ary-epiglottic folds
 vi. False vocal cords (ventricular folds)
 vii. True vocal cords
 viii. Rima glottides
 ix. The upper few rings of trachea
 x. Pyriform fossae.

The pyriform fossa are the parts of the pharynx and not of the larynx.

This mirror is also used for:

 i. Removing a foreign body by laryngeal forceps (holding type) from the base of the tongue, vallecula, pyriform fossa, etc.
 ii. Removal of small benign tumour and taking a tissue for biopsy from larynx or hypopharynx by the laryngeal forceps (cutting type).

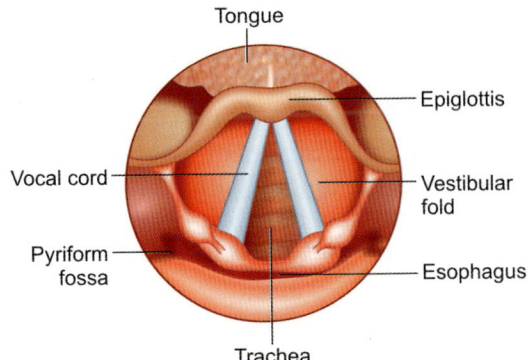

Fig. 38.1: Structures seen in indirect laryngoscopy

Technique of Indirect Laryngoscopy

Warm the mirror to avoid condensation of moisture (not for sterilization) during breathing.

After warming the mirror, touch metal side of it on the dorsum of the hand to be sure that it is not too hot. Request the patient to protrude the tongue. Hold the tongue with a piece of gauze by the left hand. Tongue depressor is not used in this procedure.

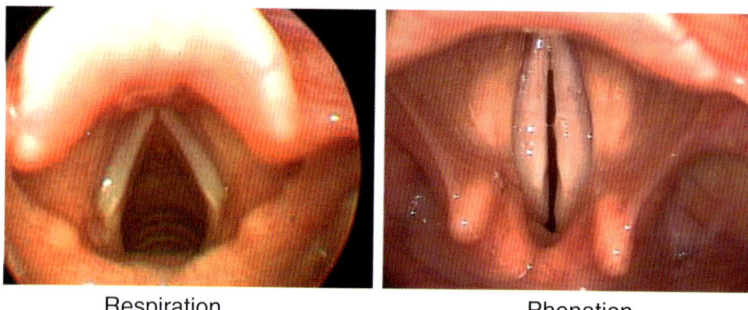

Respiration   Phonation

Fig. 38.2: Position of the vocal cords during phonation and respiration

Now hold the mirror in the same manner as you hold a pen in the right hand and pass it into the oral cavity. Push the soft palate and uvula upwards and backwards with the back of the mirror. The posterior pharyngeal wall is not touched to avoid retching. Request the patient to breathe through the mouth.

To see the movements of the vocal cords ask the patient to utter "Ah" and "Eh".

During phonation the vocal cords become adducted and during respiration the cords are abducted.

3. Laryngeal Forceps (Mackenzie's)

These are of two types:

i. Sharp or Cutting Type

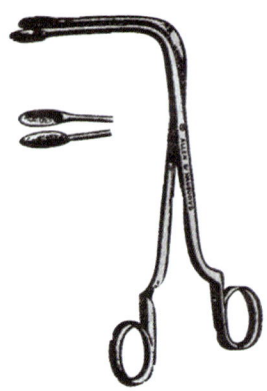

Used for taking biopsy from the larynx, base of tongue, valleculae etc., to remove small benign tumours of the larynx and hypopharynx. Local anaesthesia and laryngeal mirror are essential for using this instrument. (Assistant or the patient himself will hold the tongue with a piece of gauze instead of the surgeon.) The surgeon holds the laryngeal mirror by the left hand and the forceps by the right hand.

ii. Holding Type

It has serrations on the broadened tip. It is used for removal of foreign body from larynx, base of tongue, vallecula, pyriform fossa, etc. Here also local anaesthesia and laryngeal mirror are essential and the assistant or the patient will hold the tongue with a piece of gauze.

4. Tonsillar Haemostatic Clamp (Yorke's)

Use: To stop reactionary and secondary haemorrhage in postoperative cases of tonsillectomy.

Parts

    i. In one blade, there is a circular slab with a convex rough surface.

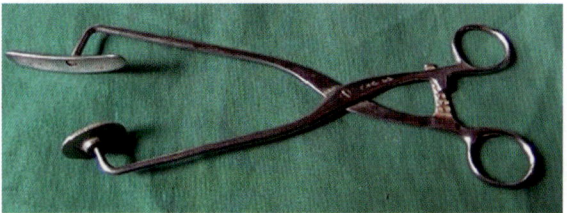

ii. In the other blade, there is a movable, narrow, long piece which is concave on one surface and convex on the other.

The convex slab covered with sterile gauze should be placed against the tonsillar fossa. The concave surface of the long blade should be placed outside on the angle of the mandible. The catches are applied gently so that the internal carotid artery is not compressed. This is to be kept for about twenty minutes at a time and the fossa is to be examined. If bleeding does not stop, catches should be tightened again.

5. Adenoid Curette with Cage (St. Clair Thomson's)

The part with the tooth-like projections is the cage and that with the sharp edge is the curette. The handle of the instrument is to be held like a dagger with the concavity of the instrument facing downwards. In this position it should be introduced into the oral cavity after the nasopharynx is palpated with the index finger. The curette is now pushed into the nasopharynx until it hinges against the posterior free margin of the nasal septum. Then a gentle pressure downwards and a swinging movement is applied to curette the adenoids. The nasopharynx should be palpated again after curetting the adenoids to feel whether any remnant of it is left behind or not.

The instrument should be kept strictly in the midline. If it is deviated to on side, the opening of the eustachian tube might be injured. This will give rise to permanent conductive deafness owing to subsequent healing by fibrosis.

The cage of the instrument with spring action remains closed during the use. The purpose of the cage is to catch the curetted adenoid tissue so that it does not fall back into the nasopharynx. If curetted adenoid tissue falls back into the nasopharynx, there will be difficulty in removing it from a pool of blood in the nasopharynx or it may even enter into the nasal cavity during the attempt at removal.

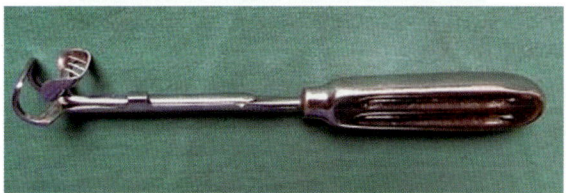

6. Draffin's Bipod

Draffin's bipods are used in place of the chest piece and rod to fix the Boyle Davis' mouth gag in dissection method of tonsillectomy under general anesthesia.

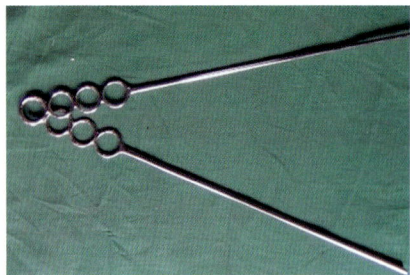

7. Boyle Davis' Mouth Gag

The whole instrument consists of the following parts:

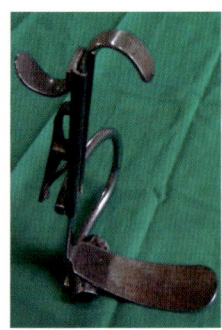

    i. Mouth gag proper with tongue blade.
    ii. Chest piece.
   iii. A rod or jack which connects the gag with chest piece for fixing the gag.

Method of holding the instrument
The instrument is to be held during use with the blade downwards and pointed at the patient. The tongue blade retracts the lower jaw with the tongue. The other projections guarded with rubber tubes are engaged on the upper incisor teeth and thus retract the upper jaw.

    This gag is used in tonsillectomy by the dissection method under general anesthesia.

8. Tonsil Holding Forceps (Denis Browne's)

This is used to hold the tonsil and to pull it medially in the dissection method of tonsillectomy.

(image of tonsil holding forceps)

9. Tonsil dissector with Pillar Retractor Beavis'

This instrument is used for blunt dissection of the tonsil from its bed. The other end with a bend is used to retract the anterior pillar to explore any bleeding point and tonsillar tag just after tonsillectomy. Sometimes the soft palate is being retracted by it to visualize the nasopharynx after removal of the adenoids.

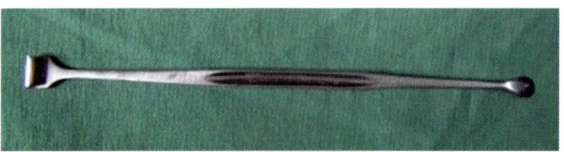

10. Tonsillar Snare (Eve's)

This is used to crush and cut the lower pole of the tonsil in the dissection method of tonsillectomy. This is the biggest of all the snares used in ENT operations. The number '2' steel wire is used in it.

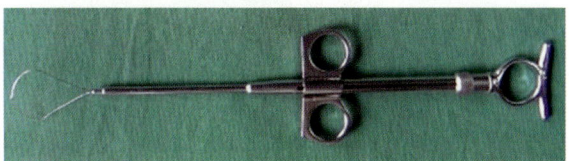

11. Negus' Artery Forceps

A pair of artery forceps with curved end. This is used at the time of applying ligatures of the bleeding points in the tonsillar bed. The bleeding point is first caught by a dissecting forceps or a straight tonsil artery forceps which is replaced by the Negus' artery forceps. Then the ligature is applied. Owing to the curved head, the thread may easily be slipped beyond the tip of the instrument. Some surgeons recommend this instrument to be used for removal of nasopharyngeal packs given after curetting the adenoids. This instrument is used also in laryngofissure operation for applying ligatures.

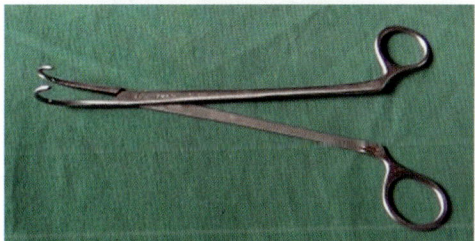

12. Knot-tier and Ligature Slipper (Negus')

This is used for slipping the ligature beyond the curved tip of the artery forceps (Negus) and also to tie the knots during an attempt to stop the bleeding points during tonsillectomy by dissection method and laryngofissure operation.

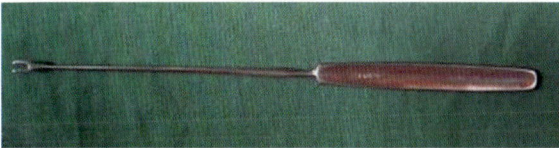

13. Tonsil Guillotine (Ballenger's)

This is used in tonsillectomy by guillotine method. Most surgeons today do not like the guillotine method of tonsillectomy because of its many disadvantages (see text). Nowadays tonsillectomy is very commonly performed by dissection method.

In the guillotine method the patient is kept in supine position with his neck slightly extended. The surgeon stands on the right side of the patient. In the dissection

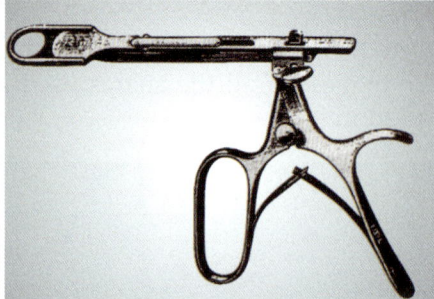

method the patient is kept in a supine position with hyper extended neck and the surgeon sits on the head end of the patient.

14. Doyen's Mouth Gag

This is used for opening the mouth during tonsillectomy by guillotine technique. This is also an important emergency instrument used to give free airway in comatose patients.

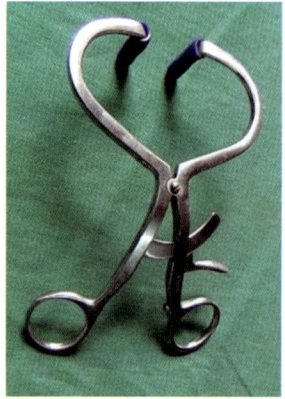

15. Peritonsillar Abscess Drainage Forceps or Quinsy Dilator (St. Clair Thomson's)

Used for draining a peritonsillar abscess.

Site of Drainage

If there is a pus point or any bulging with fluctuation at any particular point, the closed forceps is introduced at that point after giving an incision. After introduction, the blades are to be opened crosswise inside the abscess cavity for better drainage of pus. No anaesthesia is required for this operation. Other sites of incision are:

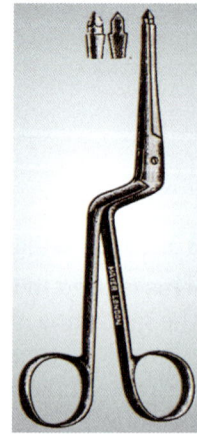

    i. One to two cm external to the point of junction of the two imaginary lines, e.g. a horizontal line along the base of the uvula and a vertical line along the medial margin of the respective anterior pillar.

    ii. About the middle of an imaginary line drawn from the base of the uvula and the respective last upper molar tooth.

Carbolic acid may be touched by a swab at the calculated point of the puncture. This helps in the following ways:

i. Marks the site of puncture

ii. Produces anaesthesia

iii. Acts as an antiseptic

16. Direct Laryngoscope (Chevalier Jackson's)

This is used for direct visualisation of the larynx (direct laryngoscopy). This operation is preferably done under local anaesthesia, may also be performed under general anaesthesia if the condition permits. It is used during the removal of foreign body, papilloma or other benign growth from the larynx and hypopharynx and also in taking tissue for biopsy from the suspected malignant growth of the larynx and hypopharynx. It is contraindicated in the diseases of cervical spines like caries spine and gross cervical spondylosis.

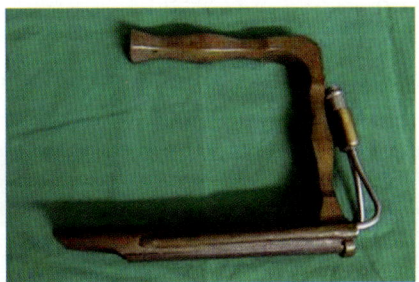

17. Laryngoscope used for Suspension Laryngoscopy and Microlaryngoscopy

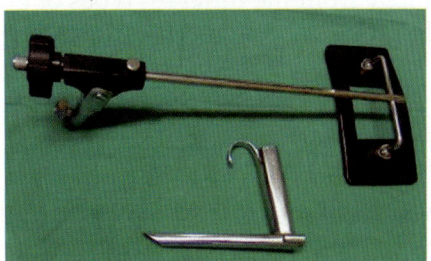

18. Paterson's Forceps

A long and narrow pair of forceps which may be passed through the endoscopes (oesophagoscope, laryngoscope or bronchoscope). There are two types:

i. Cutting type

ii. Holding type.

The cutting type is used for taking biopsy and the holding type is used for removal of foreign body.

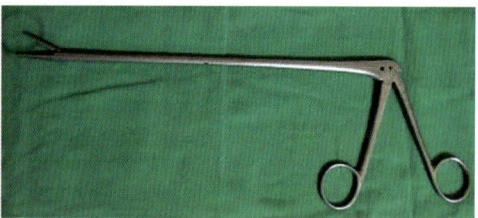

Technique of Removing Foreign Body

After visualising the foreign body, the holding variety of the forceps is introduced through the scope. If the foreign body is large after catching the foreign body the scope and the forceps are taken out simultaneously, as because the foreign body will not pass through the lumen of the scope (either oesophagoscopy or bronchoscopy).

19. Bronchoscope (Chevalier Jackson's)

This instrument may be differentiated from the oesophagoscope by the presence of holes (two on either side) near its distal end. These holes help to keep the airway patent for the ventilation of one lung during examination of the bronchioles of the other lung.

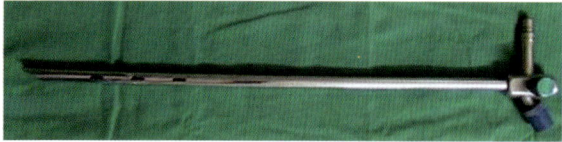

As the name suggests, the instrument is being used for the examination of the bronchus and the bronchioles (bronchoscopy). It may also be used for taking tissue for biopsy or excision biopsy from the different types of growths relating to lungs, bronchus and bronchioles, removal of foreign body and periodic aspiration of pus from the bronchiectatic and lung abscess cavities.

Oesophagoscopy may be performed by the Bronchoscope but not vice versa.

20. Oesophagoscope (Negus')

This is used for direct visualisation of the oesophageal lumen (oesophagoscopy). This may also be done under local anaesthesia. Oesophagoscopy is also of use for removal of foreign body, for taking biopsy in cancer oesophagus, diagnosis of cardiospasm, dilatation of benign stricture of oesophagus, etc.

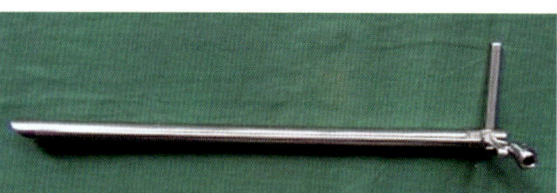

21. Tracheal Dilator (Trausseau's)

Tracheal dilator is used in tracheostomy operation. This dilates the tracheal incision for smooth introduction (cannulation) of the tracheotomy tube. The blades of this instrument spread out by approximation of the ring grips unlike the action of usual forceps. This instrument is not required if the Fuller's bivalved tracheostomy tube is used.

22. Sharp Tracheal Hook

It is used in tracheostomy operation to fix the trachea during the incision. The hook is passed through the cricotracheal membrane just below the lower edge of the cricoid cartilage. As the trachea moves up and down during respiration due to laryngeal obstruction, the incision cannot be made on the desired site unless the trachea is fixed. During tracheostomy in comatose patients and in planned tracheostomy, fixation of the trachea is not necessary during incision over it. Hence this instrument is not required.

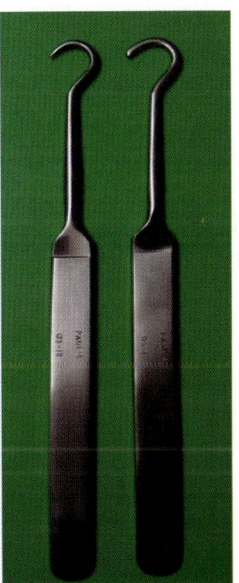

23. Blunt Tracheal Hook

It is used to retract the isthmus of the thyroid gland during tracheostomy. Some surgeons, of course, cut the isthmus in between the two clamps. Its tip is blunt. It may also be used for retracting the strap muscles of neck away from the field of operation.

24. Bivalved Metallic Tracheostomy Tube (Fuller's)

It should be kept for 48 to 72 hours because it helps in making the tracheostomy tract. If it is kept for more than that, it may cause necrosis of the cartilage of trachea.

In the outer tube there are two cusps, that is why it is called bivalved. The inner tube has an opening or hole on the top of its convexity which is helpful to aid phonation and enables us to determine whether the obstruction above has subsided or not, i.e. whether the nasal breathing is possible or not and to train or educate the patient to breathe through nose because he develops the habit of respiring through this tube. The outer opening of the tube is closed during this procedure.

During introduction, take out the inner tube. Press the two cusps of the outer tube to appose them and then introduce with its concavity directed downwards. After fixing the outer tube with tapes around the neck, introduce the inner tube through the outer one and cover the opening of the tube with a piece of wet sterile gauze.

As the inner tube always projects out of the outer tube, the outer tube never gets blocked by tracheobronchial secretions.

The advantage of double tubing is that if the inner tube gets blocked by the tracheobronchial secretion it can be taken out for cleaning. During that time the outer tube serves the purpose and keeps the tracheal opening patient. Moreover, the bicuspid outer tube helps in avoiding tracheal dilator during introduction.

For other details of tracheostomy see text.

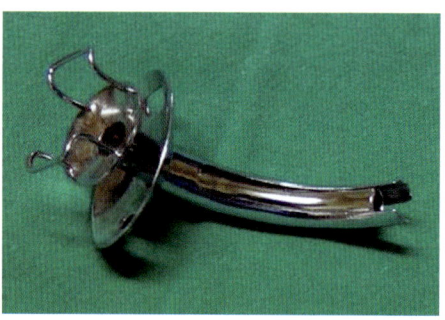

25. Doughty's Mouth Gag

Doughty's mouth gag with slotted tongue blade is used in tonsillectomy and repair of cleft palate operation.

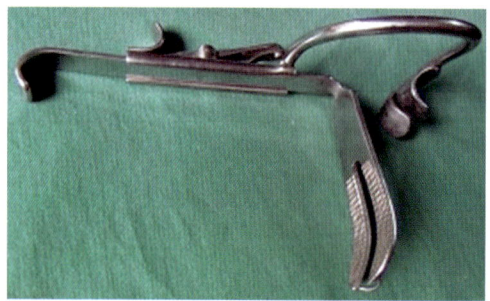

Section

7

Radiology and Imaging

39. Radiology and Imaging

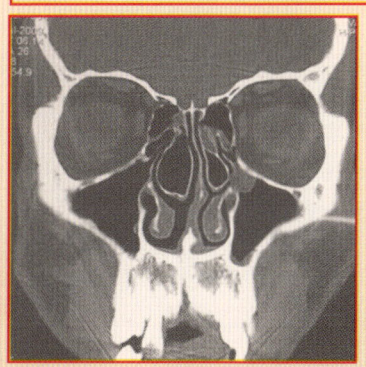

Radiology and Imaging

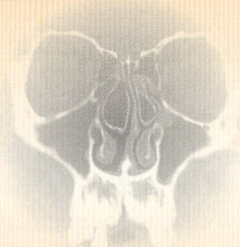

I. Cardiospasm

A barium swallow X-ray of the oesophagus showing enormous fusiform dilatation with a fluid level. There is a smooth constriction of the oesophageal wall at the level of diaphragm (Fig. 39.1). Had it been a case of carcinoma, there

   i. Would have been an irregular filling defect,

   ii. Would not have enormous dilatation above the constriction.

Clinical Features

See text. The diagnosis is confirmed by oesophagoscopy.

Treatment

a. Medical and

b. Surgical (*see* text).

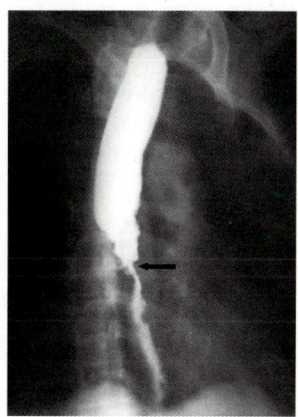

Fig. 39.1: Cardiospasm

II. Carcinoma of the Oesophagus

A barium swallow X-ray of the oesophagus showing irregular filling defect in its lower third with shouldering (Fig. 39.2). There is minimal dilatation of the oesophagus above the site of filling defect. The area of irregular filling defect is also called malignant stricture of oesophagus. Cardiospasm is to be excluded by the following points:

   Had it been a cardiospasm, there would have been

   i. Regular filling defect,

   ii. Enormous dilatation above it,

   iii. Cardiospasm of the oesophagus occurs always at the level of the diaphragm and never in the upper, middle or lower third of it.

   Diagnosis is confirmed by oesophagoscopy and biopsy.

Fig. 39.2: Carcinoma of the lower third of the esophagus

III. Foreign Body in the Oesophagus

A straight X-ray of the chest showing a coin (a radiopaque shadow) in the PA view with the flat surface projecting anteroposteriorly. The lower end of the coin is at the level of fourth thoracic vertebra. A linear radiopaque shadow is visualised in the lower part of the neck in lateral view. Had it been in the trachea the flat surface would not be seen anteroposteriorly in a PA view. The impression of the coin would be a linear one in this view. A coin can enter into the trachea through the larynx with the rim of it lying only anteroposteriorly because of the anteroposterior position of the glottic chink. That position is maintained by the deficiency of the tracheal rings posteriorly. But in case of oesophagus the hard vertebral column as such lies behind it and no space is left posteriorly. Moreover, the oesophagus remains collapsed anteroposteriorly (Fig. 39.3).

For clinical features, complications and treatment *see* text.

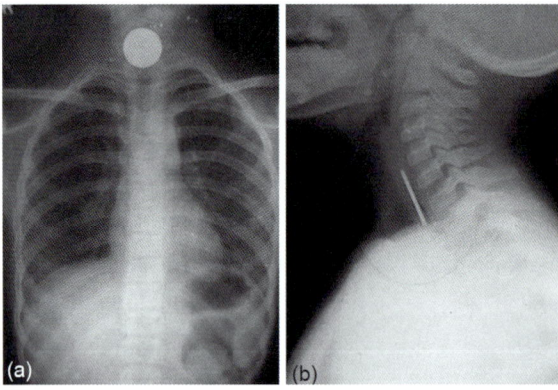

Fig. 39.3: Foreign body in the oesophagus. (a) PA view; (b) Lateral view

IV. Foreign Body in Trachea and Bronchi

This plate is not usually given in examination because such a plate is rarely available. Usually, if at all, what is given is a safety pin in the trachea or a melon seed in the right bronchus. Owing to wide lumen, less angulation with trachea and more entry of inspiratory air, the foreign body commonly enters into the right main bronchus.

Clinical Features

At the time of accident cough and dyspnoea occur. The patient may have expectoration, which may sometimes be bloodstained. Asthmatoid wheeze is a common symptom. If the foreign body is of non-vegetable nature, it produces a little or no inflammation of the bronchial mucosa. Later on hoemoptysis may occur from granulation formation. Atelectasis occurs if the obstruction is complete which may be followed by lung abscess formation. In partial obstruction emphysema may develop due to ball-valve type of mechanism, i.e. during inspiration air enters as the bronchial wall is dilated and during expiration air cannot come out due to contraction of bronchial wall on to the foreign body.

In vegetable foreign body there is intense inflammatory reaction of bronchial mucosa. Bronchial obstruction becomes marked resulting in atelectasis and lung abscess or a localized pneumonitis. A valvular emphysema may result in partial obstruction.

Diagnosis

From pulmonary TB, acute tracheobronchitis, pneumonia and other causes like bronchiectasis and lung abscess.

Points in Favour of Diagnosis

AP and lateral view X-ray may show a radiopaque shadow in the trachea or right main bronchus with or without collapse and/or emphysema of the ipsilateral lung.

Treatment

Removal of foreign body through bronchoscope.

V. Maxillary Sinusitis

X-ray (Occipitomental view) of the para-nasal sinuses (see the frontal and maxillary sinuses of both sides) showing:

Opacity of left maxillary antrum with normal bony outlines.

The side of the X-ray plates is determined by seeing the impression 'L' or 'R' in one corner of the plate. If it is not present the side cannot be ascertained. The opacity may be due to gross mucosal thickening, the sinus being filled up with a cyst, a polypus, tumour, blood, or mucopus or any combination of these (Fig. 39.4).

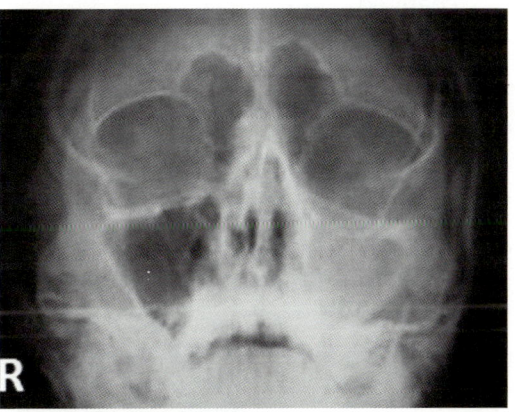

Fig. 39.4: Left maxillary sinusitis

This may be a case of acute sinusitis, which can only be diagnosed radiologically if the clinical features are known.

In allergic sinusitis usually both the antra become hazy or opaque. If the opacity is unilateral or more in one side than the other, the pathology is usually of infective type.

By diagnostic antral lavage (proof puncture) and the bacteriological examination of the returning fluid, the disease may be confirmed. For details of sinusitis, *see* text.

VI. Bilateral Sinusitis

It shows a fluid level in both the maxillary antra. The opacity is due to fluid and not due to any soft tissue. This may be confirmed by two ways:

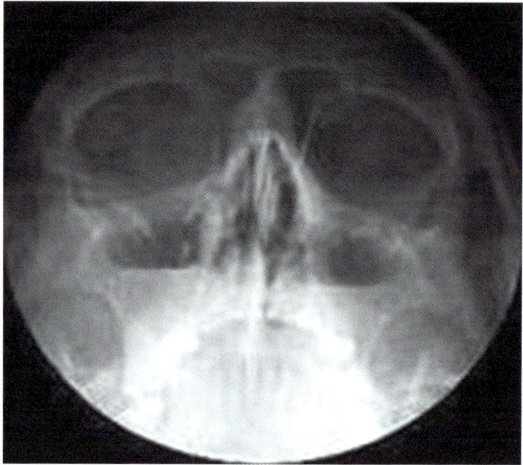

Fig. 39.5: Bilateral sinusitis

   i. By taking a second X-ray in a tilting position in which the fluid level will be changed,

  ii. By antral washout. This indicates an acute process. This may be due to acute sinusitis, acute coryza, acute allergy, a blood or fluid level secondary to a fracture maxilla. Correct diagnosis is only made if the clinical features are known (Fig. 39.5).

VII. Malignant Growth in the Maxillary Antrum

CT scan of the paranasal sinuses showing heterogeneous opacity of the left maxillary antrum with destruction of the posterior bony wall extending into the infratemporal fossa (Fig. 39.6).

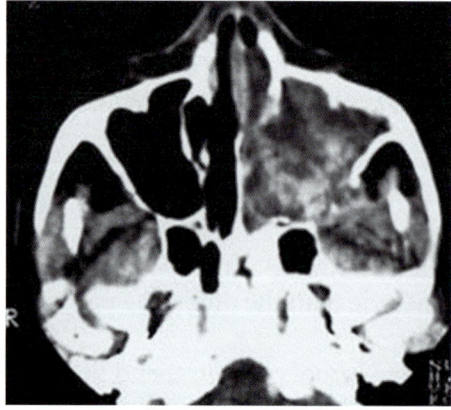

Fig. 39.6: Malignant growth in the maxillary antrum

VIII. X-ray of the Mastoids

X-ray of the mastoids shows either pneumatic or sclerotic type of mastoids in normal cases. In 80% of the population, the mastoid is highly pneumatised in which the sigmoid sinus plate and dural plate are clearly demarcated in the lateral oblique views. In acute mastoiditis the air cells are seen hazy and sometimes a cavity is seen when mastoid abscess is developed. In chronic mastoiditis, bone necrosis is seen and the mastoid antrum may be widened with clean-cut sclerosed margin if cholesteatoma is present (Fig. 39.7).

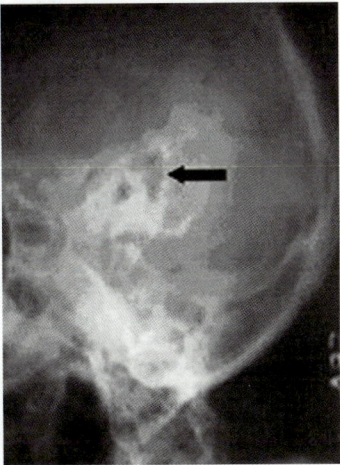

Fig. 39.7: Lateral-oblique view of the left mastoid showing bone destruction (cholesteatoma)

IX. CT Scan of the Temporal Bones

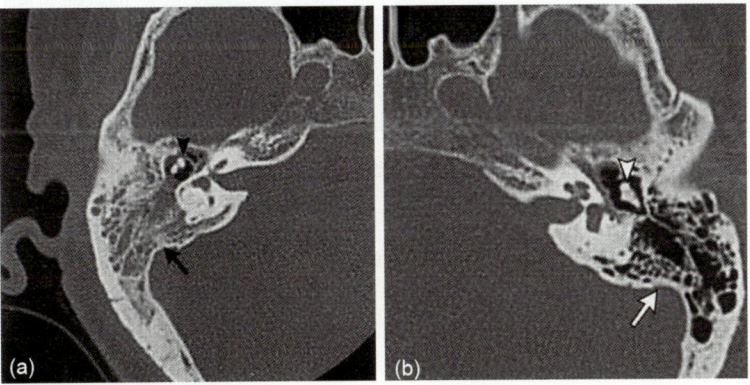

Fig. 39.8: CT scan of the temporal bones shows normal internal auditory canals, pneumatic mastoid right and soft tissue in the mastoid cavity left side

X. CT Scan of the Nasopharyngeal Angiofibroma

CT scan shows nasopharyngeal angiofibroma involving nasal cavity nasopharynx and maxillary sinus (Fig. 39.9).

XI. CT Scan of Nose and Paranasal Sinuses

CT scan of the paranasal air sinuses showing deviated nasal septum and mucosal thickening of maxillary antrum (Fig. 39.10).

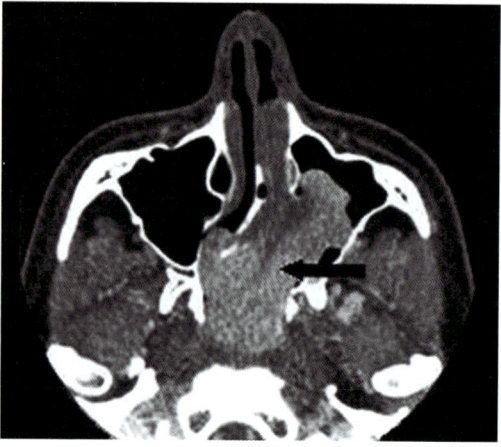

Fig. 39.9: CT scan of the nasopharyngeal angiofibroma

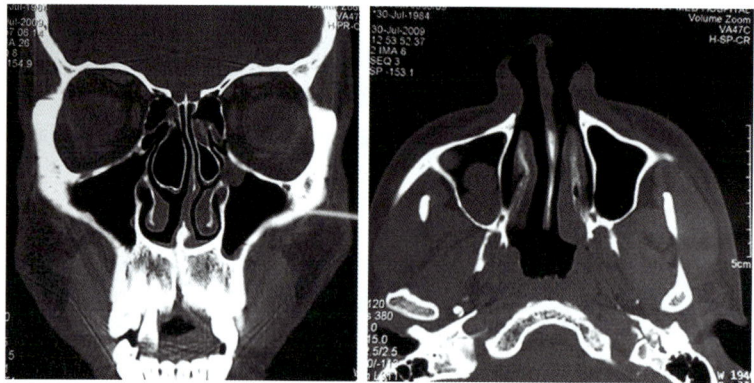

Fig. 39.10: CT scan of nose and paranasal sinuses

XII. X-ray of Skull Base Reverse Towne's View

X-ray of skull taken in reverse Towne's position exploring the infratemporal fossa. It shows hugely enlarged styloid processes. Diagnosis is stylalgia (Eagle's syndrome). Advantage of this plate is that both the styloid processes are visualised in one plate (Fig. 39.11).

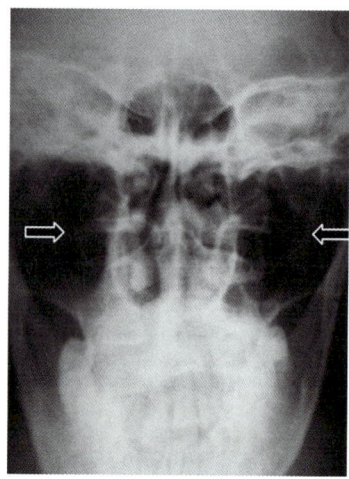

Fig. 39.11: X-ray of the elongated styloid process

Recent Advances

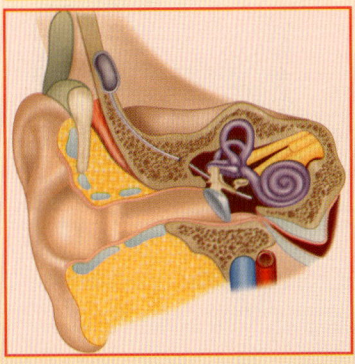

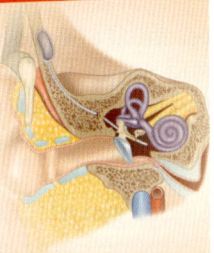

Recent Advances

40

1. Cochlear Implants

A cochlear implant is an electronic device. It is used in patients who have bilateral severe to profound sensorineural deafness and who are not benefited by hearing aids. It works by stimulating the auditory nerve directly.

A cochlear implant has two components:

1. External, e.g. speech processor and transmitter
2. Internal: Surgically implanted and it has the electrode array and the receiver stimulator.

The speech processor has a microphone, which picks up the sound, analyses and codes the sound into electrical impulses. The electrical impulses from the speech processor via radiofrequency go to the surgically implanted receiver stimulator through the transmitting coil. The receiver stimulator decodes the signal and transmits it to the electrode array placed in the scala tympani of the cochlea. The electrodes of the implant stimulate the spiral ganglion cells. Thus the auditory nerve is stimulated and sends the electrical impulse to the brain, which is finally interpreted as sound.

The cochlear implants of multichannel electrodes are used nowadays. Postlingual children or adults and prelingual children are mostly benefited. Postlingual or prelingual candidates are defined as those who become severe to profoundly deaf after or before acquisition of speech and language respectively. Rehabilitation is

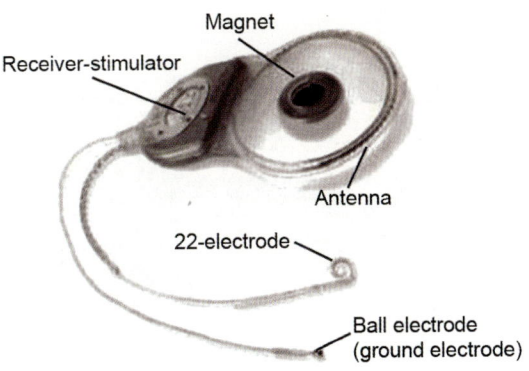

Fig. 40.1: Internal parts of a cochlear implant

essential after cochlear implantation. The children listen and speak like a normal person after rehabilitation by qualified speech and language therapist.

Operation

Under general anaesthesia, a cortical mastoidectomy is performed after elevation of a large musculoperiosteal flap with anterior base. A pocket is created under the periosteum posteriorly to place the receiver stimulator. A well is drilled in the bone posterior to the mastoid cavity, which was marked before the incision was planned.

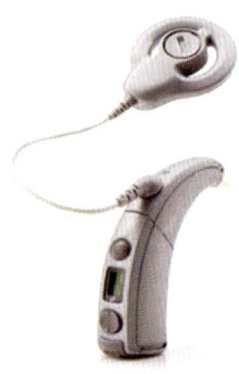

Fig. 40.2: External parts of a cochlear implant

After identification of the lateral semicircular canal and the short process of the incus the facial recess is opened, i.e. a posterior tympanotomy is performed. Facial recess is a collection of air cells lateral to the second genu of the facial nerve. It is bounded medially by the facial nerve, laterally by the chorda tympani nerve and superiorly by the fossa incudis where the short process of the incus remains attached. After identification of the round window through the posterior tympanotomy, cochleostomy is performed anteroinferior to the round window membrane. The diameter of the cochleostomy should be about 1.4 mm. The receiver stimulator is placed into the subperiosteal pocket and in the "well" created earlier and fixed with ties of monofilament sutures.

The electrode array is then inserted gently through the cochleostome into the scala tympani. The wound is closed in layers. Then the qualified and experienced audiologist specially trained for this purpose does the NRT (neural response telemetry) test to ascertain the electrode impedances and to know that the electrodes are functioning normally.

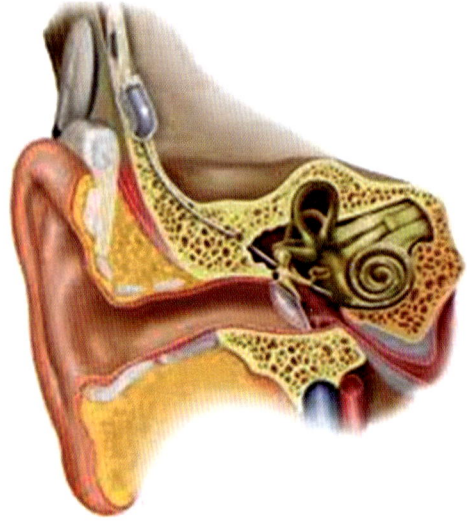

Fig. 40.3: An implant

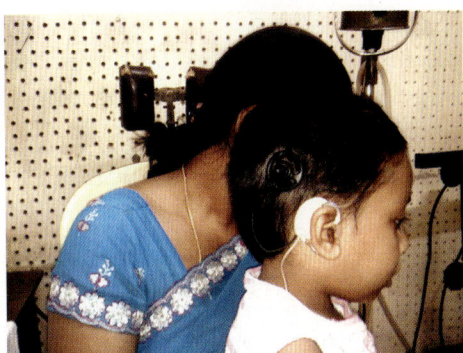

Fig. 40.4: A candidate after implantation of right ear

After NRT test final closure of the wound is done and a mastoid bandage is applied.

The electrode array is switched on after healing of the wound usually 1 week to 3 weeks (Switch-on ceremony) after the operation is done.

2. Bone Anchored Hearing Aids (BAHA)

BAHA is a bone conduction aid. It has three components:

   i. Titanium fixture, which is surgically embedded in the skull bone behind the ear.
  ii. Titanium abutment which remains exposed outside the skin
 iii. Sound processor: It is attached to the abutment. This is done after the titanium fixture is fixed with the tissue around it, which is called osseointegration. Osseointegration is completed within 2 to 6 months after implantation.

The sound processor transmits vibrations to the abutment, thereby transmitting vibration into the cochlea through the skull bone bypassing the external auditory canal and middle ear.

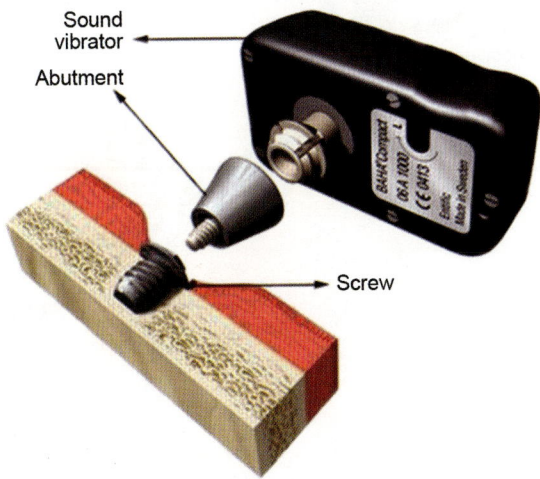

Fig. 40.5: Different parts of BAHA

Indications

1. In external auditory canal atresia (congenital or acquired)
2. In chronic ear discharge when air conduction hearing aid cannot be used
3. In single sided hearing loss
4. In otosclerosis and tympanosclerosis where surgery is contraindicated.

3. Vibrant Sound Bridge (Middle ear implants)

It is a semi-implantable device. It has two components like cochlear implant: an external and an internal component. Internal component has three parts: the receiver, Floating mass transducer (FMT) and a conductor linking the other two. The floating mass transducer (FMT) is connected to the incus. The external part is called the sound processor containing a microphone, which picks up sound and transmits across the skin by radiofrequency waves to the internal receiver.

It is used in adults above 18 years of age with moderate to severe sensorineural deafness.

The procedure is the same as cochlear implant surgery. The receiver is positioned under the skin over the mastoid. Standard cortical mastoidectomy and posterior tympanotomy are performed as they are done in cochlear implantation. The FMT is clipped with the long processes of the incus. After 6 to 8 weeks of surgery, the patient is fitted with the external audio processor. This is attached magnetically with the internal receiver exactly like in cochlear implants.

The advantages are:

It bypasses the ear canal and tympanic membrane and eliminates the inherent problems of conventional hearing aids such as occlusion, feedback, discomfort and wax related conditions.

It improves the quality of sound in noisy environments.

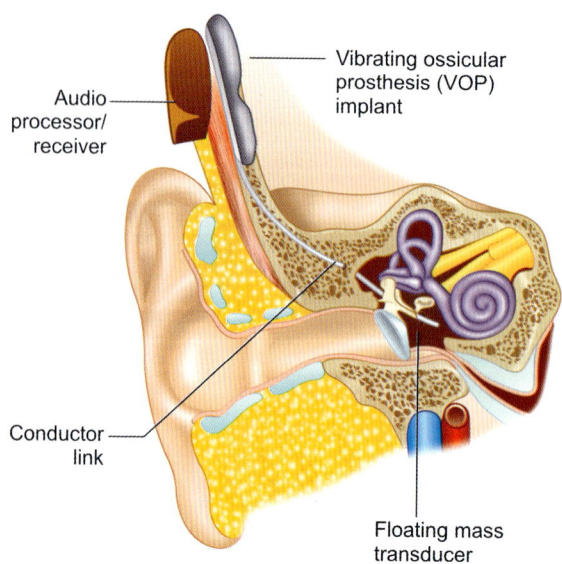

Fig. 40.6: Showing the vibrant sound bridge in middle ear

4. Auditory Brainstem Implants (ABI)

ABI is applied in the fourth ventricle. It stimulates the cochlear nuclei in the brainstem. ABI is needed in patients with bilateral auditory (VIII cranial nerve) damage, which is common in removal of vestibular schwannoma (acoustic neuroma). This implant (multichannel cochlear implant) is used in such a way that the electrode array is attached to a Dacron mesh on the brainstem. ABI helps in recognition of the environmental sounds. ABI is not as efficient as cochlear implants. It has limited use and is not performed as frequently as cochlear implants.

5. Computerized Tomography

Computerized tomography (CT) is the most important contribution to the medical

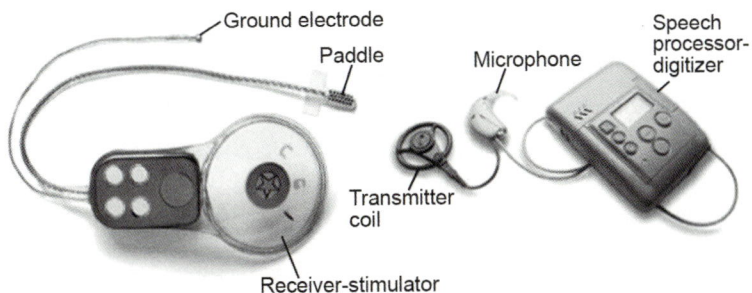

Fig. 40.7: Different parts of auditory brainstem implants (ABI)

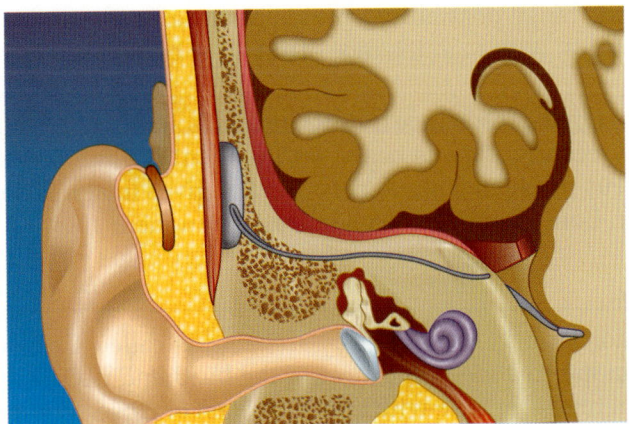

Fig. 40.8: ABI *in situ*

diagnostic imaging technique. Computerized axial tomography (CAT) was introduced in 1971 by GN Hounsefield, a British scientist, who won the Nobel Prize for this pioneering work. Since then this technique, which is non-invasive one, has made a revolutionary impact on neuro-radiology throughout the world.

The technique involves the idea of examining soft tissue structures in the human body by means of X-rays detected by sodium iodide crystals instead of conventional film. The computer processes the detector findings and reconstructs a cross section of the soft tissue examined. Plain X-ray is simple, fast and inexpensive. It produces sharp images of high contrast structures (air, fluid and bone). High contrast objects can obscure low contrast objects and the presence of overlying objects can sometimes be misleading. Polytomography is aimed at improving visualization of localised areas of the body, which has at least two limitations:

1. Background blur of structures above and below the focal plane and
2. A good amount of the radiation is scattered from the patient, whereas computerized tomography allows the reconstruction of tissue contrast in true cross sections (i.e. without being influenced by nearby or distant tissues in the section) and excellent tissue contrast discrimination.

Advantages of CT in diagnostic radiology are as follows:

1. Blurred background and superimposed overlying structures are removed.
2. A true tomographic section is obtained.
3. The CT image is stored and displayed digitally.
4. The transverse plane axial CT provides exquisite soft and hard tissue details, which is otherwise unavailable.
5. CT is more sensitive than film in the detection of areas of varying X-ray absorption by different soft tissue structures.

By using an IV contrast medium iophandylate (pantopaque), the vascular structures may be better differentiated from the adjacent tissues by virtue of their contrast enhancement. The new generation high resolution scanners, with a smaller pixel (picture element) and with the combination of thin section (1 to 1.5 mm.) and the extended bone range possibility provide clear definition and differentiation of soft tissue structures, with maintenance of superior bone detail to complex motion tomography.

The nuclear magnetic resonance (NMR) imager is another radiological technique developed very recently. This is based on the identification of the hydrogen ion spin of the nucleus producing a magnetic field. It gives image of soft-tissues better than CT scanner. Bone is not seen well in this technique.

6. Cryosurgery

Tissue destruction due to cell death by freezing is called Cryosurgery. It is an important tool in the treatment of cancer of the head and neck. Liquid nitrogen at –196°C is used in this technique with either an open or closed cryoprobe. The tissue to be destroyed must reach a temperature of at least –20°C. Open probe causes much deeper and rapid penetration than that of a closed cryoprobe. But closed cryoprobe is commonly used, as it is a more precise instrument and good for small tumours.

The critical temperature for cell death lies between 0°C and –10°C. The majority of living tissues undergo cryogenic death in a temperature of –20°C or below if exposed for more than 1 minute. The cells are protected by super cooling.

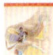

Degrees of Cryonecrosis and the Size of the Cryolesion

These depend on the following factors:

1. Temperature of the probe.
2. Size of the tip of the probe.
3. Duration of freezing.

Duration of freeze is rarely necessary for longer than 5 minutes. The body temperature and vascularity of the area affect the speed and extent of freezing. Greater tissue necrosis is achieved if the tissue is less vascular and the rewarming phase is longer. The density of the tissue also affects the size of the cryolesion. High water content of the tissue facilitates freezing. Bone, having low water content, is little affected by freezing.

Mechanism of tissue destruction

1. Rupture of cell membrane occurs due to formation of intracellular ice crystals. Ice crystals form in the rewarming phase on reaching about –2.2°C. It is therefore important that the rewarming phase should be slow. During treatment of neoplastic tissue the cycle of rapid freezing and slow rewarming (thawing) should be repeated at least two or three times. ,
2. Intracellular dehydration results in a raised and toxic concentration of electrolytes.
3. Denaturation of cell proteins affects the nucleus and mitochondria.
4. Destruction of cell metabolism leads to enzyme inhibition. Local ischaemia and microthrombosis result after a few hours producing anoxia and PH changes.

Clinical course: After cryosurgery the area appears the same as before treatment, but gradually it becomes hyperemic and congested and an inflammatory reaction surrounds the treated area. After a few days, a definite necrosis is evident and a slough forms. On separation of the slough, a clean, granulating area is found, which heals rapidly with a new epithelium and there is often remarkably little scarring or distortion.

Lesions of the head and neck due to their easy accessibility offer good scope for the use of cryoprobe. Cryosurgery has been tried for almost every type of lesion with variable success rate. Nowadays it is used as a therapeutic tool in many conditions.

7. Fibreoptic Endoscopy In ENT

Fibre-bundles are used in this system. These bundles transmit light and images through an optical system without electrical connections. Light is transmitted from a light source through the fibre-optic bundle to the distal end of the instrument. The system may be rigid or flexible. Suction, anaesthesia or the introduction of biopsy instruments is possible if a separate, parallel multipurpose channel is incorporated in it. Photography is also possible. A separate side observer attachment can be incorporated for demonstration and teaching.

In ENT the most promising areas for fibre-optic endoscopy are the postnasal space, ears and the larynx. Fibreoptic examination is valuable in bedridden patient, patients with trismus (inability to open the mouth) and in patients with lesions of the palate or tongue.

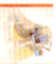

The nasopharynx, maxillary sinus, larynx, oesophagus, bronchus, trachea, mediastinum and even the intracranial structures can be visualised and biopsy and photography, etc. can be taken by the help of fibreoptic endoscopic instruments.

8. LASER Surgery

LASER means Light Amplification by the Stimulated Emission of Radiation. It is an electro-optical device containing a lasing medium, which is usually a gas or crystal. When stimulated by an extrinsic energy source, these atoms emit electromagnetic radiation or photons in a narrow, intense beam. Simply, a laser emits organised light rather than the random pattern light that is emitted from the common light bulb. The key to this organisation is stimulated emission.

In a stable atomic system an atom can interact with a photon and rise to a higher energy state. This process is called absorption. Similarly, this same atom in the high-energy state can emit a photon and decay to a more stable atomic state. This is called spontaneous emission. If a photon interacts with an atom, which is already in a high-energy state, and decay of that atomic system occurs, then two photons are released. That is, the original photon and the second photon emitted by decay of the high-energy system. These two photons are of equal wavelength and are coordinated in time and space (coherent). This process is called stimulated emission. This is the underlying principle of laser physics.

Lasing medium: The following are the laser medium:
1. CO_2—wavelength of light is 10.6 mm. Therefore it is invisible.
2. Argon—used in the treatment of Otosclerosis. Its wavelength is 0.488 to 0.514 mm. Therefore it is visible light and blue-green in colour.

The Wound of CO_2 Laser

There is a centre area of tissue ablation. Surrounding this is an area of protein denaturation approximately 50 mm in diameter. Next is an area of tissue oedema usually not more than 250 mm, which will remain as viable tissue. Small vessels, nerves and lymphatics are sealed in the area of protein denaturation. The minimal mechanical trauma and the "sealed" area probably account for the notable absence of postoperative oedema and pain characteristic of laser wounds.

Denaturation of protein occurs at a temperature of 60 to 65°C. The tissue becomes blanched in this state. Vaporization of intracellular water occurs with resultant vacuolization, cratering and tissue shrinkage at a temperature of 100°C.

CO_2 laser causes ocular damage, skin and mucous membrane burns. Protection of those and the endotracheal tube by an aluminium foil is essential. Smoke evacuation from the endoscopes or oral cavity should be done for visualization of the operative field.

Tracheal perforation, laryngeal web formation, subglotic stenosis, vocal cord fibrosis, arytenoid perichondritis, delayed bleeding and delayed postoperative airway obstruction may develop after using laser.

Role of KTP Laser in Revision Stapedectomy

In revision stapedectomy the poor results are due to dissection of scar tissue. Laser surgery with KTP Laser allows the safe removal of scar tissue covering the oval window and accurate placement of the new prosthesis. The results are very convincing. Air-bone gap closure to within 10dB is achieved in 80.5% of the patients.

Using the Laser to remove scar tissue and to open the oval window improves safety and efficacy of revision stapes surgery.

9. Evoked Response Audiometry (*see* text)

10. Radiosurgery (Surgery without knife)

It is the technique of using radiation in a high dose, which kills the tumour cells in a single session. The radiation must be precisely delivered. Delivery of a high radiation in a single session needs extreme precision and planning by the neurosurgeon, radiation oncologist and radiation physicists.

11. Radiofrequency (RF)

Radiofrequency techniques use high frequency alternating current to cut or coagulate tissue by inducing thermal lesions and tissue necrosis. By applying radiofrequency energy, a thermal lesion is created followed by scar formation, which results in stiffening or shrinking of that tissue. Radiofrequency is used to treat patients with problems of snoring and obstruction of upper airway. It is usually used in the hypertrophied inferior turbinates, soft palate, hypertrophied base of tongue and enlarged tonsils.

12. Robotic Surgery

Robotic surgery is known for more than 50 years. Medical application of robot assisted procedures was first used in 1985 for neurosurgical and transurethral biopsies. The FDA (Food and Drug Administration) of the USA had approved the first medical application of robot in 1992. During that time the concept of telepresence battlefield surgery during the "golden hour" of trauma in the battlefield was evoked. In a robotic setup, surgery can be performed remotely on an injured person, by a team of expert surgeons from a distant place and safe zone.

Robotic surgery is a telesurgery. The feasibility of robotic telesurgery was established in 2001 by surgeons in New York performing a cholecystectomy on a patient in Paris.

In ENT and head-neck surgery the da Vinci system (Fig. 40.9) is used. It consists of two major components. The first one is a master control where the primary surgeon sits to manipulate the robotic arms. The second one is the robotic cart, which is manipulated remotely by the operating surgeon. The robotic instruments are designed to mimic and even exceed the natural range of movements of the surgeon's wrists, giving 7° of freedom. The robotic telescope incorporates two separate cameras in the distal tip, offset by 15°, giving a true stereoscopic, three-dimensional high-definition view of the field. The combination of the wristed movement, distal dexterity and three-dimensional views makes this tool well suited for surgery within a confined space.

The first reported case in ENT and head-neck surgery in a live patient was the excision of a benign vallecular cyst. Shortly after, Weinstein and colleagues described

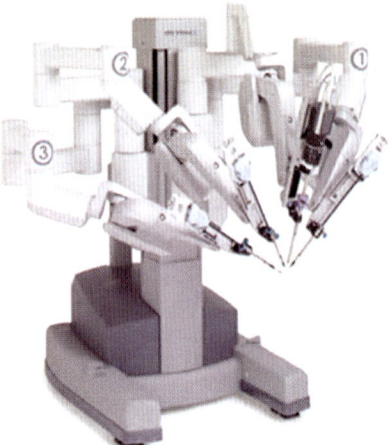

Fig. 40.9: Robot for ENT surgery

the first transoral robotic surgery (TORS). Vocal cord stripping, partial cordectomy, resection of tongue base, arytenoidectomy, thyroidectomy, etc. are the procedures which can be performed precisely with the help of this technology. Tonsils and base of the tongue cancer resections are the more commonly performed procedures with TORS.

As the procedures continue to evolve and the technology improves further and further, robotic surgery will play a big role in the treatment of diseases of ENT and head-neck surgery.

IMPORTANT SYNDROMES IN ENT

a. *Alport's syndrome:* Neurosensory (perceptive type) deafness. Nephritis: Keratoconus and corneal dystrophy

b. *Behçet's syndrome:* Ulceration of oral mucosa and anogenital region. Iritis, choroiditis and retinitis

c. *Cogan's syndrome:* Sensorineural deafness may be unilateral or bilateral. Vertigo, vomiting and tinnitus. Interstitial keratitis with vestibular dysfunction because of degenerative changes found in the vestibule and spiral ganglion

d. *Collet-Sicard syndrome:* Unilateral paralysis of lower four (IX, X, XI, XII) cranial nerves resulting in hoarseness, nasal intonation, regurgitation of food, speech defect and reduced taste sensation. Causes are: Skull base tumours or trauma, neoplastic extension in the jugular foramen, basal meningitis, and cervical 1st vertebrae fracture.

e. *Costen's syndrome:* It is a malocclusion syndrome involving temporomandibular joint due to the absence or extrusion of lower molar teeth. It causes pain in TM joint, ear and tinnitus.

f. *Crocodile tear syndrome:* It commonly occurs after facial nerve paralysis where the salivary gland nerve fibres of the facial nerve are damaged and regrow into the lacrimal gland during regeneration. It causes spontaneous lacrimation during eating along with normal salivation.

g. *Crouzon's syndrome:* It is a hereditary disorder characterized by conductive deafness due to bony ankylosis of stapes and craniofacial dysostosis with small maxilla. It may be associated with ectropion and districhiasis, additional row of eyelashes at the inner margin, hyperteleorism and oxycephaly.

h. *Down's syndrome:* Craniofacial dysostosis. It is characterized by mental retardation, mongolism and hypotonia.

i. *Frey's syndrome (Auriculotemporal syndrome):* Localised facial sweating and flushing in the area of auriculotemporal nerve during mastication of food. It follows parotidectomy. It is due to cross innervation between the postganglionic secretomotor fibres (parasympathetic) to the parotid gland and the postganglionic sympathetic fibres supplying the sweat glands of the skin.

j. *Horner's syndrome:* One eye enopthalmos, ptosis of the same side, miosis (constricted pupil) of that eye and anhydrosis (lack of sweating) of the affected side of the face. It is due to involvement of the cervical sympathetic plexus.

k. *Gradenigo's syndrome:* It is due to petrositis in cases of CSOM. Features are: i) Otorrhoea, ii) Diplopia and internal squint due to VI cranial nerve palsy iii) Retro-orbital pain due to involvement of trigeminal ganglion (V cranial nerve).

l. *Heerfordt's syndrome:* Bilateral facial paralysis with uveitis, parotitis and fever. It occurs in Sarcoidosis.

m. *Jaccoud's syndrome:* Blindness opthalmoplegia and pain (retrorbital) in the distribution of V cranial nerve.

n. *Kartagener's syndrome:* Sinusitis, dextrocardia, bronchiectasis, situs inversus and cystic fibrosis are the features due to developmental abnormalities.

o. *Klippel-Fiel syndrome:* Atresia of the ear and deafness, cervical and thoracic vertebral anomalies leading to short neck and low hairline. It occurs due to hereditary disorders.

p. *Lermoyez syndrome:* Deafness and tinnitus are the symptoms, which disappear after an attack of vertigo. It is supposed to be spasm of the internal auditory artery.

q. *Waardenburg's syndrome:* Features are Heterochromia iridis, white forelock and lateral displacement of eye and sensorineural deafness. An autosomal dominant condition.

r. *Treacher Collin's syndrome:* It is the mandibulo facial dysostosis. Features are obliquity of palpabral fissure, depressed cheekbones, deformed pinna, receding chin, hypoplastic mandible, coloboma eyes and conductive deafness. An autosomal dominant condition.

s. *Melkersson-Rosenthal syndrome:* Features are recurrent orofacial swellings, relapsing facial paralysis and fissured tongue. It is common in children and a relapsing condition.

t. *Mikulicz's syndrome:* It is usually associated with Sarcoidosis. The features are: symmetrical enlargement of the salivary glands, narrowing of the palpabral fissure and dryness of mouth.

u. *Mondini's syndrome:* It causes congenital deafness due to partial aplasia of both the osseous and membranous labyrinths.

v. *Pendred's syndrome:* Neurosensory (perceptual) deafness associated with goiter.

w. *Stevens-Jonson syndrome:* Stomatitis with ulcers, purulent conjunctivitis and fever due to hypersensitivity reaction following intake of drugs such as sulfonamides, thiacetazones, isoniazide and tetracyclines.

x. *Meniere's syndrome:* See text.

y. *Ramsay Hunt syndrome:* See text.

SOME IMPORTANT SIGNS IN ENT

i. *Holman Millar sign:* It is seen on X-ray paranasal sinuses as anterior bowing of the posterior wall of maxillary sinus; commonly seen in juvenile angiofibroma, schwannoma and carcinoma of the nasopharynx.

ii. *Delta sign:* It is seen in CT scan with contrast study in cases of lateral sinus thrombophlebitis as a filling defect as an enhancement due to a clot.

iii. *Rising sun sign:* It is seen in glomus tympanicum in the inferior portion of tympanic membrane and external auditory canal due to dilatation of tympanic vessels.

iv. *Brown's sign:* Blanching of tumour mass while examining with Seigle's pneumatic speculum or pneumatic otoscopy in cases of glomus tympanicum.

v. *Thumb sign:* It is a radiological sign seen in acute epiglottitis on lateral neck X-ray.

vi. *Schwartz's sign:* See text.

vii. *Griesinger's sign:* See text.

Appendix

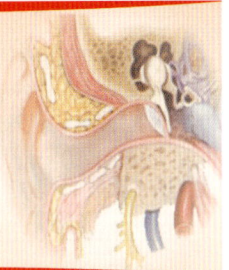

PRESCRIPTIONS

For Nose and Paranasal Sinuses

1. Sodium bicarbonate

   Sodium biborate } ... ... aa 30 gm

   Sodium chloride ... ... 60 gm

   M. Ft. pulv.

   Sig: One teaspoonful to be dissolved in a half pint (280 ml) of water.

   Use: As nose wash.

2. Anhydrous glucose ... ... aa 8 gm

   Glycerin ... ... 30 ml

   Use: In ozeana.

3. Ephedrine hydrochloride, 1 per cent in normal saline.

   Use: As nose drops or spray to produce decongestion.

4. Xylometazoline–nose drop as decongestant (0.1%)

5. Oxymetazoline–nose drop as decongestant (0.05%)

6. Ung. hydrargyri nitratis

   Paraffino mollis flavi } ... ... aa 4 gm

   Use: In dermatitis of nasal vestibule.

7. Sodium chromoglycate.

   Use: As nasal spray in allergic rhinitis.

8. Kemicetine antiozaena

   Use: As nasal drop or spray in atrophic rhinitis.

For Pharynx

1. Sodium bicarbonate ... ... 2 gm

   Liq. thymol

   Glycerin } ... ... aa 30 ml

   Sin: One teaspoonful in a cup of warm water for mouth wash and gargle.

   Use: In acute tonsillitis and after tonsillectomy.

2. Mandl's pain ... ...

   Iodine ... ... 375 mg

Potassium iodide	... ...	750 mg
Aq. Dest.	... ...	0.75 ml
Ol. Menthae Piperitae	... ...	0.12 ml
Alcohol 90 per cent	... ...	1.125 ml
Glycerin	... ...	to 30 ml

Sig: Throat paint.

Use: In chronic pharyngitis and chronic tonsillitis.

3. Solution of silver nitrate, 10 per cent

Use: As a paint for superficial ulcers of the pharynx and in vincent's angina.

4. Solution of iron perchloride ...   ...   4 ml

Glycerin   ...   ...   to 30 ml

Sig: Throat paint

Use: In chronic pharyngitis

5. Tab mycostatin 5,00,000 units

Use: Fungus infection of the oral cavity. One tablet to be allowed to dissolve in mouth three times daily.

6. Chlotrimazole 0.1% solution

Use: As a paint in oral thrush.

For Larynx

1. Tinct. Benzoin Co.

Sig: One teaspoonful in a pint (560 ml) of steaming water as an inhalation of vapour.

Use: In acute laryngitis.

2. Pulv. orthoformi

Sig: Use as insufflation.

In dysphagia of tuberculous ulceration.

For Ears

1. Icthamol 10 per cent in glycerin.

Use: A strip of ribbon gauze to be soaked with the solution and packed into the external ear canal in furuncle of the ear.

2. Sol. aluminium acetate, 8 percent.

Use: A strip of ribbon gauze to be soaked in the solution and packed into the external auditory canal in furuncle of the ear.

3. Amphotericin B (fungilin)

Use: In candida infections.

4. 2 per cent salicylic acid in alochol as ear drop in otomycosis

5. Borospirit drops.

Boric acid	... ...	250 mg
Boric spirit	... ...	4 ml
Aqua	... ...	ad 15 ml

Sig: Four to five drops in the affected ear.

Use: Chronic in middle ear suppuration.

6. Enteromycetin otic solution 5%
   Use: As drops in middle ear suppuration.
7. Hydrocortisone and neomycin ear drops.
   Use: As drops in myringitis and otitis externa.
8. Genticin and Genticin-B ear drop.
   Use: As above.
9. Glycerin acid carbolic   ...   ...   8 ml
   Glycerin
   Sig: Otic drop.
   Use: In early stage of acute otitis media.
10. Guttae phenol
    Phenol   ...   ...   0.5 gm
    Rect. spirit   ...   ...   15 ml
    Aqua   ...   ...   30 ml
    Sig: Otic drop
    Use: In chronic suppurative otitis media
11. Chlotrimazole 1% in propylene glycol ear drop.
    Use: In otomycosis.
12. GSB drop (glycerine-sodibicarbonate)
    Sodium bicarbonate   ...   ...   2 gm
    Glycerin   ...   ...   ad 30 ml
    Sig: Otic drop.
    Use: To soften the wax before syringing the ear.
13. Chromic acid
    Use: As crystals fused on a silver probe in aural granulations.
14. Trichloracetic acid.
    Sig: To be applied by means of a small pledget of cotton wool on a probe.
    Use: In aural granulations and office closure of small central perforation in CSOM.
15. Iodi. resublimati   ...   ...   225 mg
    Pulv. acid boric   ...   ...   ad 30 mg
    Sig: Iodine 0.75 per cent in boric acid powder for insufflation.
    Use: In chronic suppurative otitis media with large perforation.
16. Tab. Nicotinic acid, 50 mg
    Use: Two tablets three times a day in tinnitus and vertigo.
    As vasodilator.
17. Tab. Diligan (UCB)
    Use: One tablet three times a day in labyrinthine vertigo, tinnitus and after stapedectomy in otosclerosis.
18. Prochlorperazine, 5 mg tab.
    Use: One tablet thrice a day in vertigo and migrainous headache.
19. Betahistine 8 mg tabs.
    Use: One or two tablets thrice a day in Meniere's disease or in vertigo due to vasoconstriction.

20. Dimenhydrinate 50 mg tabs.

Use: One or two tablets thrice a day in Meniere's disease or in vertigo due to vasoconstriction.

21. Promethazine theoclate 25 mg tabs.

Use: Labyrinthine sedative in vertigo.

22. Cinnarizine 25 mg tabs

Use: Labyrinthine sedative in vertigo, tinnitus and Meniere's disease.

Index